100054

Bonnie Balzer

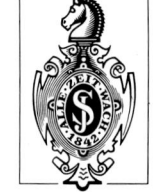

Gisela Dallenbach-Hellweg   Hemming Poulsen

Atlas of Histopathology of the Cervix Uteri

With 221 Figures, Most in Color

Springer-Verlag Berlin Heidelberg New York
London Paris Tokyo Hong Kong Barcelona

Dr. Gisela Dallenbach-Hellweg
form. Professor of Pathological Anatomy
Hospital for Women of Mannheim
University of Heidelberg
Institut für Pathologie, A 2, 2
6800 Mannheim 1, Germany

Dr. Hemming Poulsen
Professor of Pathological Anatomy
Department of Pathology
Hvidovre Hospital
University of Copenhagen
2650 Hvidovre, Denmark

ISBN 3-540-52295-6 Springer-Verlag Berlin Heidelberg New York
ISBN 0-387-52295-6 Springer-Verlag New York Berlin Heidelberg

Library of Congress Cataloging-in-Publication Data
Dallenbach-Hellweg, G. (Gisela) Atlas of histopathology of the cervix uteri / Gisela Dallenbach-Hellweg, Hemming Poulsen. p. cm. Includes bibliographical references.
ISBN 0-387-52295-6 (U.S. : alk. paper)
1. Cervix uteri-Histopathology-Atlases. 2. Cervix uteri-Cytodiagnosis-Atlases. I. Poulsen, H. E. (Hemming Engelund) II. Title. [DNLM: 1. Cervix Diseases-diagnosis-atlases. 2. Cervix Uteri-pathology-atlases. 3. Cytodiagnosis-methods-atlases. WP 17 D146aa] RG310.D35 1990
618.1'407-dc20 DNLM/DLC 90-9693

This work is subject to copyright. All rights are reserved, whether the whole or part of the material is concerned, specifically the rights of translation, reprinting, reuse of illustrations, recitation, broadcasting, reproduction on microfilms or in other ways, and storage in data banks. Duplication of this publication or parts thereof is only permitted under the provisions of the German Copyright Law of September 9, 1965, in its current version, and a copyright fee must always be paid. Violations fall under the prosecution act of the German Copyright Law.

© Springer-Verlag Berlin Heidelberg 1990
Printed in Germany

The use of general descriptive names, registered names, trademarks, etc. in the publication does not imply, even in the absence of a specific statement, that such names are exempt from the relevant protective laws and regulations and therefore free for general use.

Product Liability: The publisher can give no guarantee for information about drug dosage and application thereof contained in this book. In every individual case the respective user must check its accuracy by consulting other pharmaceutical literature.

Typesetting, printing and binding: Appl, Wemding
2123/3145-543210 - Printed on acid-free paper

Preface

During the past decade our understanding of the histopathology of the cervix uteri has changed greatly. Because of the life-styles of the modern permissive society, cervical viral infections have become epidemic, resulting in inflammatory and precancerous lesions that were uncommon but now are seen mainly in the younger age groups with increasing frequency. Then too, progress in molecular biology and immunohistochemistry has enabled us to distinguish subtypes of papilloma viruses, to proceed in understanding their action within the genome, and to trace the infected metaplastic and neoplastic-transformed cells to their histogenetic origins. The resultant refined classification of cervical neoplasias has helped to predict clinical outcome and to choose type of therapy.

This atlas is intended for all pathologists, to aid them in their routine diagnostic work. We hope it explains just how comprehensive, important and complex the histopathology of the cervix uteri has become during the last few years. It covers all pertinent differential diagnostic aspects and describes in detail how to reach the correct diagnosis. The atlas is also meant for the clinician, to guide him in his often difficult decision how to provide optimal care for the frequently young patient, who desires children but is at risk for cancer. In particular, the atlas is designed to foster an improved dialogue between the pathologist and the clinician.

The microphotographs were selected from our daily diagnostic material, since they show best the technical variations confronting the clinical pathologist in his daily routine, where effects of specimen transport, differences in tissue fixation, and variations in embedding and staining often compound his diagnostic problems. The various shades of haematoxylin-eosin stains shown by our photographs reflect the differences we have experienced with our material as it comes in daily or is received as referral cases from clinics and institutes. We have not attempted to eliminate the deficiencies of these specimens, since the pathologist using this atlas is entitled to find realistic photographs rather than idealistic ones. We want him to recognize a lesion irrespective of the quality of fixation or intensity of staining.

We express our gratitude to Prof. Dr. Frederick D. Dallenbach for the subtile English translation. We also extend our thanks to the staff of the Springer-Verlag for their patience, generosity, and skill in preparing the manuscript and in reproducing our microphotographs.

We find ourselves in an exciting period of molecular biology, during which rapid developments in diagnostic techniques and concepts are clarifying relationships between molecular changes and the pathogenesis of cervical cancer. As to be expected, some of our statements will be short-lived, forced aside as new facts and information emerge to replace them. In contrast, other statements we have made may grow in importance. May both the controversial issues and those being accepted with ever-increasing favour contribute to make this atlas a source of stimulus to encourage lively discussions and rewarding ideas.

Mannheim and Copenhagen, July 1990   Gisela Dallenbach-Hellweg
and Hemming Poulsen

Contents

Methods of Obtaining and Preparing Cervical Tissue for Histological Examination 1

Operative Procedures 1
Preparation of the Cervical Specimen 2

Normal Histology, Regeneration, and Repair 4

Normal Ectocervix 4
Ascending Repair 10
Normal Endocervix 14
Descending Repair 18
Transformation Zone 24

Vestigial and Heterotopic Tissues 26

Mesonephric Duct Remnants and Hyperplasia 26
Müllerian Duct Remnants and Metaplasia 28
Heterotopic Ectodermal and Mesodermal Structures 33

Hormonally Induced Changes 35

Effects of Estrogen 35
    Parakeratosis and Hyperkeratosis of the Ectocervix 35
    Cystic Hyperplasia of the Endocervix 35
Effects of Endogenous Progesterone Under Hypersecretion 40
    Glandular and Cystic Hyperplasia of the Endocervix 40
Effects of Exogenous Gestagens 42
    Adenomatous Hyperplasia of the Endocervix 42
    Microglandular Hyperplasia of the Endocervix 47
Glandular Papillary Ectropium 48
Polyps of the Ecto- and Endocervix 48

Inflammatory Lesions 51

Nonspecific Ecto- and Endocervicitis 51
Specific Inflammations 56
    Viral Infections 56
    Bacterial Infections 61
    Parasitic Infections 64

Fungal Infections	64
Infections of Unknown Etiology	66
Irradiation Changes	66

Benign Tumors 69

Epithelial Tumors	69
Mesenchymal Tumors	72
Mixed Tumors	74

Premalignant Lesions 76

Introduction	76
Etiology and Pathogenesis	76
Histology and Immunohistochemistry	78
Dysplasia and Carcinoma In Situ	78
Squamous Cell Type	80
Reserve Cell Type	88
Adenocarcinoma In Situ	103
Biological Behavior	108

Malignant Tumors 109

Epithelial Tumors	109
Squamous and Reserve Cell Types	109
Microinvasive Carcinoma	109
Invasive Carcinoma	116
Glandular Type	128
Mucinous Adenocarcinoma	131
Endometrioid Adenocarcinoma	139
Clear Cell Adenocarcinoma	141
Serous Papillary Carcinoma	142
Mesonephric Adenocarcinoma	144
Mixed Type	148
Adenosquamous Carcinoma	148
Mucoepidermoid Carcinoma	148
Adenoid Type	153
Adenoid Cystic Carcinoma	153
Adenoid Basal Carcinoma	154
Heterotopic Type	155
Neuroendocrine Carcinomas	155
Neurogenic Tumors	157
Malignant Melanoma	158
Mesenchymal Tumors	158
Mesodermal Mixed Tumors	162
Metastatic Tumors	169

References 170

Subject Index 177

Methods of Obtaining and Preparing Cervical Tissue for Histological Examination

Operative Procedures

Histological examination of the uterine cervix is required for diagnosing a lesion which is suspicious on gross, colposcopic, or cytological examination. In such instances, the extent of the biopsy may depend on the individual situation (Anderson and Linton 1967; Hulka 1970; Selim et al. 1973; Holzner 1981), but sufficient tissue should always be removed to provide the pathologist with optimal material for examination and for consideration and evaluation of all diagnostic possibilities. Pathologists should never hesitate to ask for more tissue if they believe this will help in reaching a definitive diagnosis.

If a neoplasm or a suspicious lesion is visible, a small *punch biopsy* will suffice in most instances. As a rule, a cervical biopsy should contain tissue from the squamocolumnar junction and the border between the normal and suspicious epithelium.

If the cytology report is positive (PAP IV–V), but no lesion is visible on gross or colpo-

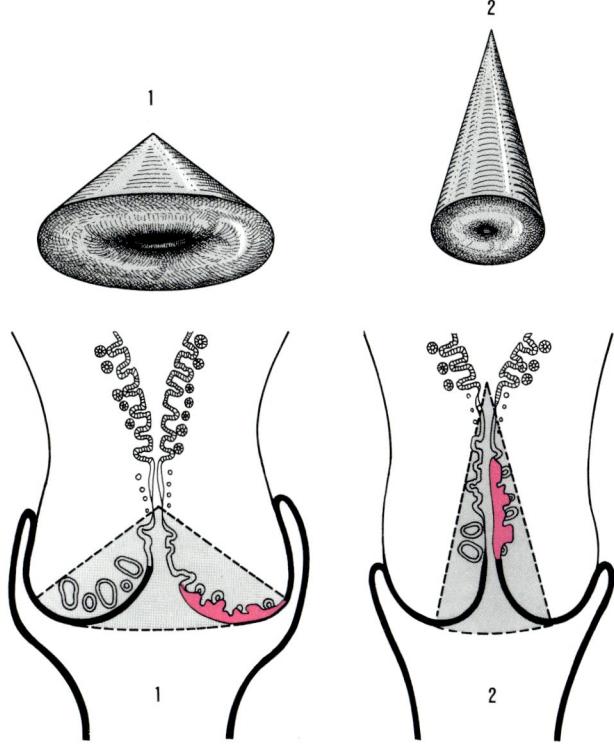

Fig. 1. Location of the squamocolumnar junction and shape of the conus required in reproductive age *(1)* and in old age *(2)* (from Dallenbach-Hellweg 1985)

scopic examination, a *cervical conization* will be necessary in order to survey the entire squamocolumnar junction. A conization must also be performed if a previous punch biopsy of a grossly suspicious lesion showed that the noninvasive precancerous epithelium had not been completely excised. A biopsy of malignant tumors can never give information about the depth of invasion. If the clinical signs fail to reveal how deeply a tumor has invaded, e. g., a crater is seen, a conization must always be performed. This is the only method on which to base the decision of whether further treatment should consist of simple surgical procedures (enlarged cone or simple hysterectomy) or involve more extensive methods (radical surgery or irradiation). A conization should always contain the entire squamocolumnar junction. Depending upon the age of the patient (Hamperl and Kaufmann 1959), that junction may be localized on the ectocervix, as during the reproductive age, requiring a flat conus, or be up in the endocervical canal, as in old age, requiring an elongated conus (see Fig. 1). Results of colposcopic examination may help the surgeon to decide whether a flat or an elongated cone biopsy is most appropriate. The cone should be marked so that the pathologist understands how it was located anatomically; the same marking procedure should be used in all cases. For example, a suture mark at "12 o'clock" will help the pathologist orient the specimen and pinpoint the site of a lesion on either the anterior or posterior lip, or both. Especially when a precancerous lesion reaches the excisional margins of the cone, correct localization of the lesion will help the gynecologist in his follow-up treatment of the patient. When a laser beam is used for excising a cone, a small coagulated zone at the margins of the specimen will be unfit for histological evaluation. The lateral margins of a cone may contain cervical glands that project deep into the tissue, possibly with precancerous lesions. Therefore, these parts of the tissue must also be carefully examined. To avoid the possibility of leaving the bottoms of glands behind, many surgeons prefer excising a more cylindrically shaped piece of cervical tissue.

In most instances precancerous lesions are totally excised by conization and no further operation will be necessary. Accordingly, diagnostic conization serves also as a therapeutic measure. Occasionally cervical conization may be required as a means of treatment, e. g., in patients with resistant vaginal discharge. Here, careful histological examination of the squamocolumnar junction is advisable to insure that possible precancerous changes are not overlooked.

A *cervical curettage* may be part of a fractionated curettage, whereby the gynecologist performs and collects the cervical scraping before carrying out the endometrial curettage. If malignant transformations are found, the pathologist should attempt from examination of the separately embedded curettings to determine whether the tumor arises only in the cervix, only in the endometrial cavity, or in both.

Preparation of the Cervical Specimen

The method used to study a uterus depends on the preceding clinical and/or histological diagnoses: If the cervix is not clinically and morphologically remarkable, a tissue section from each lip, including the squamocolumnar junction, will suffice. If a suspicious lesion is found preoperatively, both lips should be sectioned and embedded completely, like a cone specimen. If an invasive carcinoma has been diagnosed preoperatively in a cone specimen, then the extent of invasion must be determined histologically, requiring the study of all margins of the conization site, of both parametrial tissues and all lymph nodes surgically excised.

For *fixation,* a 4% neutral solution of formaldehyde is commonly used and is ideal for most diagnostic procedures. Unfixed cryostate sections may be needed in immunohistochemical studies for detecting intermediate filaments, hormone receptors, proliferation markers, or viruses. For these purposes, the tissue must be deep-frozen in liquid nitrogen or on dry ice within 30 min after excision. After fixation, a cervical biopsy must be carefully oriented so that it can be properly embedded, and biopsies as well as curettings should be completely embedded. Microtome sections are taken from various levels. Precise *orientation* of a cervical cone is essential for evaluating the entire squamocolumnar junction, where most precancerous and carcinomatous lesions originate. For this orientation different techniques have been described (Fig. 2); each has its advantages and disadvantages. We recommend either the circular or the parallel sectioning (Dallenbach-Hellweg 1985). When the anterior lip has been clearly marked, all paraffin blocks made from the cone should be numbered such that a lesion subsequently discovered on microscopic examination can be localized precisely in the cone.

Routine *staining* of all specimens should include hematoxylin-eosin and a connective tissue stain, for instance, van Gieson's. An additional PAS or alcian blue reaction may be helpful in detecting glycogen or mucopolysaccharides in squamous or glandular epithelial cells to judge the degree of cellular maturation. A reticulum impregnation can be useful in detecting interruptions of the basement membrane in early stromal invasion, or in distinguishing carcinomas from lymphomas.

For the various immunohistochemical methods with polyclonal and monoclonal antibodies we refer to detailed technical descriptions in the literature (Moll et al. 1983; Czernobilsky et al. 1984; Makin et al. 1984; Tsutsumi et al. 1984; Levy et al. 1988). For detecting subtypes of human papilloma virus infection, in situ hybridization with DNA probes is recommended (Seifert et al. 1984; Nagai et al. 1987).

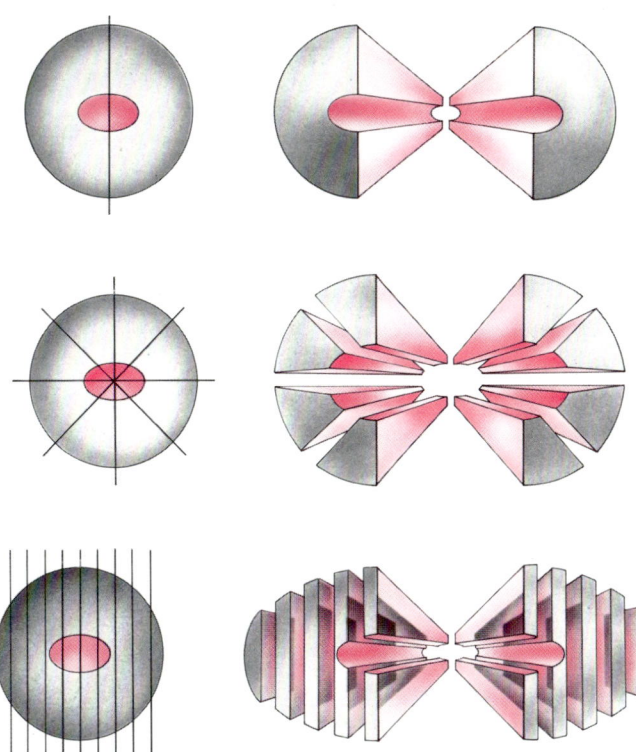

Fig. 2. Various techniques of sectioning a conus for orientation (from Dallenbach-Hellweg 1985)

Normal Histology, Regeneration, and Repair

Normal Ectocervix (Figs. 3–9)

A normal ectocervix is covered by a nonkeratinizing stratified squamous epithelium. Its height is influenced by endogenous hormone production and varies accordingly with age and hormonal stimulation.

During reproductive age (Fig. 3) the epithelium is high and well differentiated. It consists of a basal cell layer with elongated nuclei perpendicular to the basal membrane, of one or several layers of small parabasal cells, of a broad intermediate cell zone with abundant cytoplasmic glycogen, and of a covering layer of narrow, superficial cells.

In childhood and in old age (Fig. 4), because hormonal stimulation is lacking, the squamous epithelium is low. Here it consists only of a few layers of small, poorly differentiated epithelial cells. The sparse cytoplasm is devoid of glycogen; stratification may be barely visible or even absent.

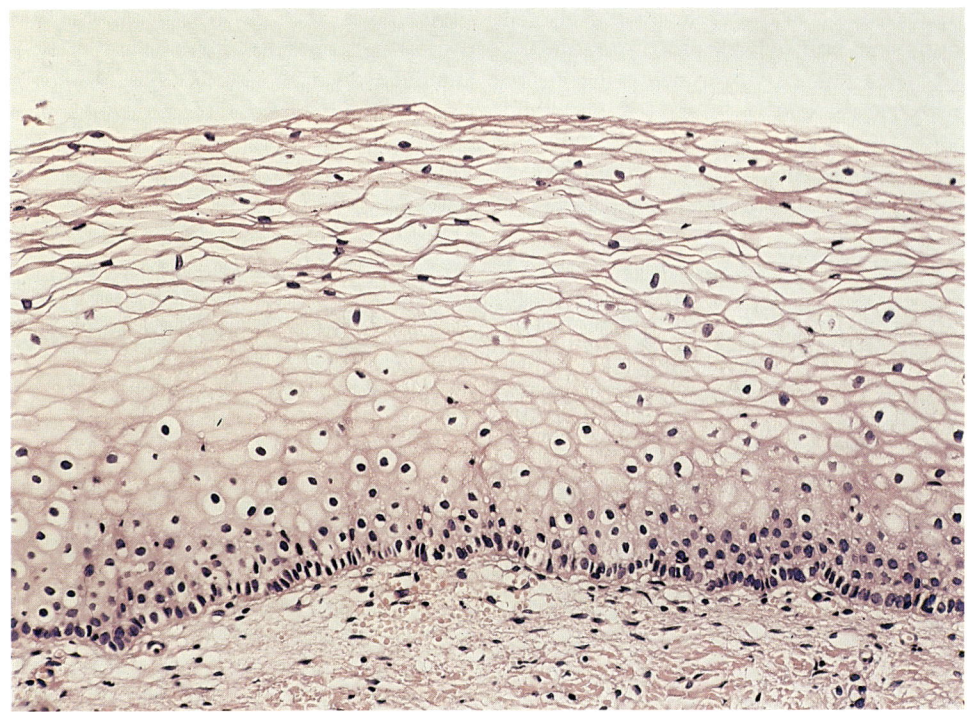

Fig. 3. Normal ectocervix during reproductive age. H & E

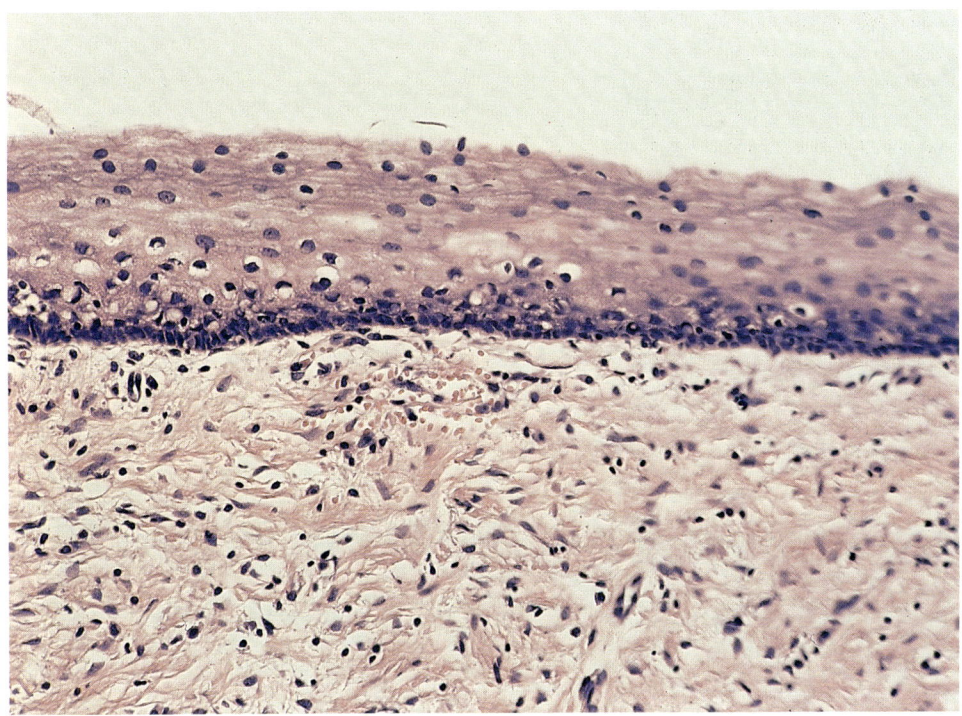

Fig. 4. Normal ectocervix in old age. H & E

Regardless of their differentiation, all cell layers stain positively for broad spectrum cytokeratins and, except for the basal cells, for cytokeratins 4 and 13 in appropriate immunohistochemical studies (Fig. 5). Cytokeratin 4 and 13 are normal constituents of epithelial cells in squamous differentiation. Furthermore, the cell membranes, but not the basal membrane, stain positively with antibodies against desmoplakin (Fig. 6). In contrast, the basal cells express cytokeratins of the simple (glandular) epithelial type: PKK 1, 18, and 19 (Fig. 7; Franke et al. 1986).

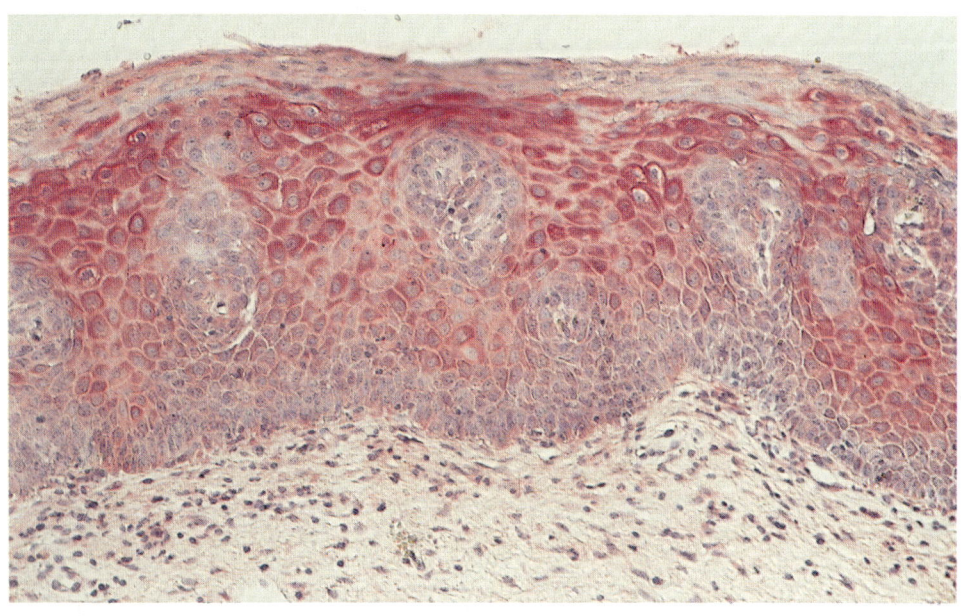

Fig. 5. Normal ectocervix. Immunohistochemical reaction with anticytokeratin 13

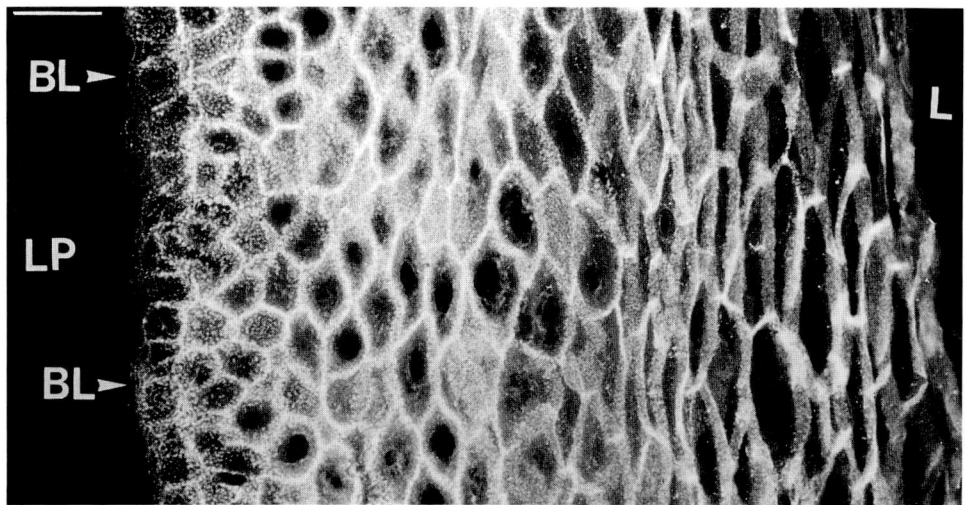

Fig. 6. Normal ectocervix. Immunohistochemical reaction with antidesmoplakin. *BL*, basal lamina; *LP*, lamina propria; *L*, lumen (from Franke et al. 1986)

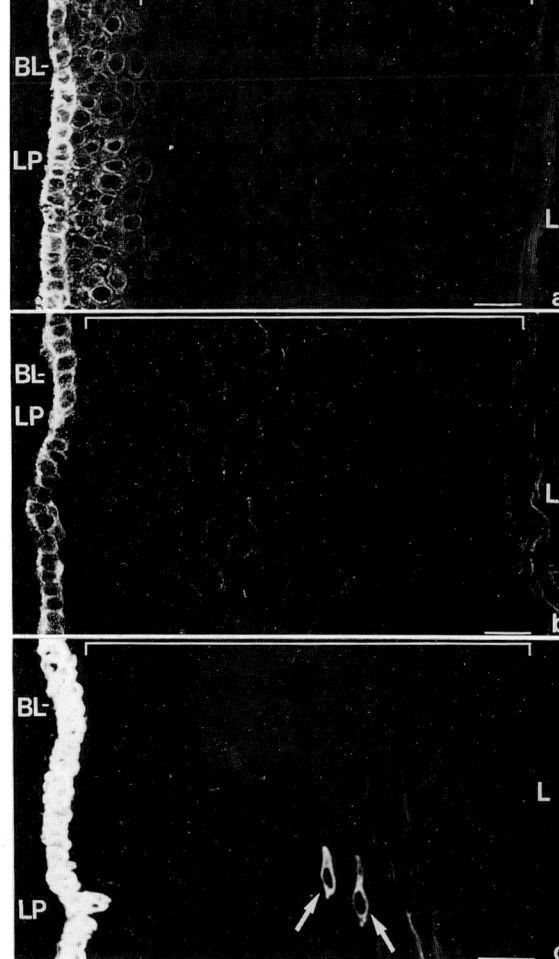

Fig. 7. Normal ectocervix. Immunohistochemical reaction with anticytokeratin PKK 1 (**a**), 18 (**b**), and 19 (**c**). *BL*, basal lamina; *LP*, lamina propria; *L*, lumen (from Franke et al. 1986)

This variation in the expression of cytokeratins by the basal cells may explain their potential for glandular differentiation and for functioning as germinal layer of the squamous epithelium (Fig. 9). It may also explain their potential to elongate and ramify as protrusions downwards into the underlying fibrous stroma (Fig. 8).

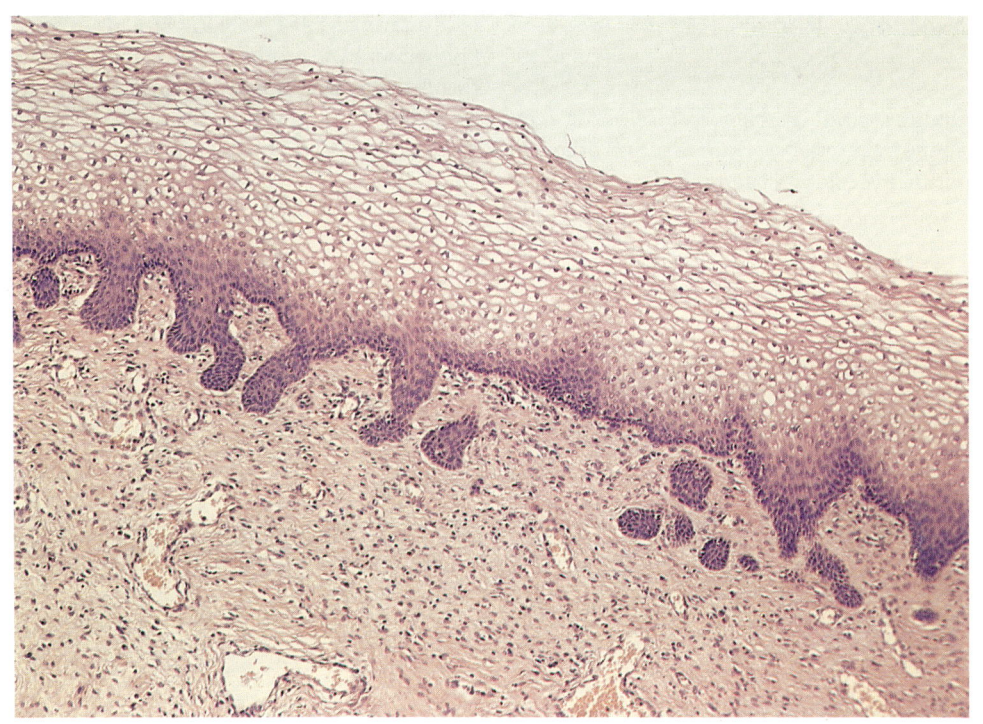

▲
Fig. 8. Ramifying protrusions from basal layer into the underlying fibrous stroma. H & E

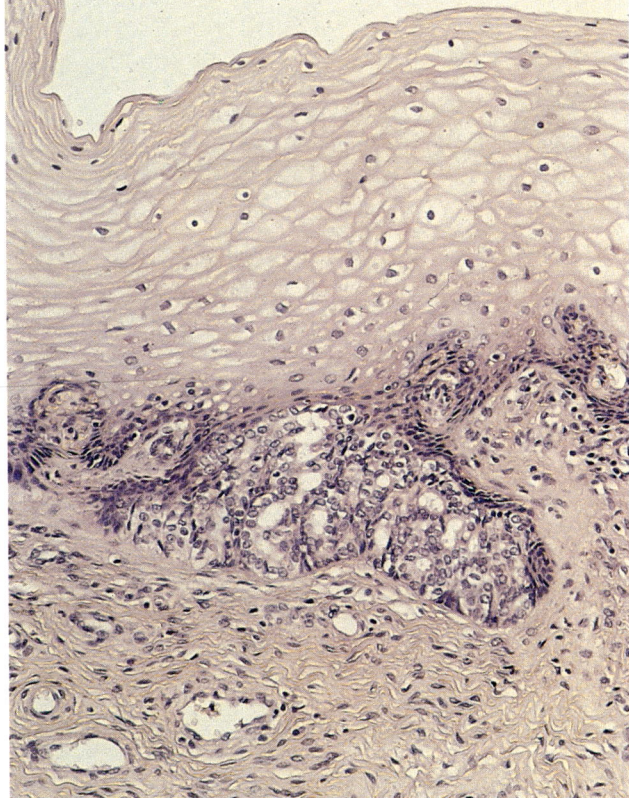

Fig. 9. Formation of glands from the basal layer of the ectocervical epithelium. H & E

Ascending Repair (Figs. 10-13)

During reproductive life, and following eversion of the endocervical mucosa onto the portio, the ectocervical epithelium is capable of overgrowing the vulnerable endocervical epithelium by ascending repair (Figs. 10, 11), thereby often occluding the openings of endocervical glands, which may then become cystically dilated with inspissated mucus (Fig. 11).

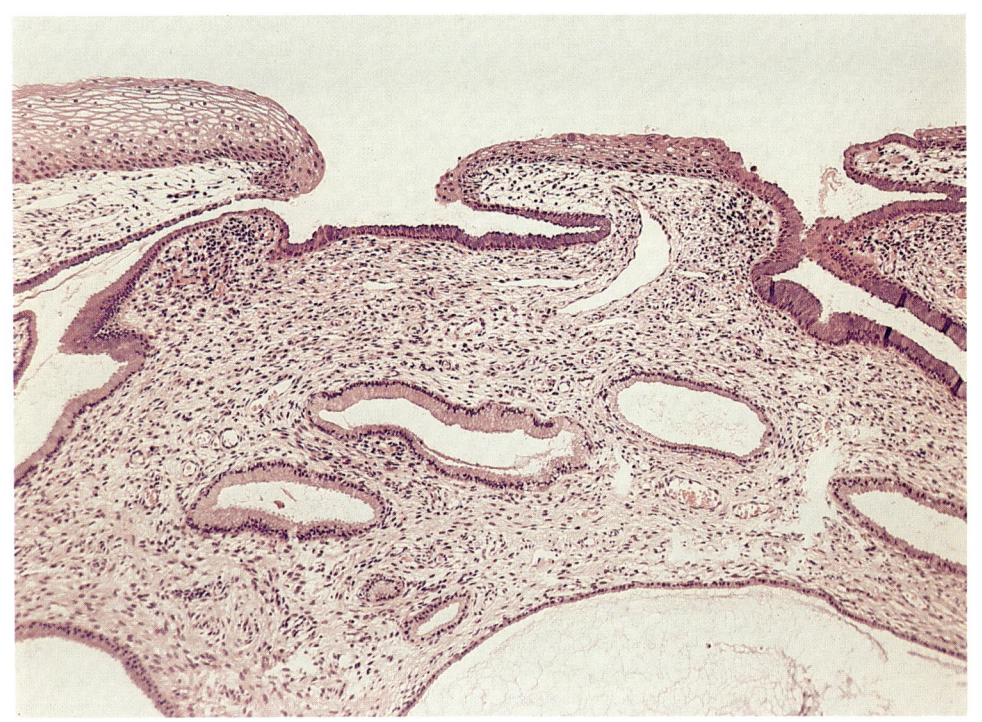

Fig. 10. Ascending repair following eversion of the endocervical mucosa onto the portio, early stage. H & E

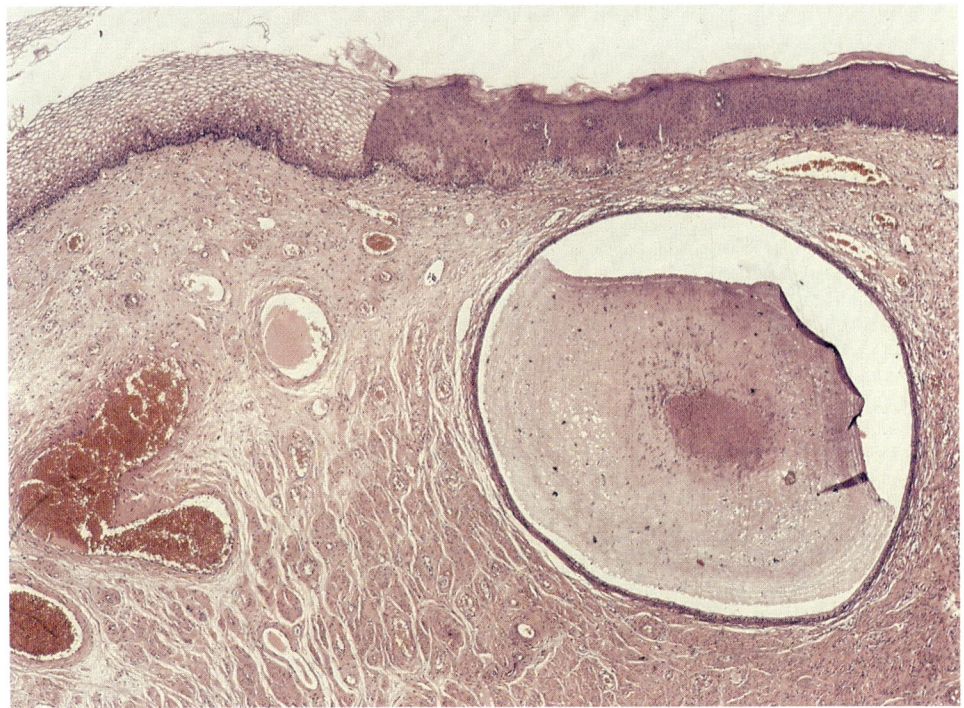

Fig. 11. Ascending repair following eversion of the endocervical mucosa onto the portio, advanced stage. H & E

In the early stages this regenerative epithelium consists of regular, but incompletely differentiated epithelial cells devoid of glycogen (Figs. 12, 13). Later, it cannot be distinguished from the original ectocervical epithelium (see p. 25, Fig. 31).

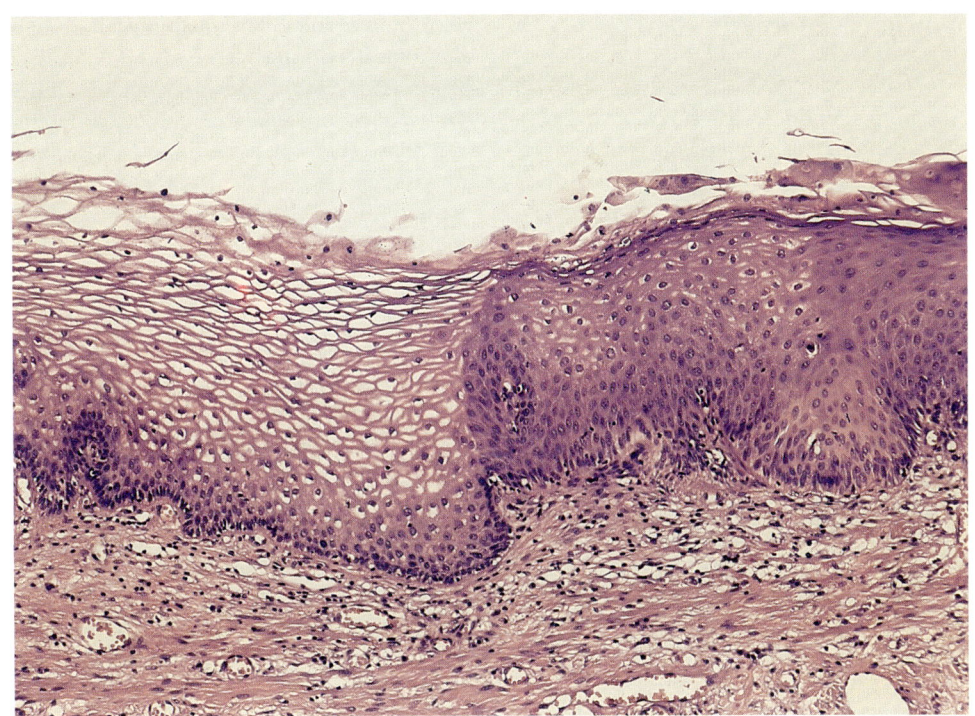

Fig. 12. Regenerative ectocervical epithelium sharply delineated from the original epithelium. H & E

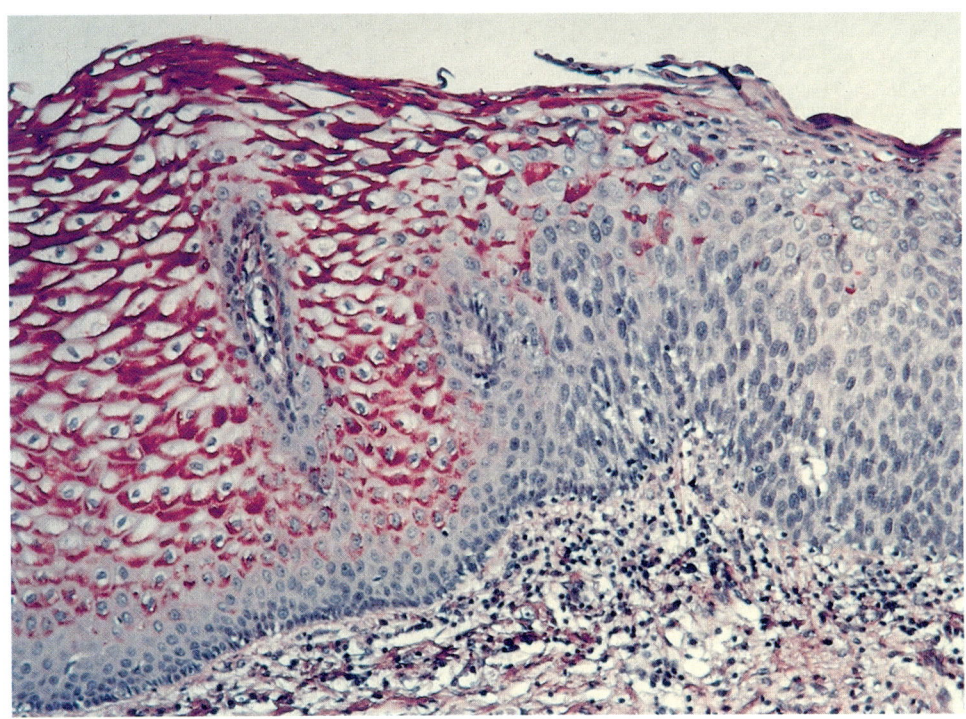

Fig. 13. Sharp line between original and regenerative epithelium. PAS reaction

Normal Endocervix (Figs. 14–19)

The normal endocervical mucosa consists of mucus-producing tubules and clefts (mucosal infoldings, usually called glands), loosely arranged in a fibrous stroma. A single layer of tall, columnar epithelial cells covers the mucosal surface and lines the intricate folds, clefts, and tubules. The small nuclei are basally placed during the early proliferative phase. The clear cytoplasm contains abundant mucus, especially in the late proliferative phase (Fig. 14). Where the endocervical mucosa merges with the isthmic mucosa, endometrial-type glands intermingle with endocervical glands (Figs. 15, 16).

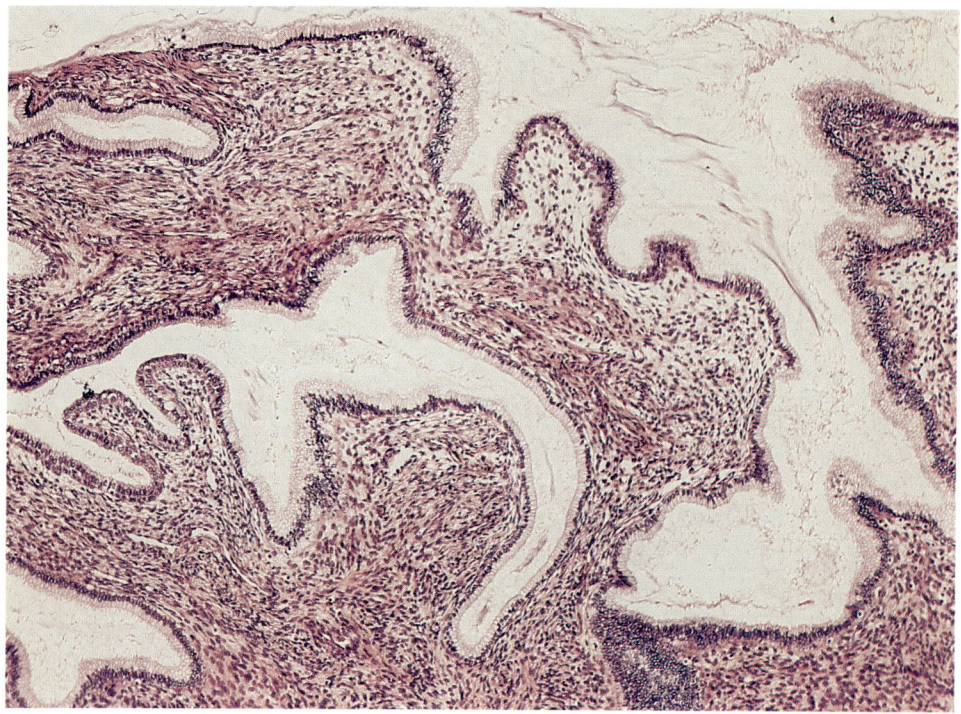

Fig. 14. Normal endocervical mucosa. H & E

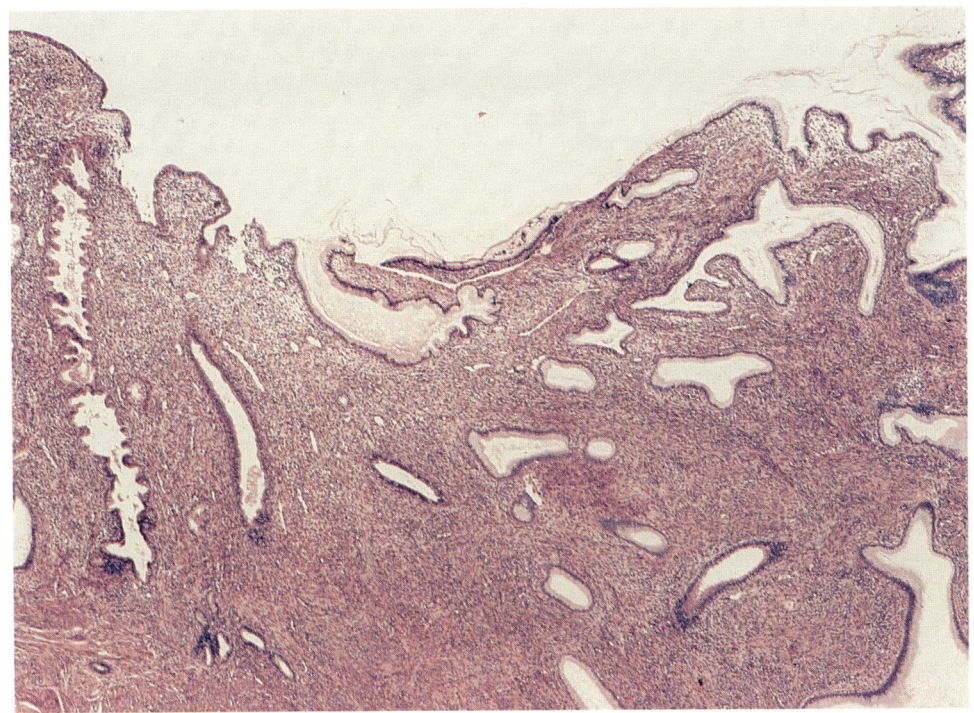

Fig. 15. Border between endocervical *(right)* and isthmic mucosa *(left)*. H & E

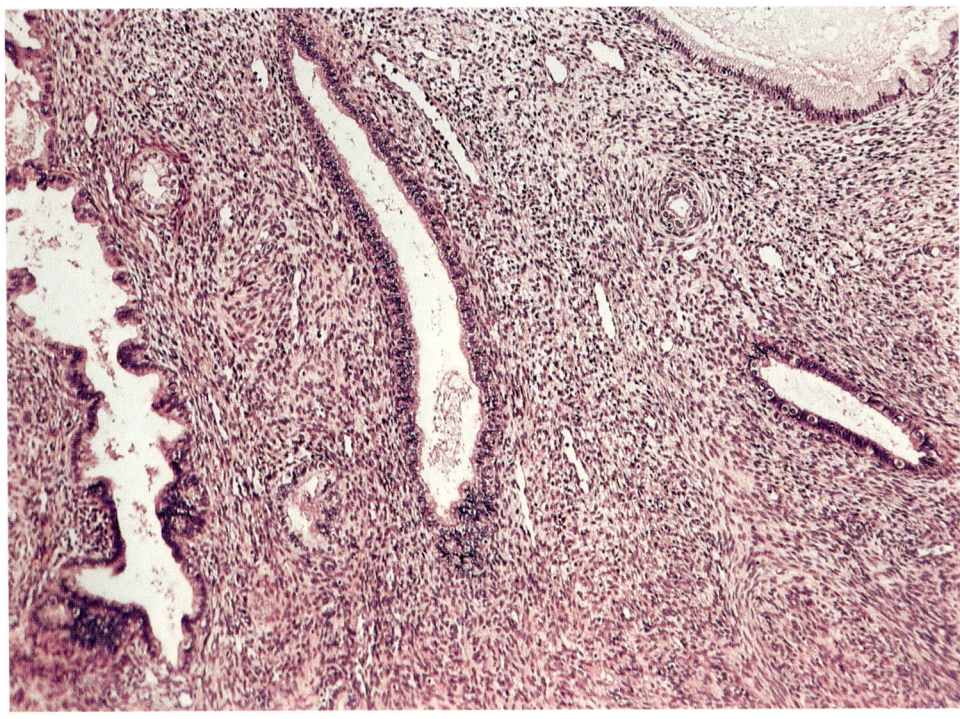

Fig. 16. Border between endocervical *(right)* and isthmic mucosa *(left)*. H & E, higher magnification

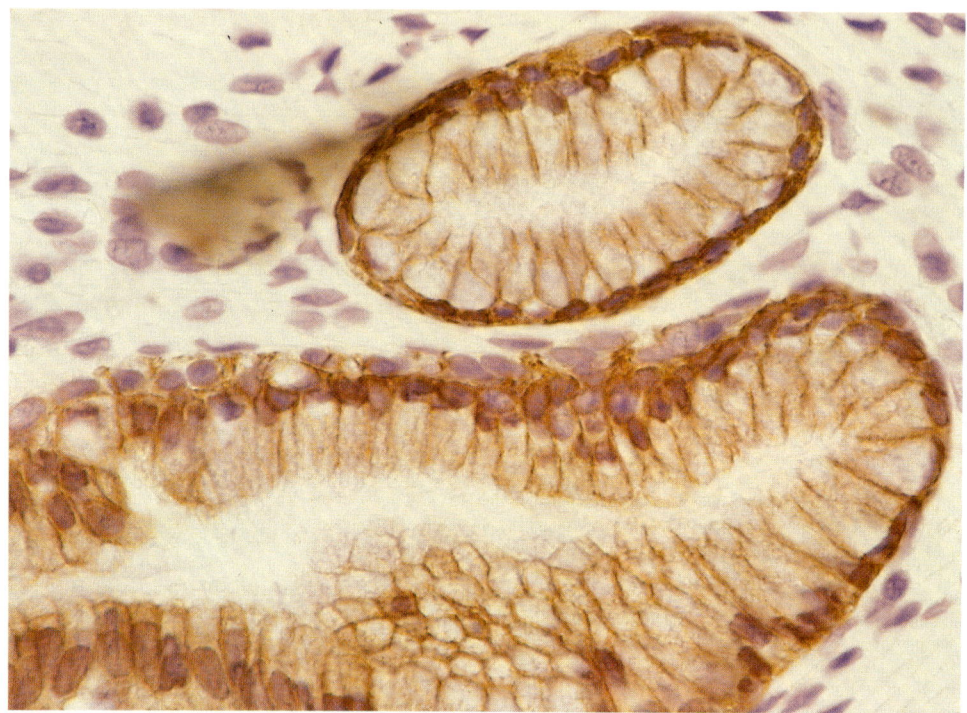

Fig. 17. Endocervical glands surrounded by a single layer of reserve cells. Immunohistochemical reaction with anticytokeratin 18

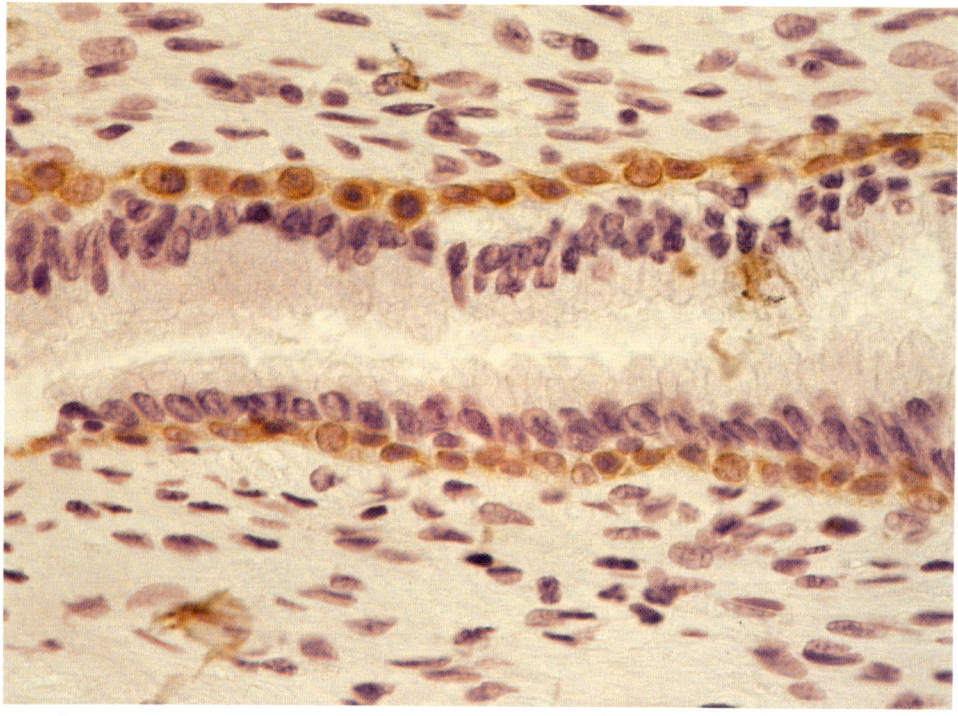

Fig. 18. Positive reaction of reserve cells with anticytokeratin KA 1, columnar cells negative

Beneath the endocervical columnar epithelium a small single layer of reserve cells can often be detected (Figs. 17-19). Immunohistochemically, these reserve cells differ in their cytoskeleton from the columnar cells: Although both cell types stain positively with broad-reacting cytokeratin antibodies, reserve cells remain unstained with antibodies against cytokeratin 18 (Fig. 17), but do react positively with antibodies against KA 1, a reaction characteristic of squamous epithelium (Fig. 18). In contrast, the columnar cells stain with antibodies against cytokeratin 18 (Fig. 17), and 8 (Fig. 19), but do not with antibodies against KA 1.

Consequently, the reserve cells of the endocervical epithelium differ immunohistochemically from the columnar cells covering them, much like the basal cells of the ectocervix differ from the cells overlying them, but in different ways. The basal layer of the ectocervix expresses cytokeratins characteristic for single (glandular) epithelial cells, yet is covered by squamous epithelium. The reserve cells of the endocervix contain cytokeratins characteristic for epithelial cells with squamous differentiation and are covered by a simple, glandular epithelium. Although the reserve cells are bipotential and capable of producing either keratin or mucin, they are not essentially precursors of the columnar cells, which can themselves proliferate by mitotic activity (Hiersche and Nagl 1980).

This distinctive endowment of cytokeratins of the basal and reserve cells and their bipotential capacities to differentiate in two different directions may explain how and why both epithelia at the squamocolumnar junction respond so characteristically to regenerative and metaplastic influences initiated by the eversion of the endocervix during the reproductive years.

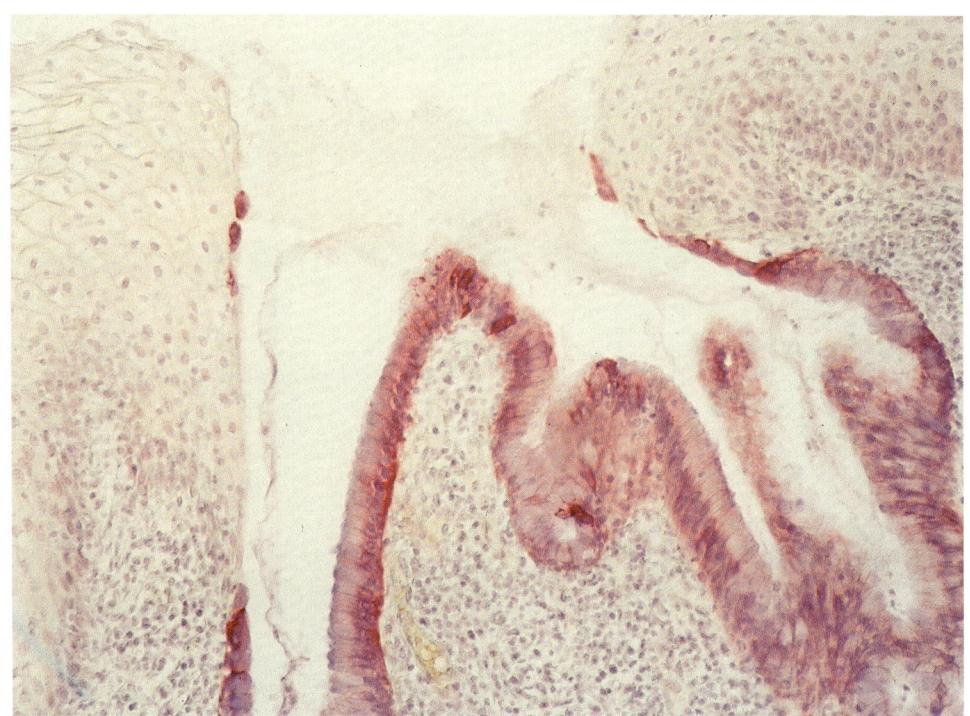

Fig. 19. Positive reaction of columnar endocervical cells with anticytokeratin 8, squamous epithelium negative

Descending Repair (Figs. 20–28)

Endocervical mucosal surface epithelium that everts out onto the portio may become replaced by squamous epithelium in two ways: (1) by overgrowth from adjacent regenerative ectocervical epithelium, as in ascending repair (Figs. 10–13), or (2) by squamous metaplasia of the reserve cells of the endocervical epithelium, as in descending repair. Both processes may occur simultaneously or separately. In general, ascending repair is stimulated by endogenous or exogenous estrogens, whereas descending repair predominates under endogenous or exogenous gestagenic stimulation (Dallenbach-Hellweg 1981). Descending repair is preceded by a double- or multilayered hyperplasia of the reserve cells, (Figs. 20, 21) which, in accordance with their cytokeratin endowment, undergo metaplastic change and differentiate into squamous epithelium (Figs. 22, 23). Some of these metaplastic cells, however, may retain their bipotential capacity and produce mucin, thereby being responsible for the monocellular mucin formation occasionally seen in squamous cell metaplasia of the endocervix (Figs. 24, 25).

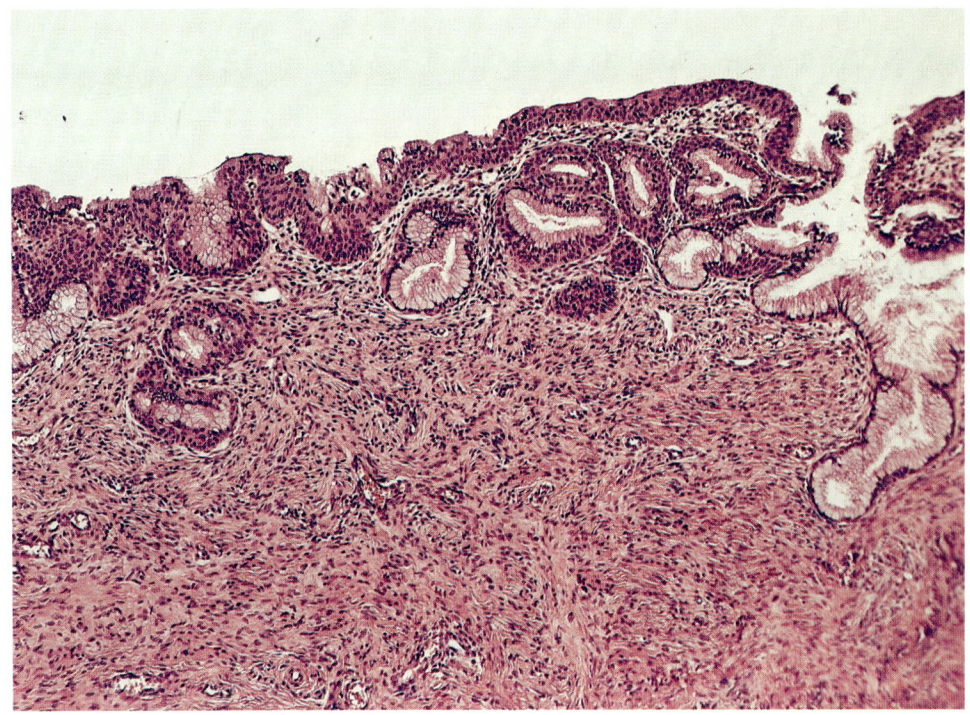

Fig. 20. Hyperplasia of reserve cells in descending repair. H & E

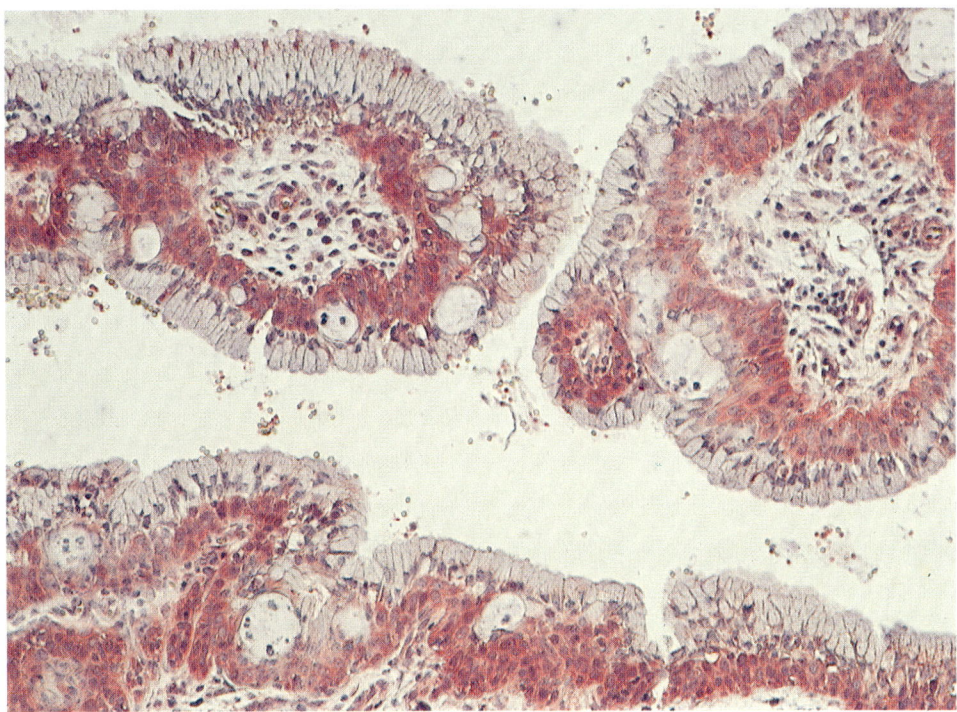

Fig. 21. Hyperplasia of reserve cells. Immunohistochemical reaction with anticytokeratin 13

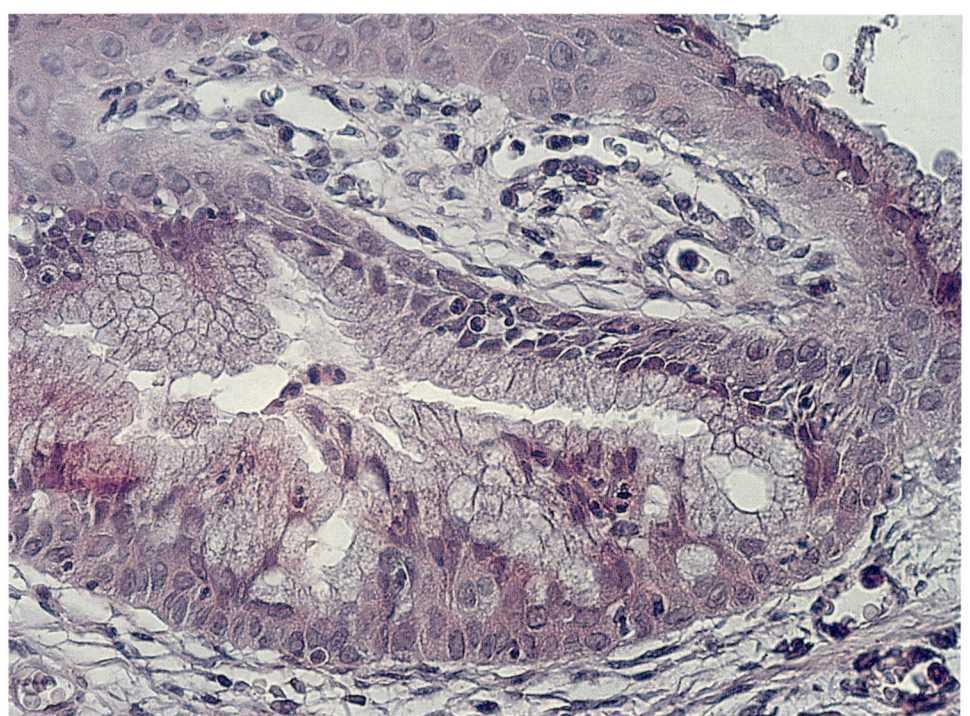

Fig. 22. Hyperplasia of reserve cells differentiating into squamous metaplasia. H & E

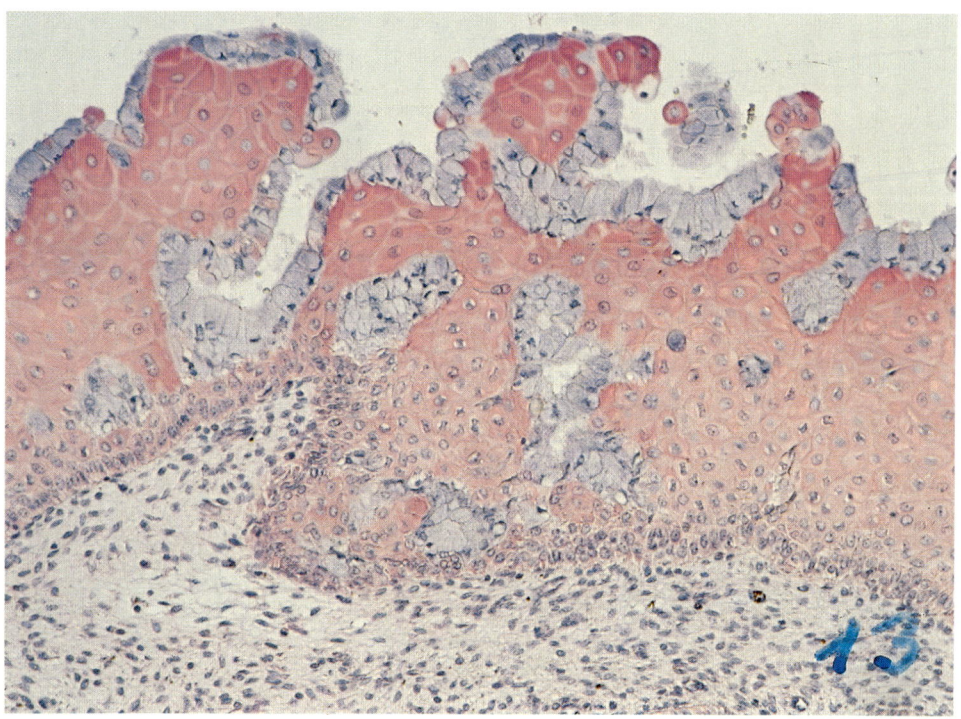

Fig. 23. Hyperplasia of reserve cells differentiating into squamous metaplasia. Immunohistochemical reaction with anticytokeratin 13

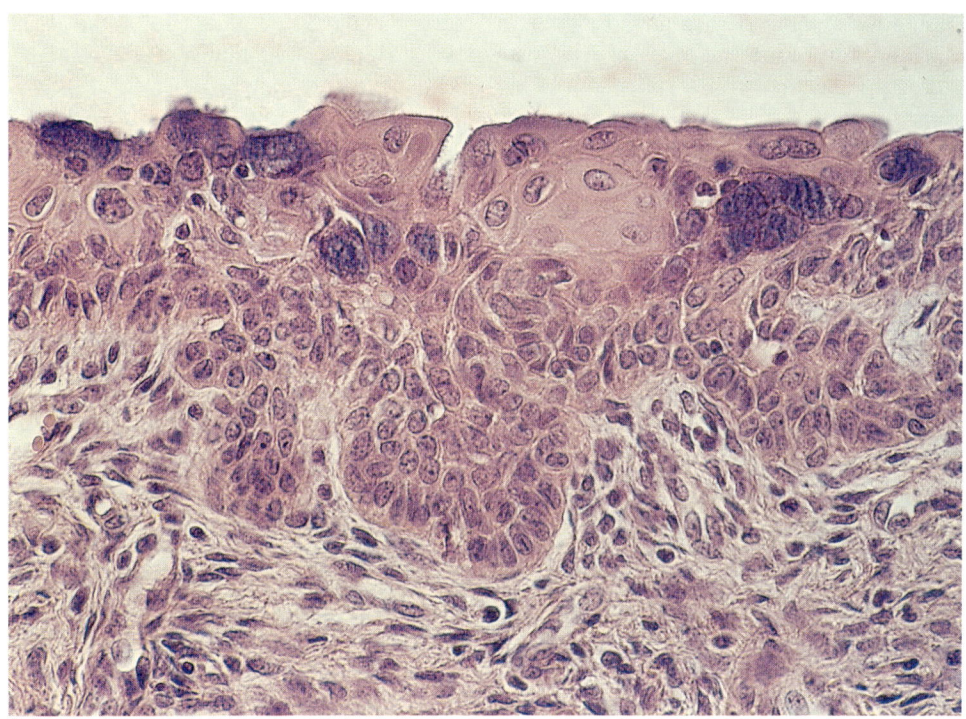

Fig. 24. Monocellular mucin formation in squamous metaplasia. H & E

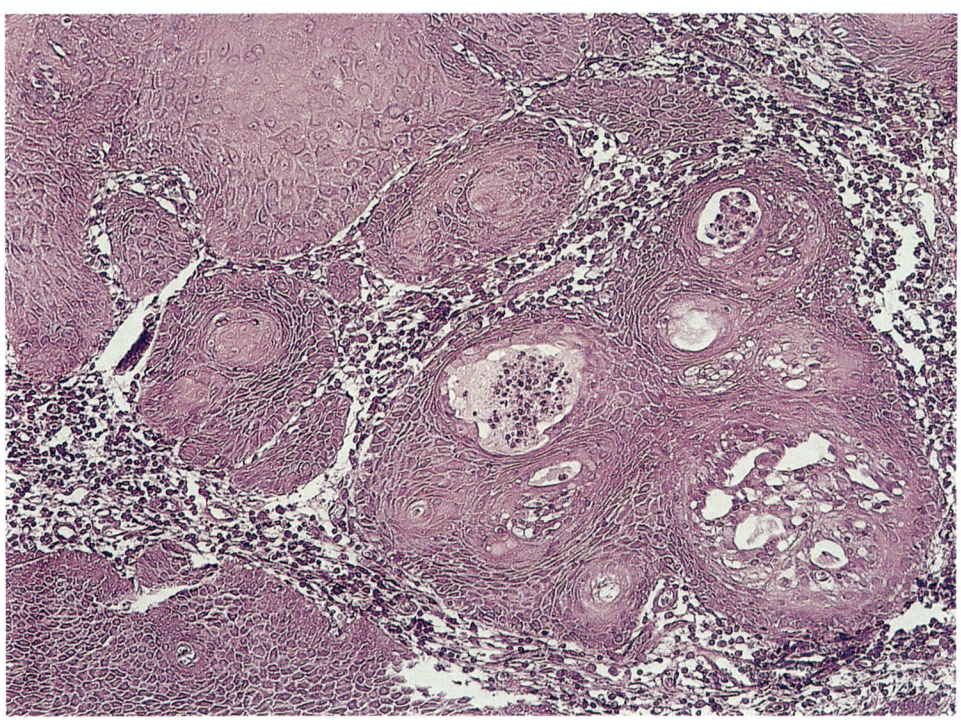

Fig. 25. Monocellular and multicystic mucin formation in squamous metaplasia. H & E

During maturation to squamous cells, their capability to produce mucin is usually lost. In contrast, the squamous epithelium adjacent to the endocervical epithelium expresses cytokeratins of the squamous epithelium type in all layers, whereas the columnar epithelium neighboring it exhibits a positive reaction only in the underlying reserve cell layer (Fig. 26). With mucin stains, a faint positive reaction may be detected in the superficial cell layer which may include the flattened atrophic remnants of columnar cells that originally covered the reserve cells (Figs. 27, 28).

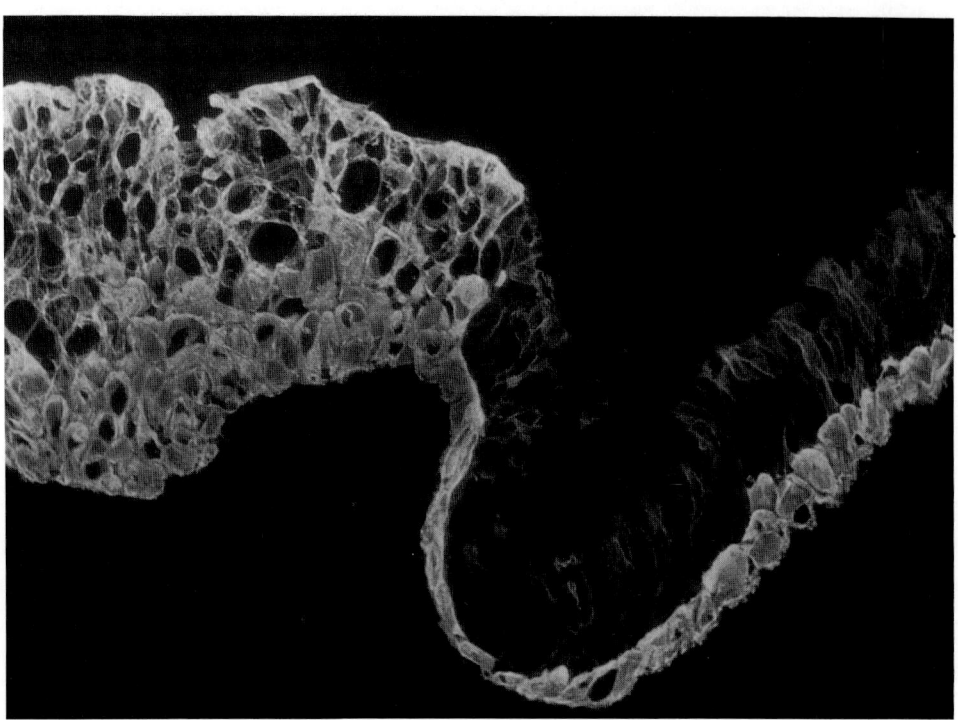

Fig. 26. Squamocolumnar junction with original squamous epithelium and adjacent reserve cell hyperplasia underneath the columnar epithelium. Immunohistochemical reaction with anticytokeratin KA 1 (from Franke et al. 1986)

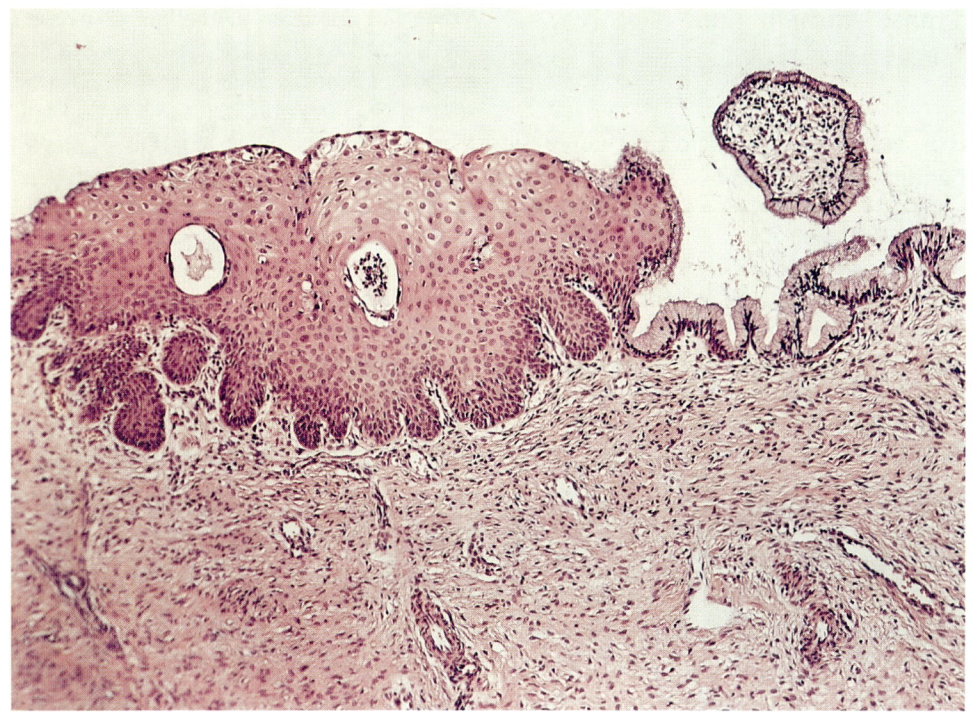

Fig. 27. Junction between squamous metaplasia and columnar epithelium. H & E

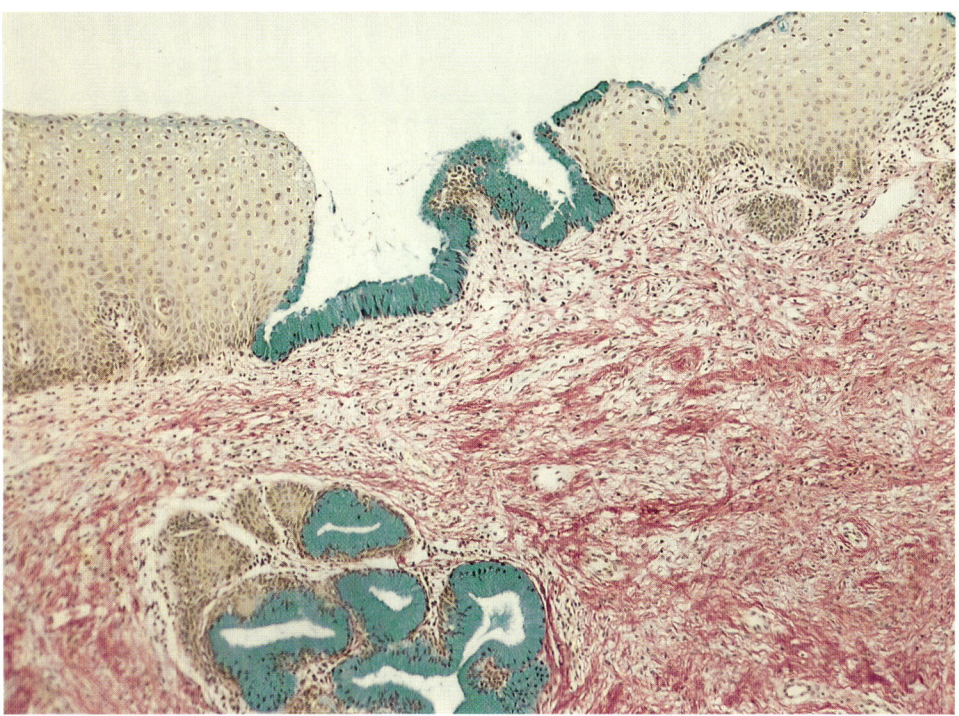

Fig. 28. Junction between squamous metaplasia and columnar epithelium. Alcian blue reaction

Transformation Zone (Figs. 29–31)

It is important to recognize and locate the transformation zone since most, if not all, cervical neoplasias arise at or above this squamocolumnar junction. In their developmental stage they usually are limited to the transformation zone. Both epithelia that participate in repair and compose this zone stain with antibodies to TPA, a tissue polypeptide antigen occurring in cancer cells and associated with cell proliferation (Löning et al. 1983).

When the squamous epithelium that covers this repair zone (Figs. 29, 30) does not undergo precancerous change, but, as in most instances, matures normally and completely, then at the end stage of repair it is impossible to distinguish the regenerative and metaplastic squamous epithelia from the adjacent primary ectocervical epithelium (Fig. 31). This "third mucosa" can only be recognized by the pinched off and often cystically dilated endocervical glands underlying the squamous epithelium. When these become large retention cysts, they may be recognized grossly as rounded protruberances (Ovula Nabothi, nabothian cysts).

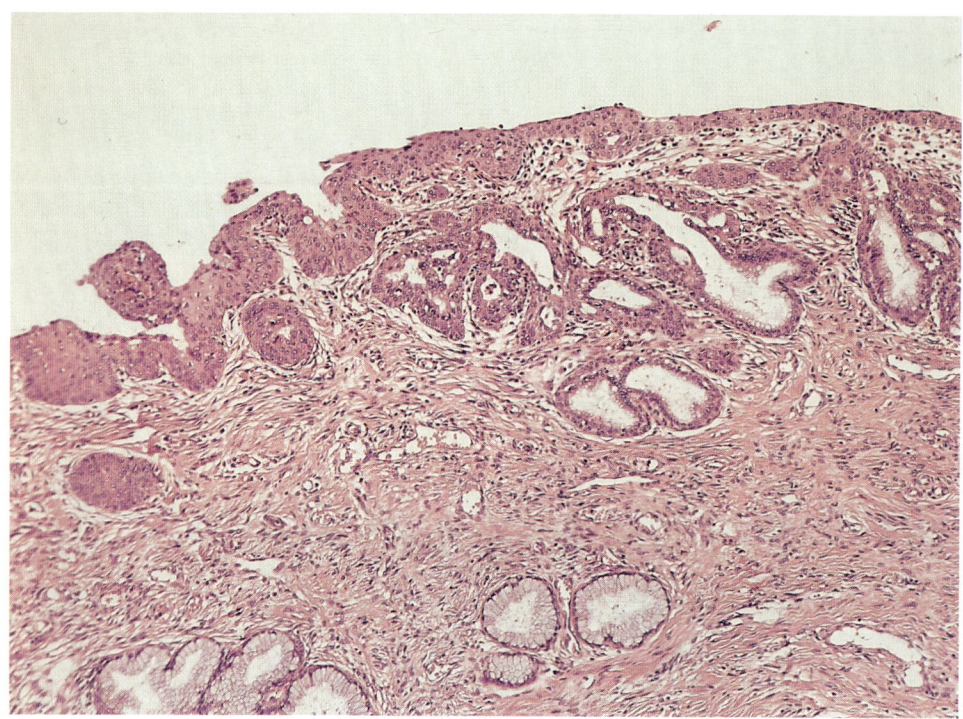

Fig. 29. Transformation zone covered by squamous metaplasia in descending repair, early stage. H & E

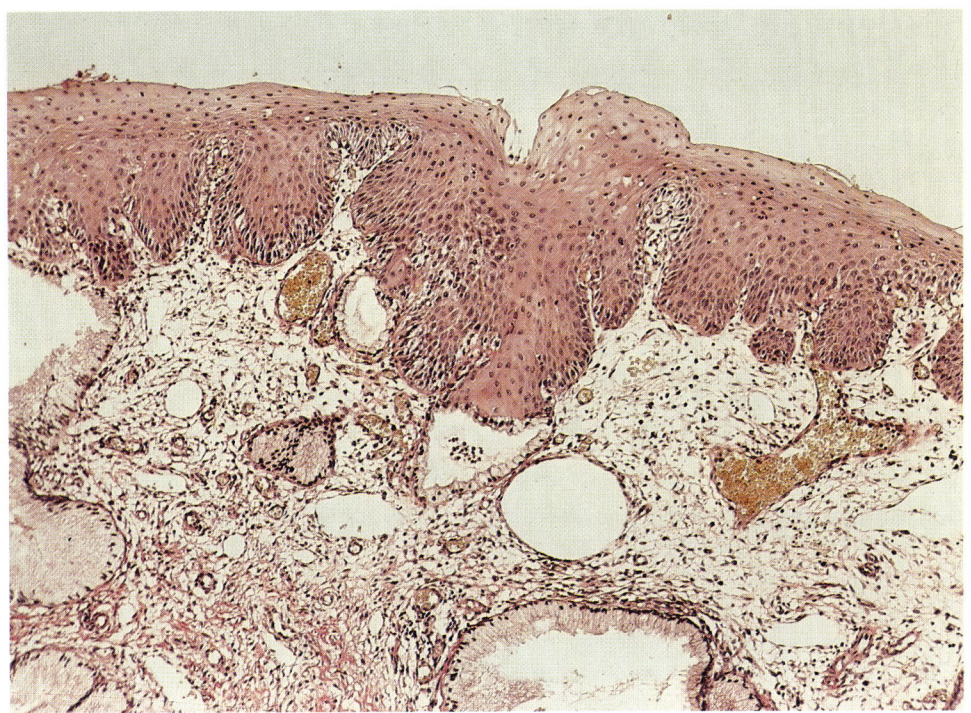

Fig. 30. Transformation zone covered by squamous metaplasia, intermediate stage. H & E

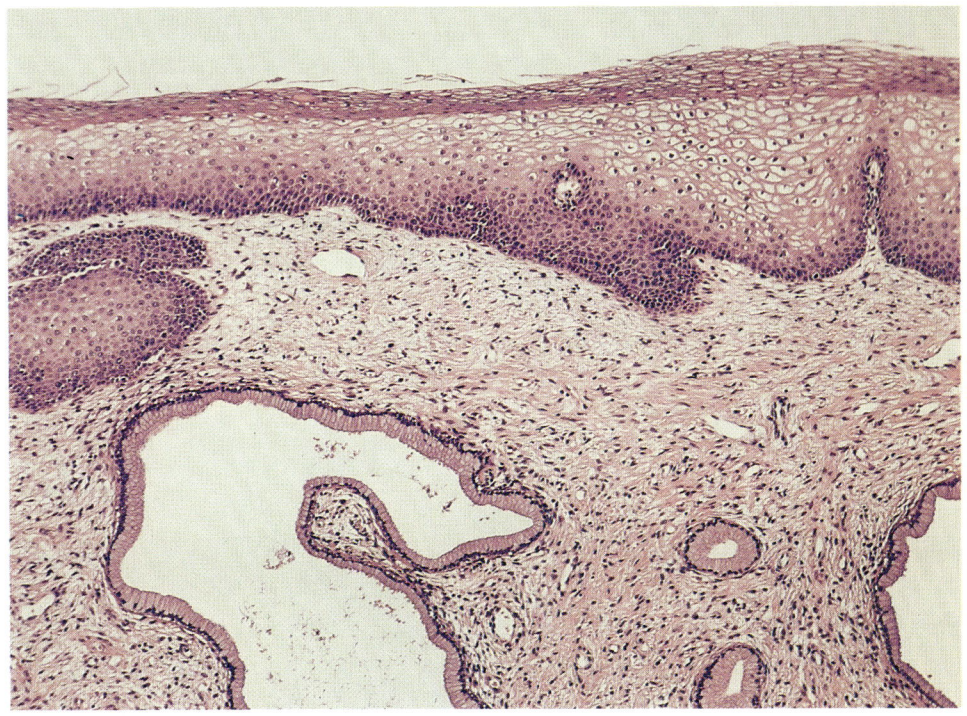

Fig. 31. Transformation zone covered by mature squamous epithelium, late stage. H & E

Vestigial and Heterotopic Tissues

Mesonephric Duct Remnants and Hyperplasia (Figs. 32–34)

Remnants of the mesonephric duct (Gartner's duct) are occasionally found deep in the lateral cervical wall (Fig. 32). They consist of small round tubules lined by a single layer of low cuboidal epithelium which contains no glycogen or mucin, whereas in the lumina one often finds eosinophilic PAS-positive homogenous material (Fig. 34). The tubules are often arranged in clusters, occasionally around an elongated remnant of a larger tubule (Fig. 33). Mesonephric duct *hyperplasia* consists of larger aggregates of such tubules which may even penetrate the entire cervical wall (florid type).

Differential Diagnosis. Hyperplasia must be carefully distinguished from: (a) mesonephric adenocarcinoma, which shows hobnail cells with cytological atypia, intraglandular epithelial papillae, and frank stromal invasion; and (b) minimal deviation adenocarcinoma of the endocervix, which shows intracellular mucin formation, a positive reaction with CEA, periglandular edema with mucin pools, a desmoplastic stromal reaction

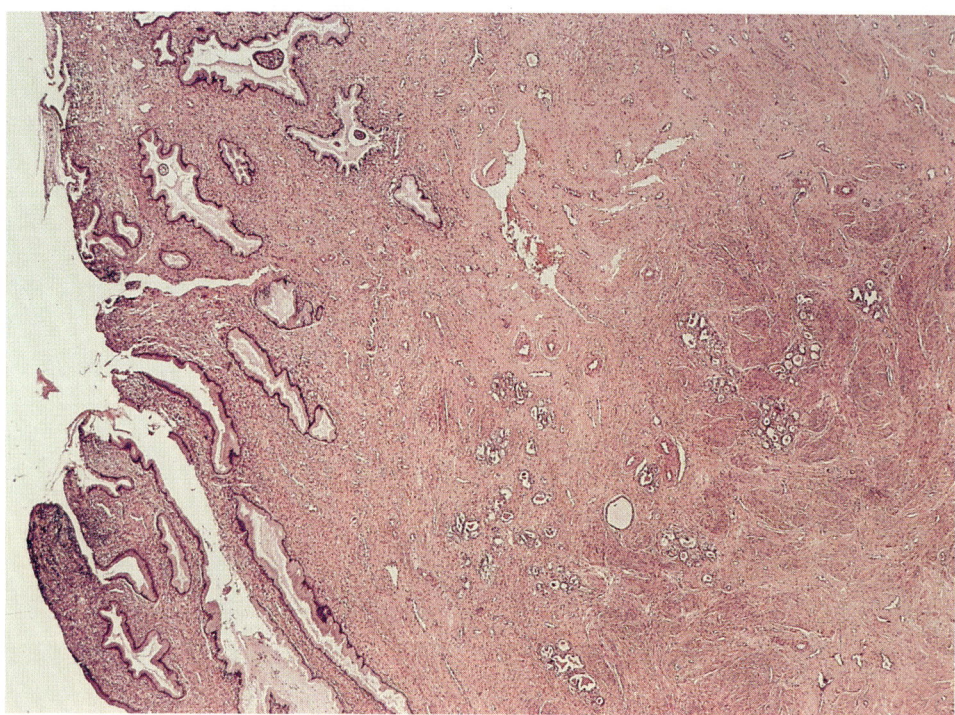

Fig. 32. Remnants of mesonephric duct in the cervical wall. H & E

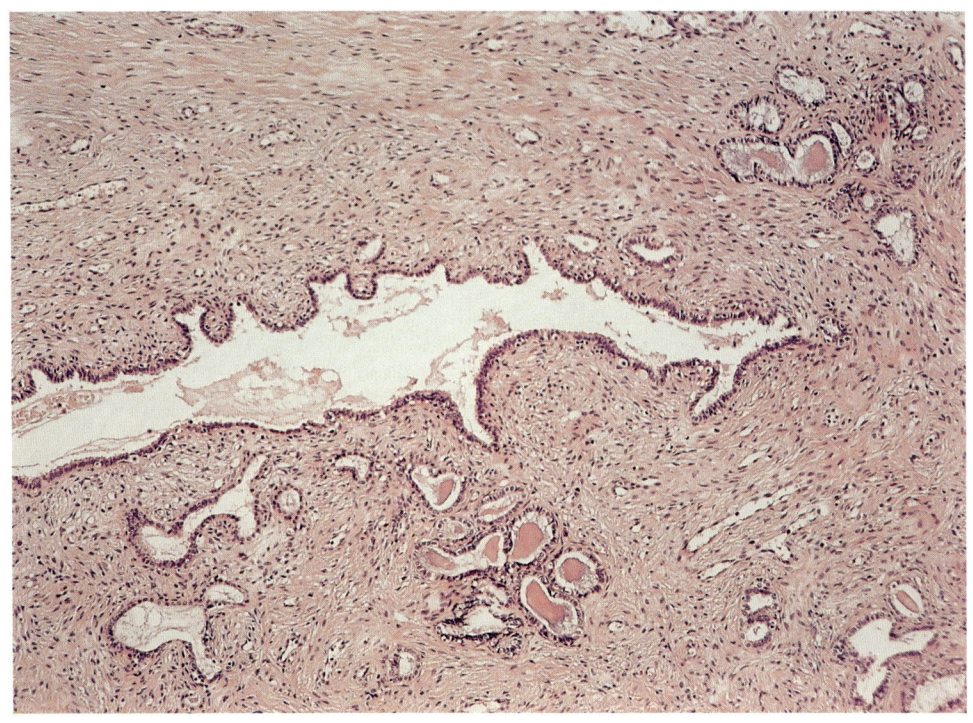

Fig. 33. Remnants of mesonephric duct in the cervical wall. H & E

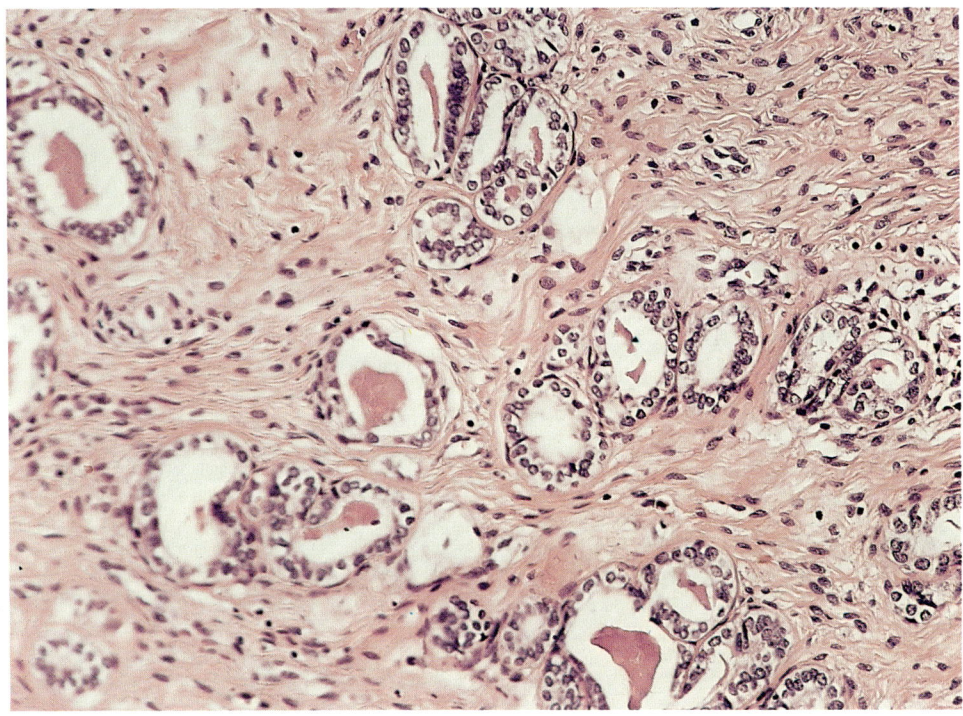

Fig. 34. Remnants of mesonephric duct in the cervical wall. H & E, higher magnification

around the invading tubules, and a histological transition between normal endocervical glands and the carcinomatous tubules (Shah et al. 1980; Ayroud et al. 1985).

Müllerian Duct Remnants and Metaplasia (Figs. 35-40)

Foci of ectocervical *endometriosis* may be located beneath the ectocervical epithelium and bulge forth as nodules (Fig. 35), grossly recognizable by the old and fresh hemorrhages in and around them (Figs. 35, 36), or be located deep in the cervical wall (Figs. 37 and 38). These deep foci correspond in their location and structure to adenomyosis of the myometrium. The glands are characteristically surrounded by an endometrial-type stroma.

In some instances, endocervical glands may be lined by columnar ciliated cells resulting from an *endosalpingial (tubal) metaplasia* (Figs. 39, 40). Such glands are devoid of surrounding endometrial-type stroma and correspond to the foci of endosalpingiosis occasionally found scattered about the small pelvis (Wells and Brown 1986). Foci of *intestinal metaplasia* may also be observed within endocervical glands.

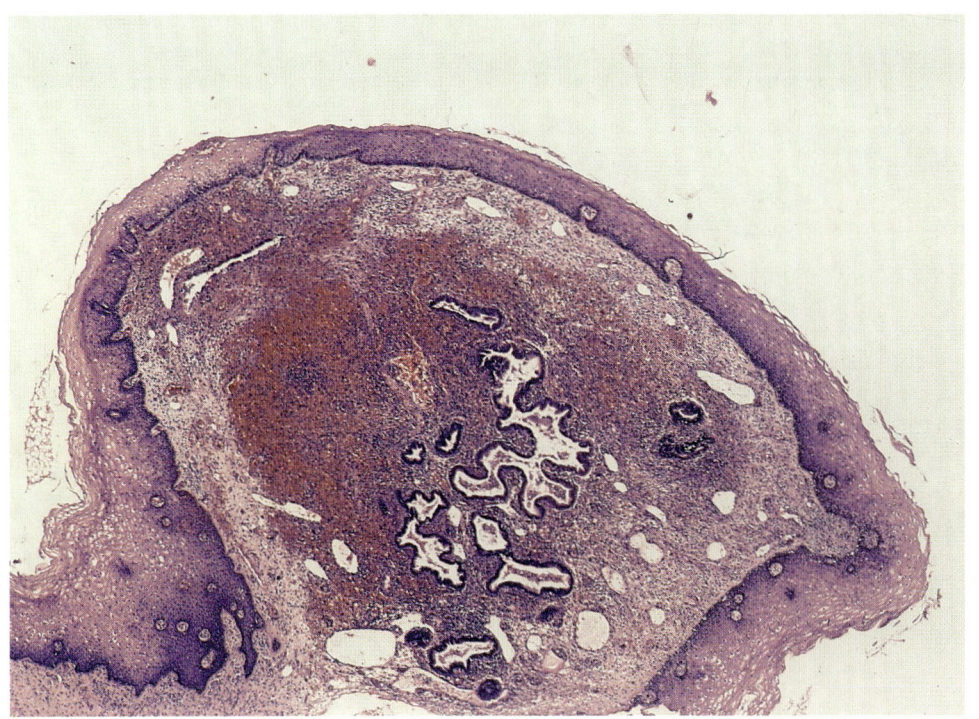

Fig. 35. Focus of endometriosis underneath ectocervical epithelium. H & E

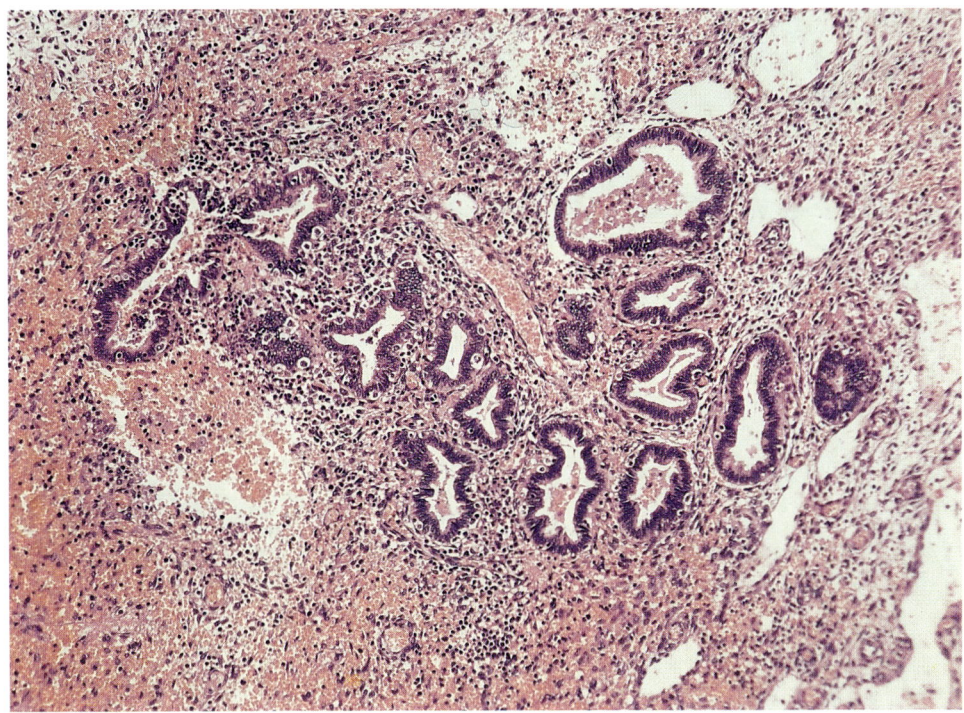

Fig. 36. Focus of endometriosis underneath ectocervical epithelium. H & E, higher magnification

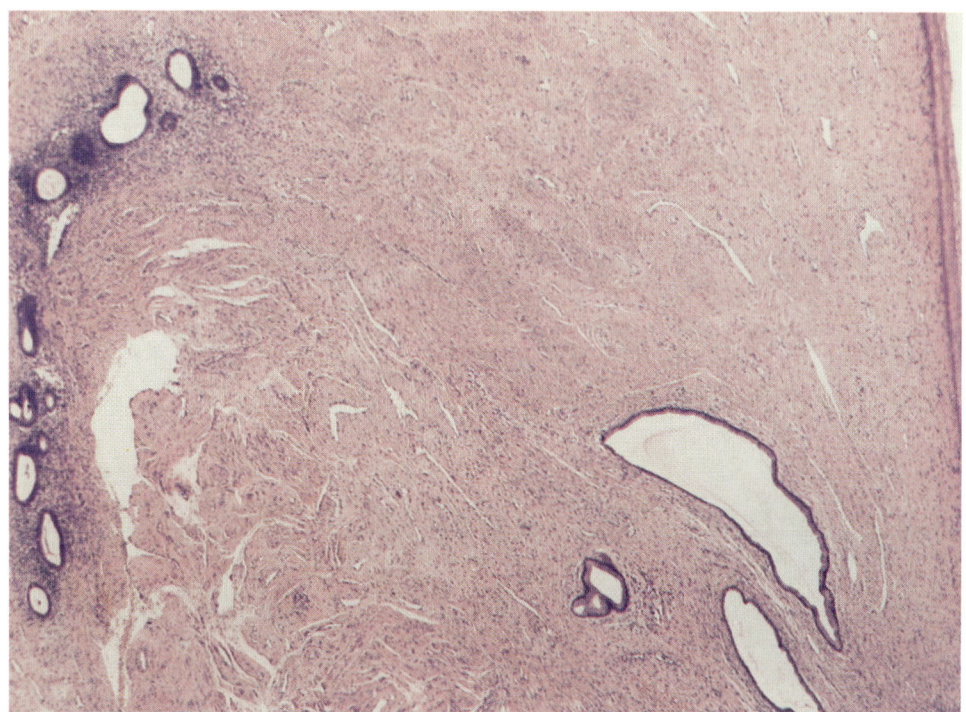

Fig. 37. Focus of endometriosis in the cervical wall. H & E

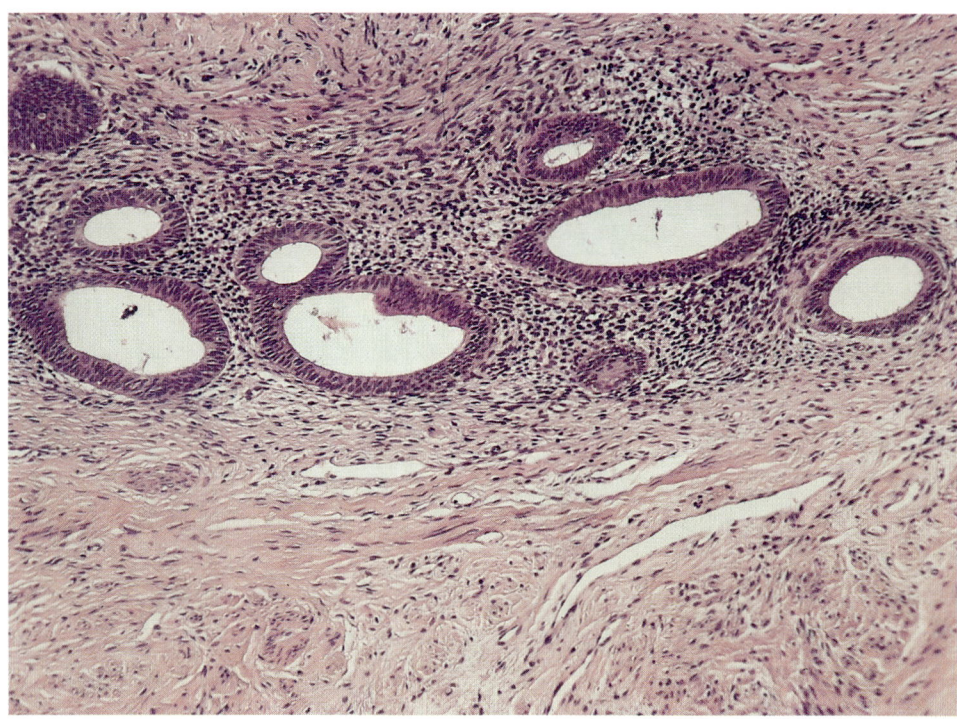

Fig. 38. Focus of endometriosis in the cervical wall. H & E, higher magnification

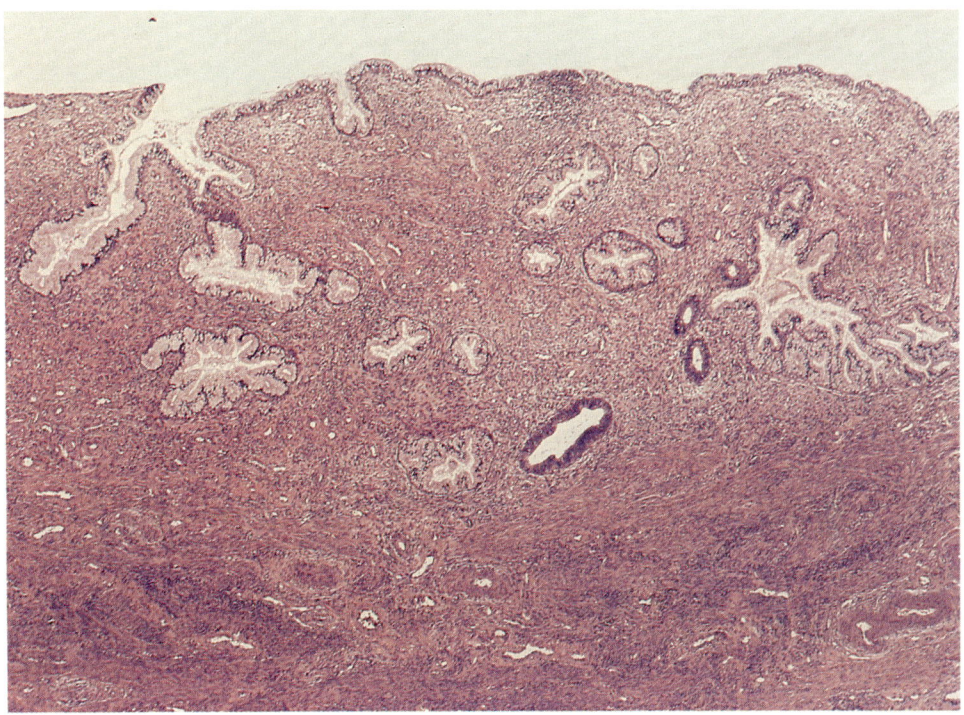

Fig. 39. Endosalpingeal metaplasia of endocervical glands. H & E

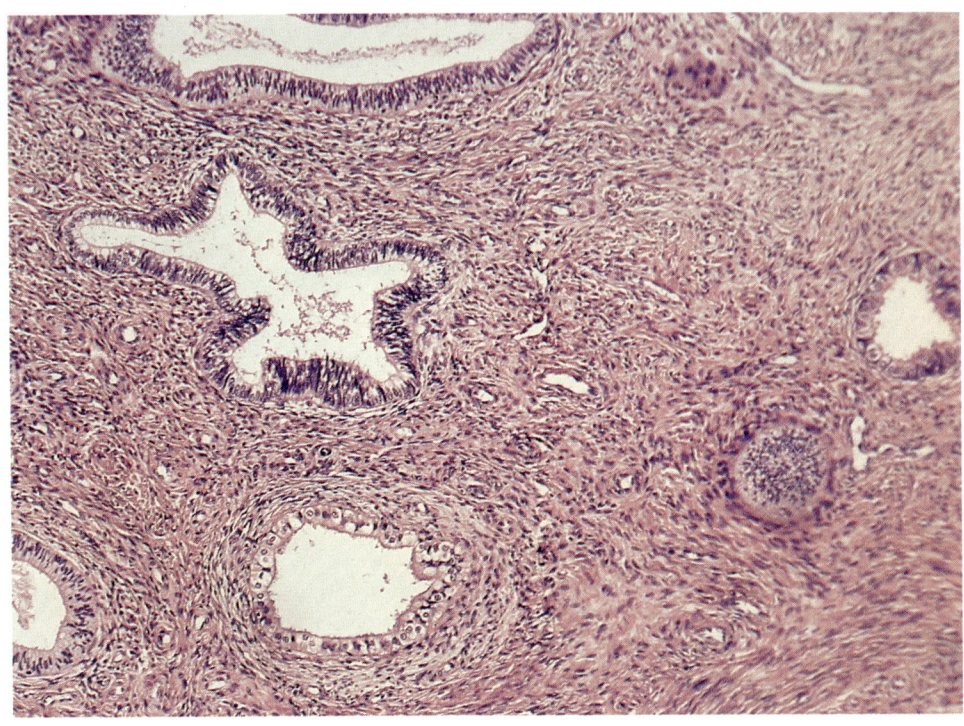

Fig. 40. Endosalpingeal metaplasia of endocervical glands. H & E, higher magnification

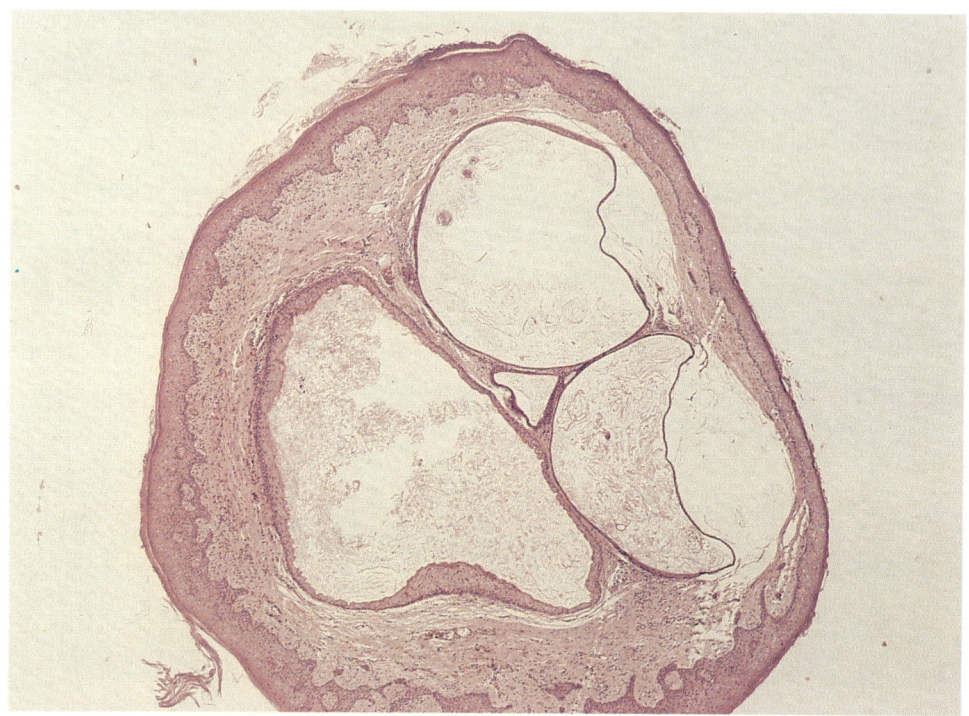

Fig. 41. Epidermoid cyst of ectocervix. H & E

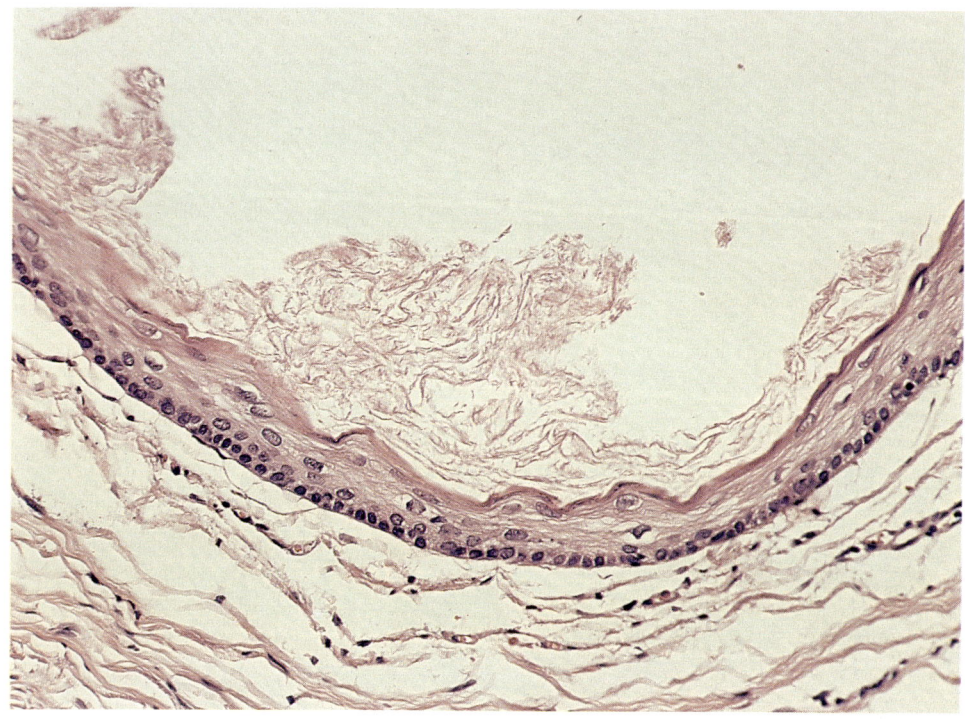

Fig. 42. Epidermoid cyst of ectocervix. H & E, higher magnification

Heterotopic Ectodermal and Mesodermal Structures (Figs. 41–45)

Rarely, heterotopic "neometaplasia" (Young et al. 1981) may result in the formation of epidermoid or dermoid cysts (Figs. 41–43) or give rise to sebaceous or sweat gland formations beneath the ectocervical epithelium (Figs. 44, 45; Dougherty et al. 1962). These structures have no clinical significance.

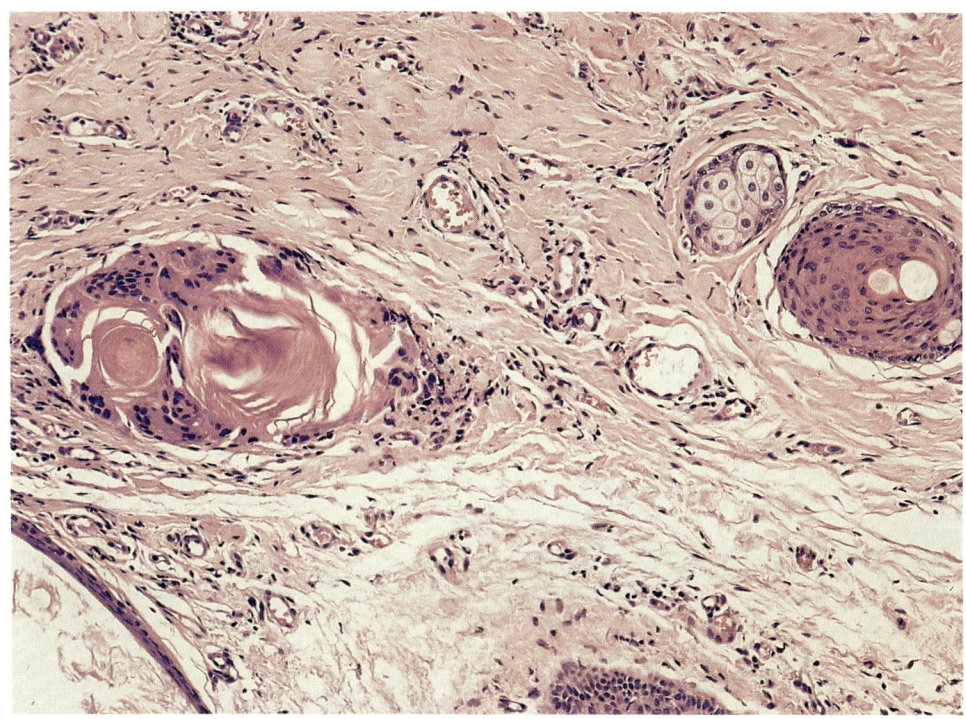

Fig. 43. Epidermoid cyst of ectocervix. Foreign body reaction around squamous cells. H & E

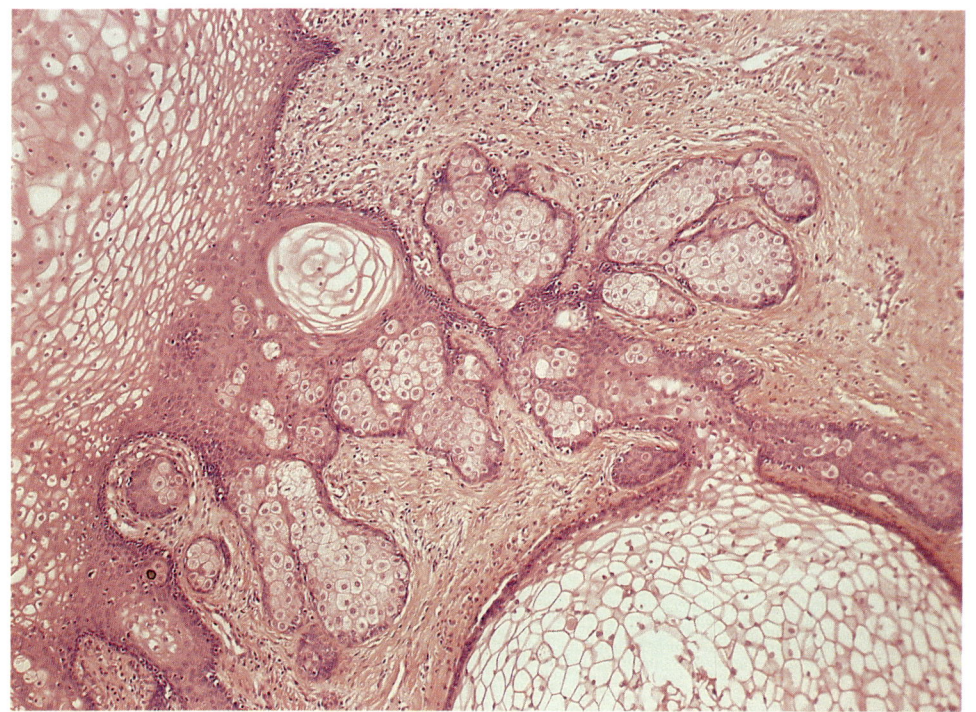

Fig. 44. Formation of sebaceous glands beneath ectocervical epithelium. H & E

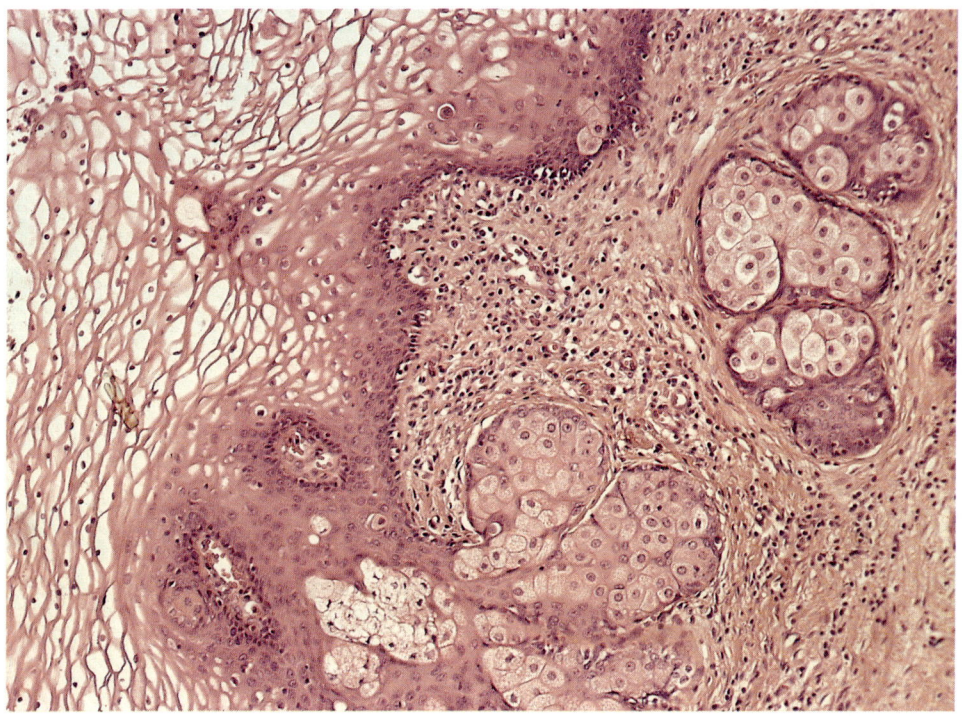

Fig. 45. Formation of sebaceous glands beneath ectocervical epithelium. H & E, higher magnification

Hormonally Induced Changes

Estrogens and gestagens act as antagonists not only on the endometrium but also on the ecto- and endocervix (Dallenbach-Hellweg 1981; Table 1).

Effects of Estrogen (Figs. 46–53)

Parakeratosis and Hyperkeratosis of the Ectocervix

Estrogens stimulate proliferation of the squamous epithelium of the ectocervix, resulting in a well-developed superficial cell layer often covered by a fairly thick layer of parakeratotic cells (Figs. 46, 47) which become keratinized prematurely. In endogenous or exogenous hyperestrogenism the keratinization may become exaggerated, whereby a thin (Fig. 48) or thick (Fig. 49) layer of hyperkeratosis is devoid of nuclei.
The proliferative effect of estrogens, furthermore, promotes ascending repair of columnar epithelium or epithelial defects which are overgrown by regenerative epithelium of ectocervical origin (see p. 10). Similar hyperkeratinization follows the stimulatory effects induced by chronic trauma, as in uterine prolapse.

Cystic Hyperplasia of the Endocervix

Under estrogenic stimulation the epithelial cells of the endocervical glands differentiate and produce mucin, which may become excessive with long-standing unopposed estrogen. Consequently, the glands become cystically dilated with inspissated mucin (Figs. 50–53). Thereby they become closely clustered, and the glandular region enlarges by extending down into the cervical wall. Reserve cells or areas of preceding reserve cell hyperplasia may differentiate and undergo squamous cell metaplasia (see p. 18).

Table 1. The effects of ovarian hormones on the uterus

	Estrogen	Progesterone
Ectocervix	Proliferation, para- and hyperkeratosis	Differentiation, desquamation
Endocervix	Differentiation: glands: secretion of mucine; reserve cells: squamous metaplasia	Proliferation (regeneration), glandular and reserve cell hyperplasia
Endometrium	Proliferation	Differentiation: glands: secretion of glycogen; stroma: decidualization

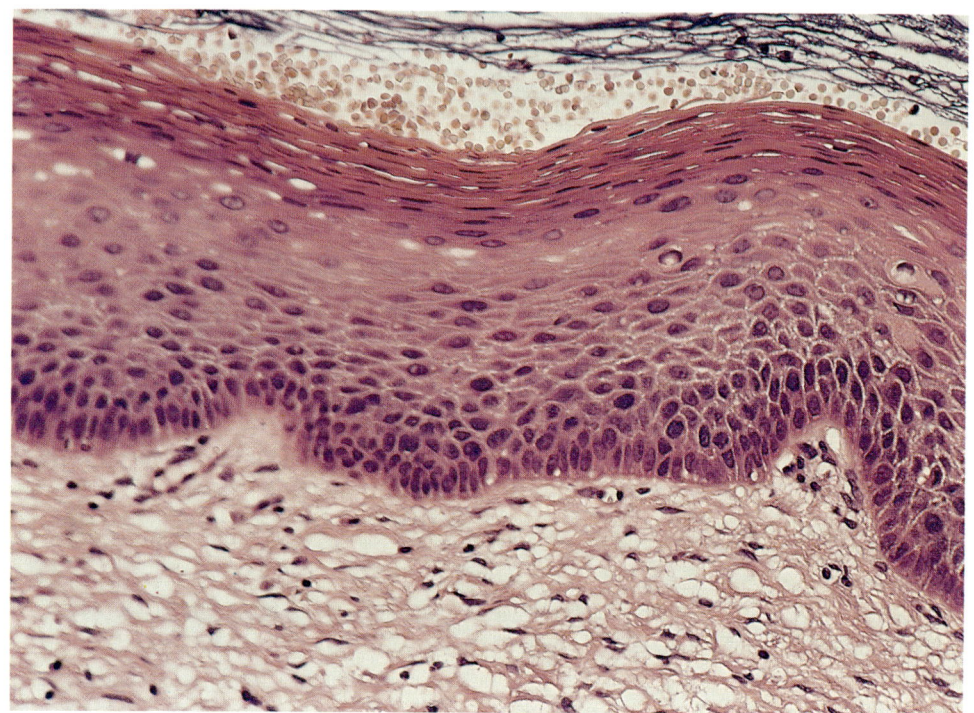

Fig. 46. Parakeratosis of ectocervical epithelium. H & E

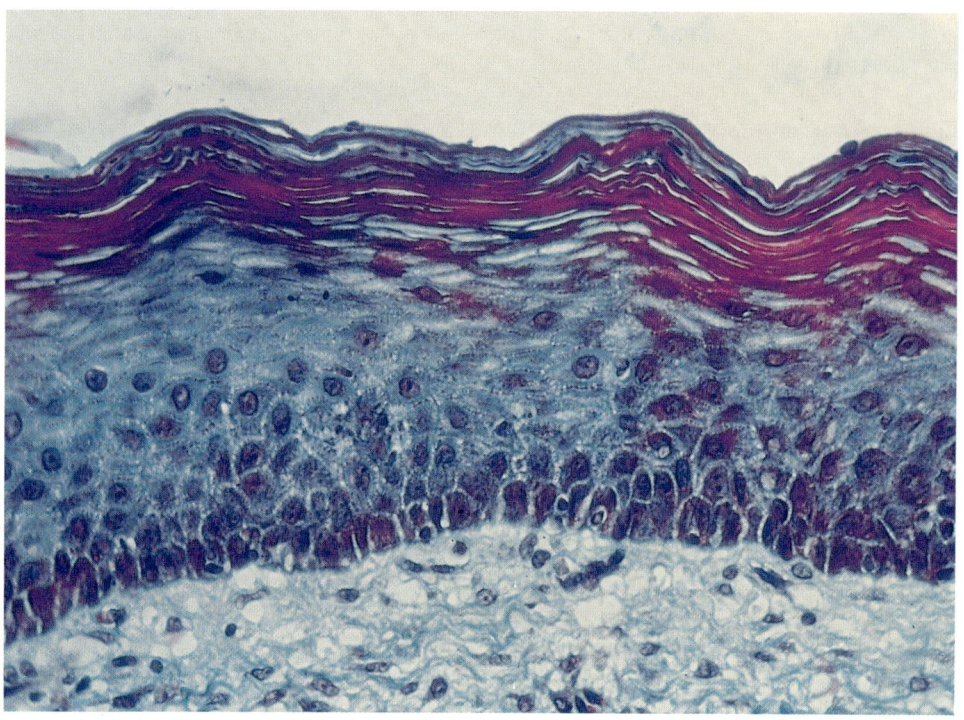

Fig. 47. Parakeratosis of ectocervical epithelium. PAS reaction

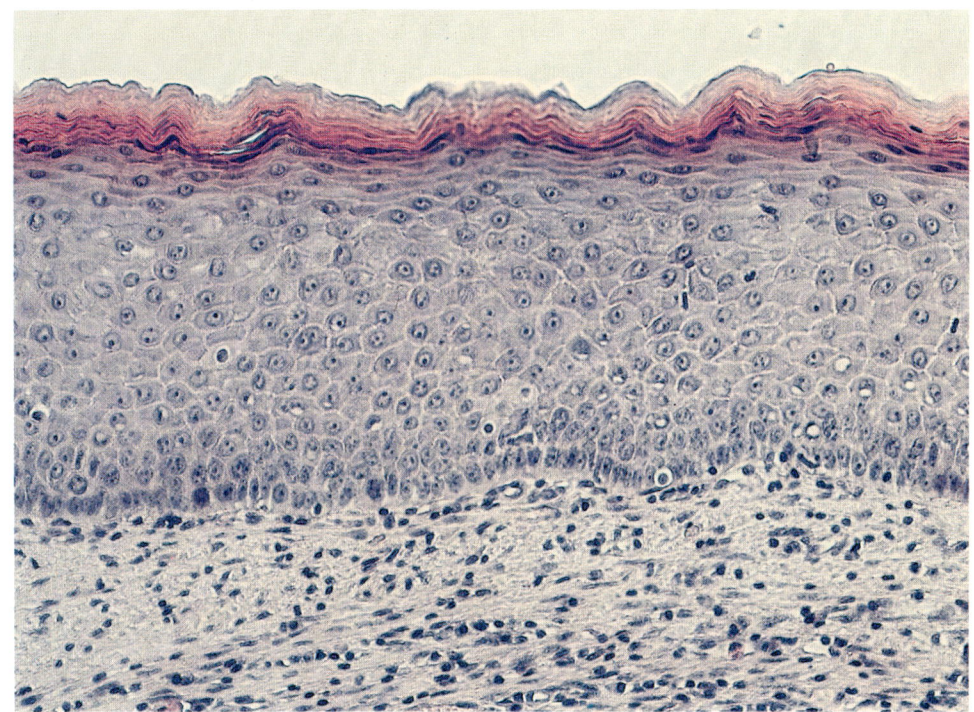

Fig. 48. Hyperkeratosis of ectocervical epithelium, mild. H & E

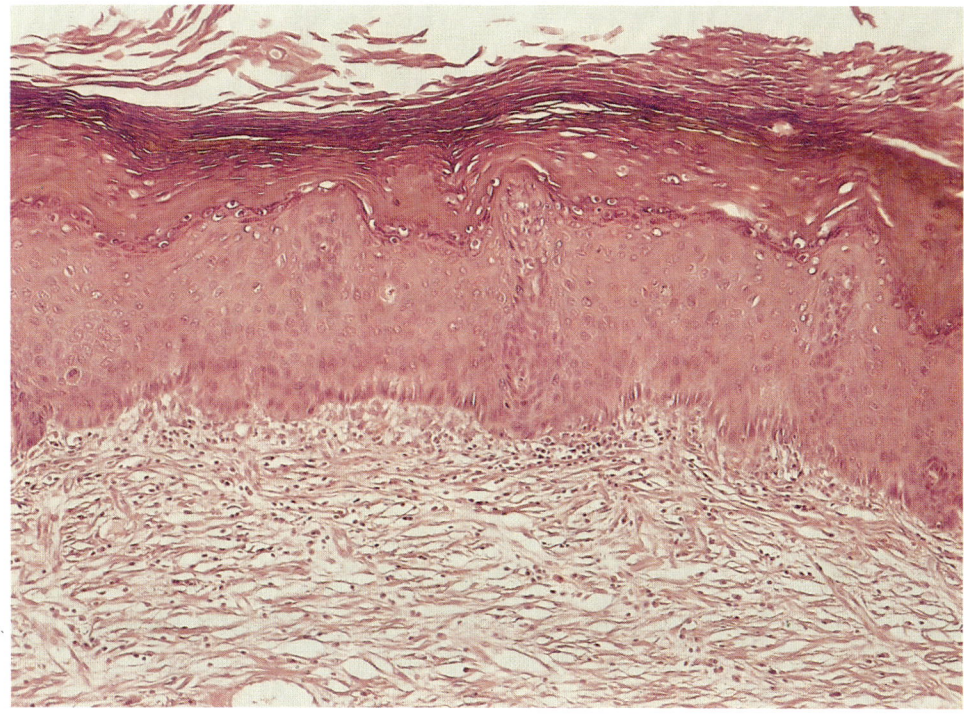

Fig. 49. Hyperkeratosis of ectocervical epithelium, extensive. H & E

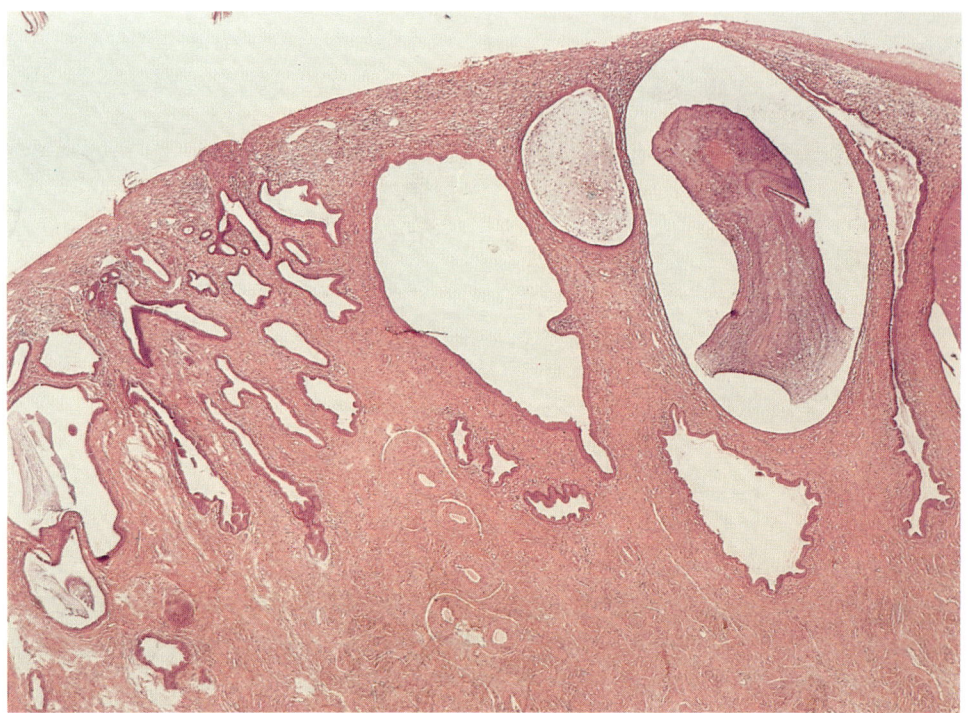

Fig. 50. Cystic hyperplasia of endocervix, mild. H & E

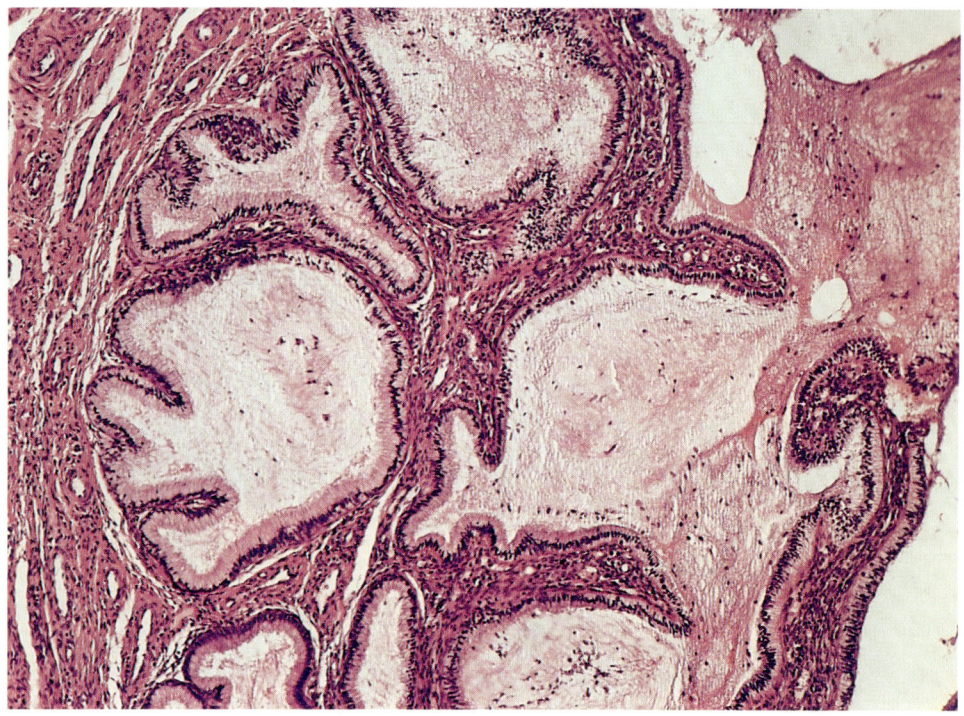

Fig. 51. Cystic hyperplasia of endocervix, mild. H & E, higher magnification

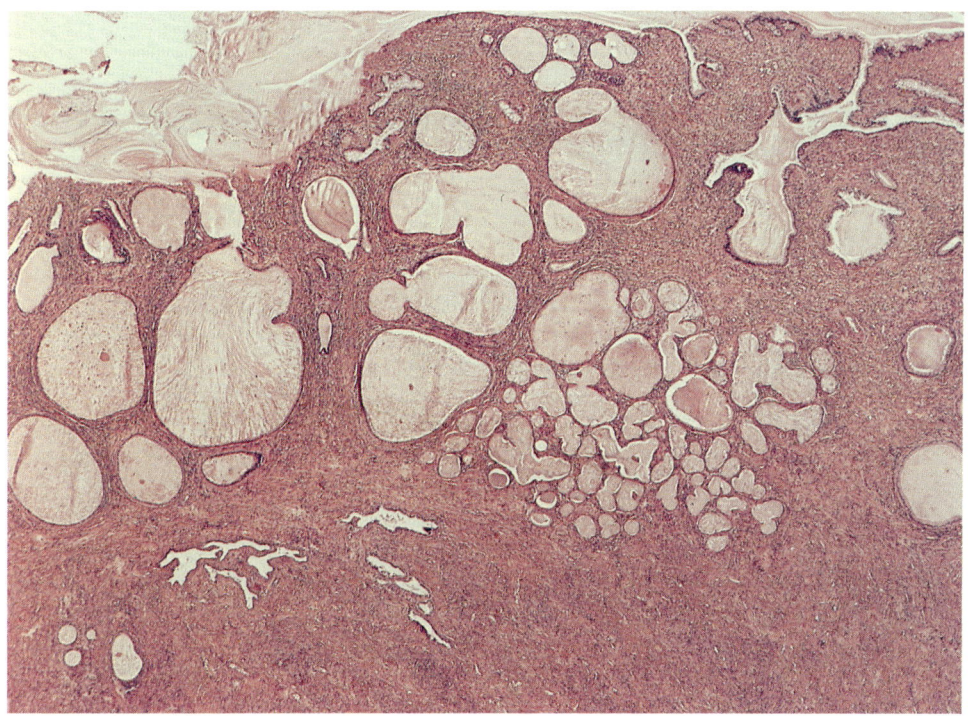

Fig. 52. Cystic hyperplasia of endocervix, extensive. H & E

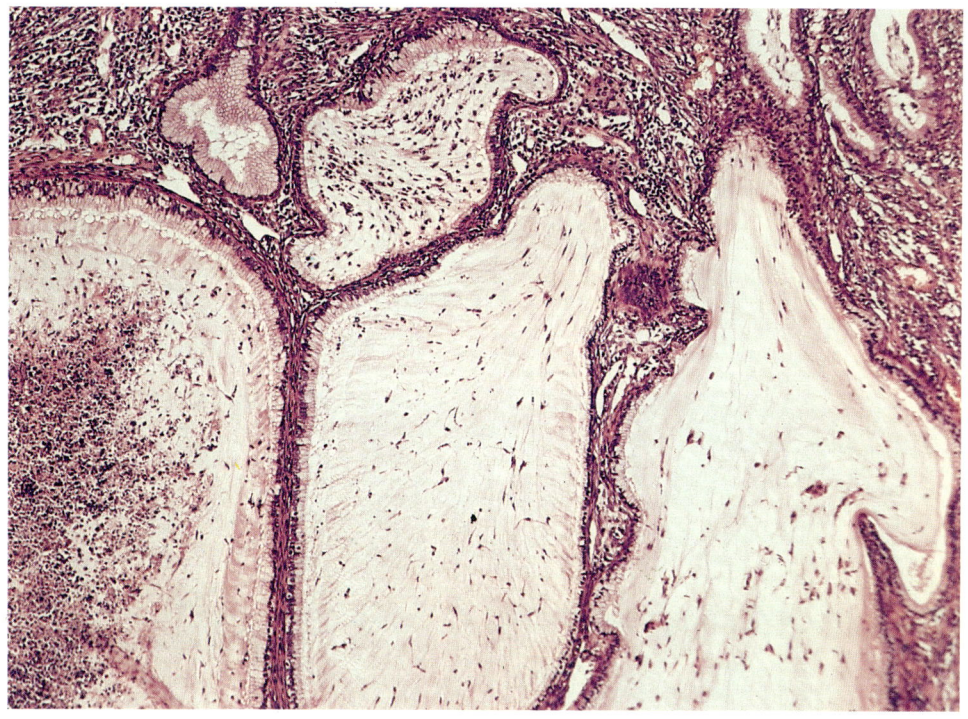

Fig. 53. Cystic hyperplasia of endocervix, extensive. H & E, higher magnification

Effects of Endogenous Progesterone Under Hypersecretion (Figs. 54, 55)

Glandular and Cystic Hyperplasia of the Endocervix

The physiologic hyperstimulation of the endocervical mucosa during gestation induces a mild or moderate hypersecretion of the glands and a proliferation of reserve cells (Fig. 55). The ectropionized mucosa usually is overgrown by an ascending regenerative epithelium (Fig. 54). Foci of ectopic decidua may be found in the endocervix and appear much like those seen at various other sites throughout the small pelvis during pregnancy. They show that they possess the inherent genetic potentialities of müllerian-derived cells. In like manner, an Arias-Stella reaction is also occasionally observed in endocervical glands.

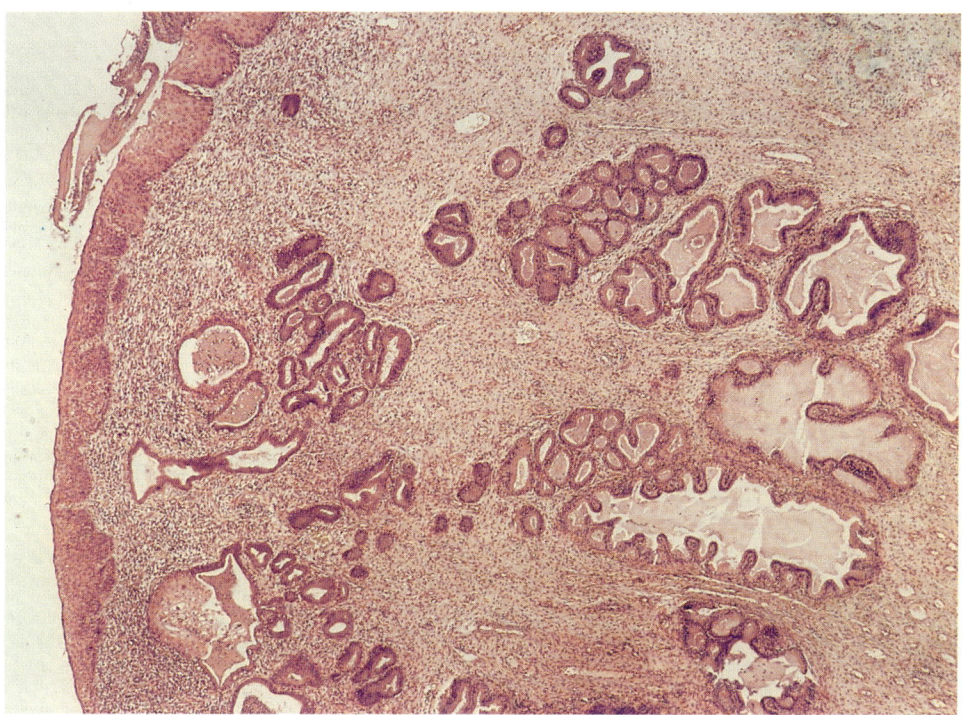

Fig. 54. Glandular and cystic hyperplasia of endocervix during pregnancy, with proliferation of reserve cells. H & E

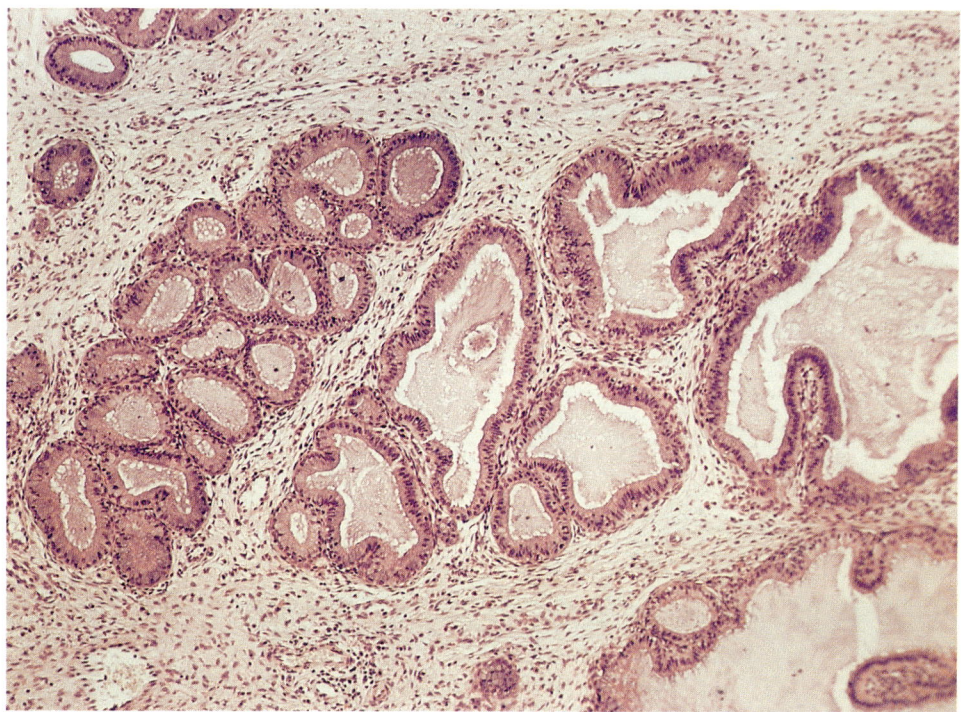

Fig. 55. Glandular and cystic hyperplasia of endocervix during pregnancy, with proliferation of reserve cells. H & E, higher magnification

Effects of Exogenous Gestagens
(Figs. 56-63)

Under the influence of synthetic gestagens the maturation of the ectocervical stratified squamous epithelium ceases at the intermediate stage, and desquamation is enhanced. In contrast, under the same hormonal stimulation, the endocervix shows proliferative changes, the intensity and histological appearance of which varies depending on the length of administration, dose, potency, and chemical structure of the gestagen given (Moltz and Becker 1977). Glandular proliferation may be either predominantly adenomatous or microglandular, the immature glandular epithelium either single- or multilayered. The proliferation of the glandular epithelium is often accompanied by a multilayered hyperplasia of underlying reserve cells.

Adenomatous Hyperplasia of the Endocervix

New glands form and the glandular epithelial cells become pseudostratified, containing elongated hyperchromatic nuclei in a less well-differentiated cytoplasm. The glands may ramify (Fig. 56) or become crowded (Fig. 57). The production of mucin is reduced or absent and occurs irregularly from one gland to another (Fig. 58) or within the same gland (Figs. 59, 60). Cells with mucin and those without may lie together. In addition, the chemical composition of the mucus is often changed (Gaton et al. 1982).

The reserve cells underneath the glandular and superficial epithelium may undergo hyperplasia to form several layers. That hyperplasia is stimulated by the gestagens. Such hyperplastic reserve cells may appear quite immature and contain depolarized hyperchromatic nuclei (Gall et al. 1969).

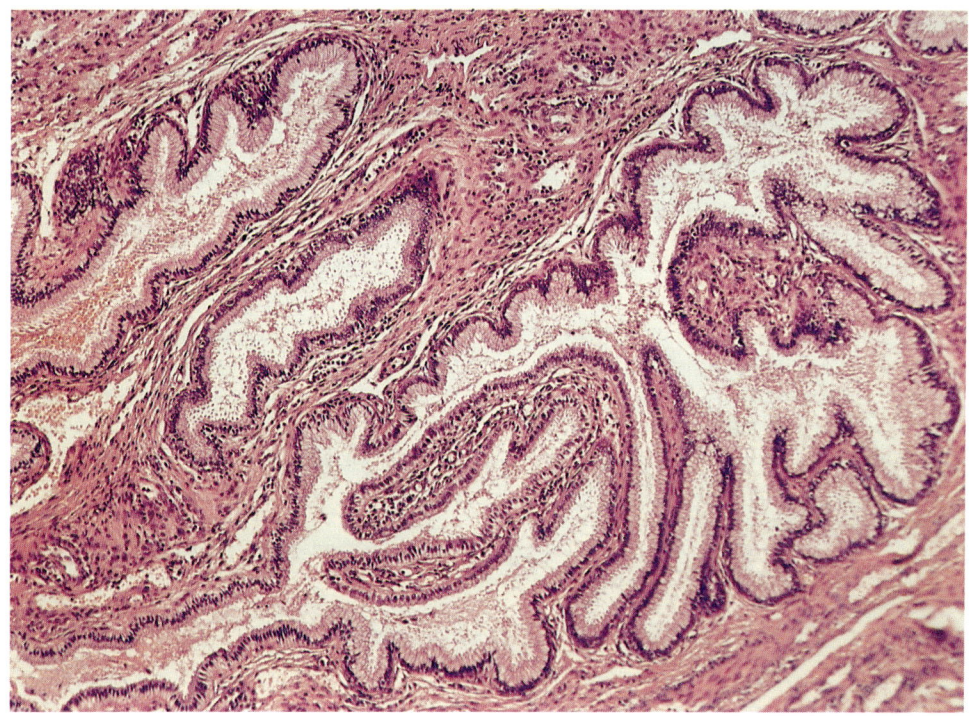

Fig. 56. Adenomatous hyperplasia of endocervix. H & E

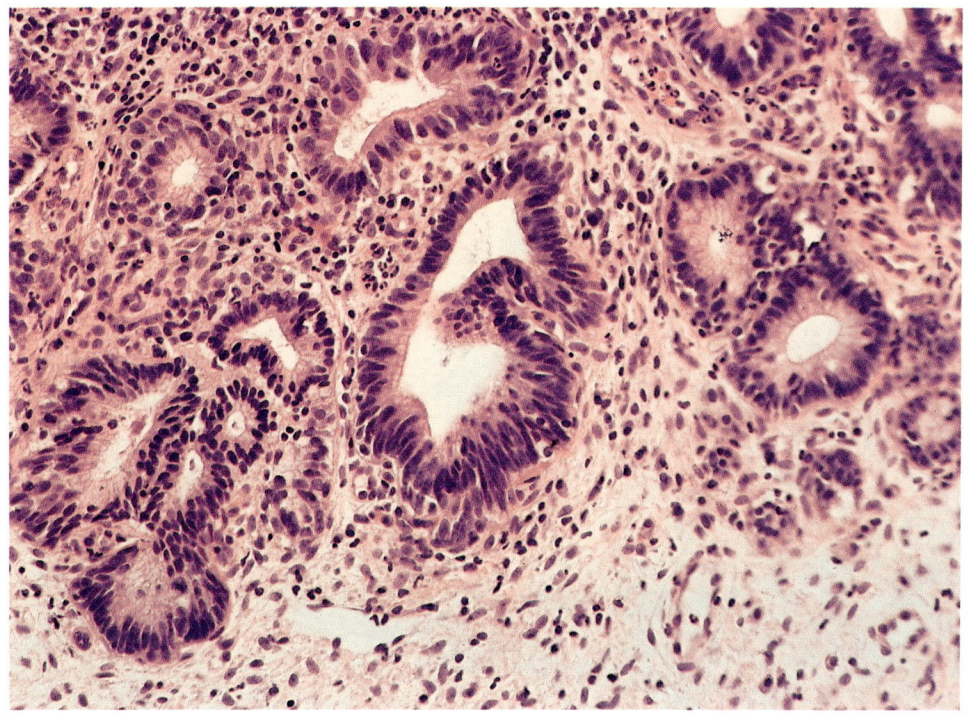

Fig. 57. Adenomatous hyperplasia of endocervix with crowding of glands. H & E

Differential Diagnosis. These adenomatous proliferations have to be distinguished from a well-differentiated adenocarcinoma of the endocervix. The invading carcinomatous glands induce, in most instances, a stromal reaction as they grow into the cervical wall. A large biopsy of the cervical wall may be required to make the distinction with H & E sections. If only a small portion of tissue is available, the immunohistochemical reaction for CEA is of great help – an adenomatous hyperplasia is negative for CEA, whereas an invasive adenocarcinoma reacts positively in most cases. An adenocarcinoma in situ can be distinguished from adenomatous hyperplasia by its cytological atypias, cellular stratification, densely arranged nuclei, and by its positive reaction with anti-CEA (Figs. 128–136).

It is well known that milder degrees of epithelial atypia may develop in some glands or parts of glands in cases of adenocarcinoma in situ and invasive adenocarcinoma of the cervix. Similar epithelial atypia may also occur alone. For these changes the term cervical glandular atypia has been proposed; they probably represent a continuum from low grade atypia to adenocarcinoma in situ (Wells and Brown 1986).

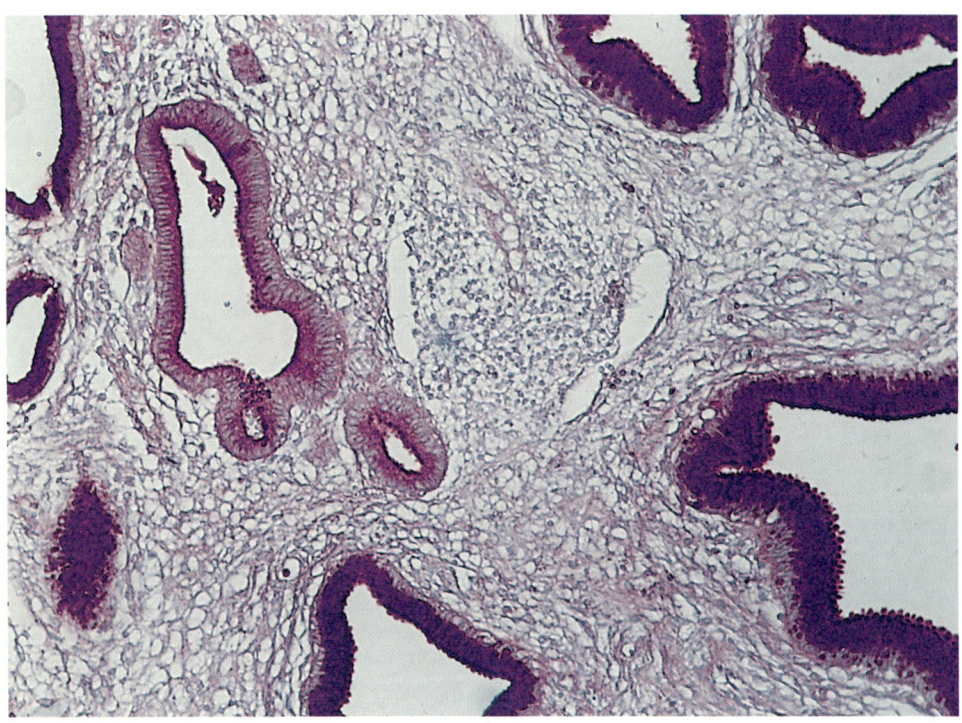

Fig. 58. Adenomatous hyperplasia of endocervix, variable content of mucin from one gland to another. PAS reaction

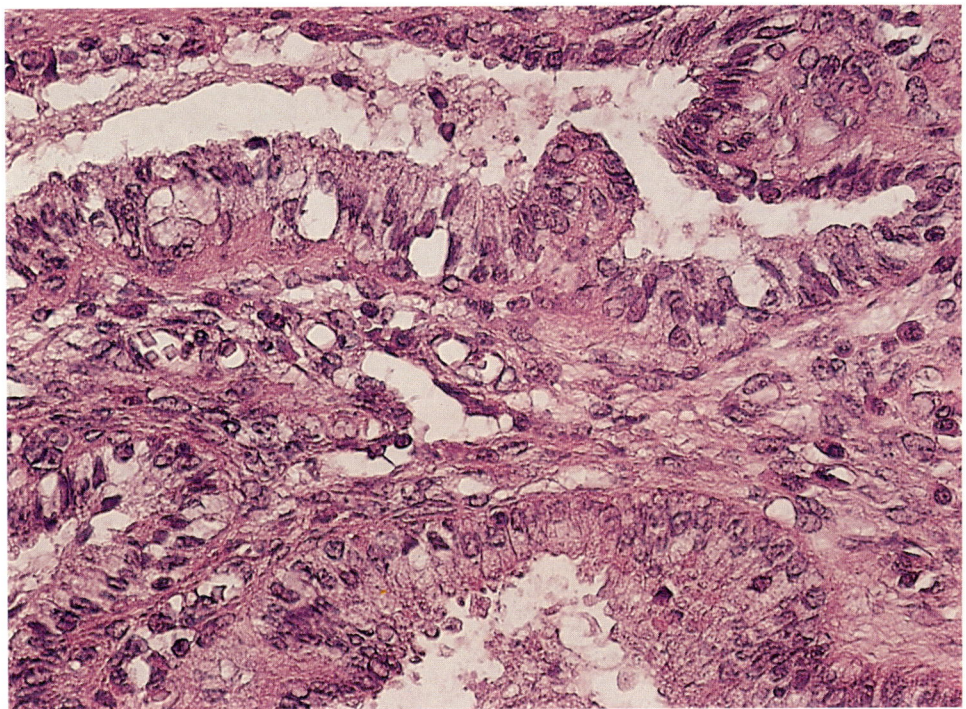

Fig. 59. Adenomatous hyperplasia of endocervix. H & E

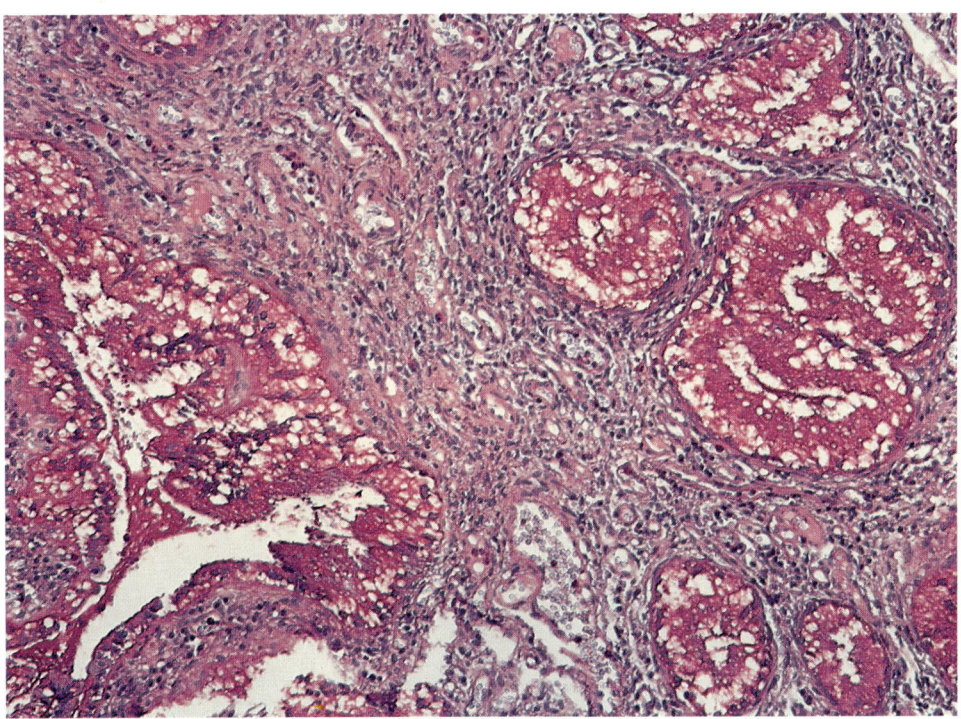

Fig. 60. Same as Fig. 59, irregular and deficient mucin formation in the glandular epithelial cells. PAS reaction

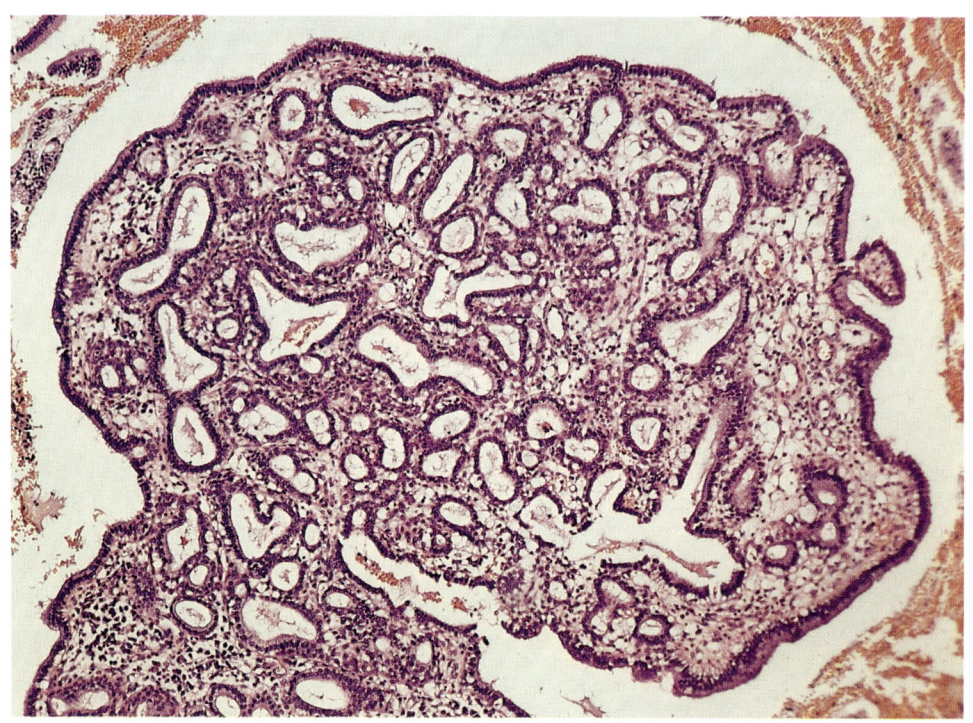

Fig. 61. Microglandular hyperplasia of endocervix. H & E

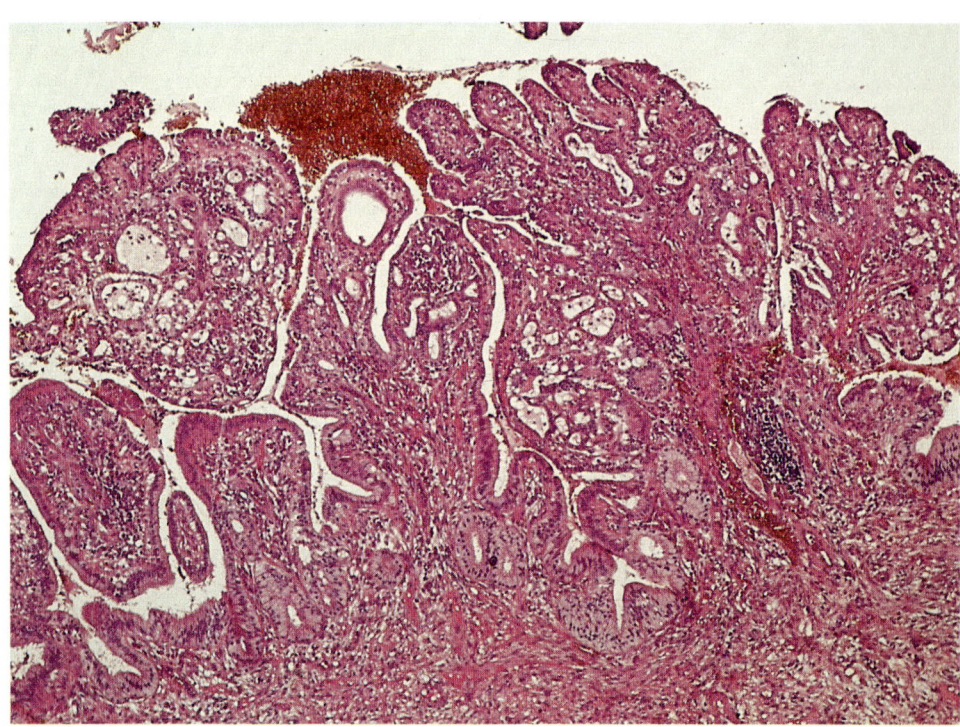

Fig. 62. Microglandular hyperplasia of endocervix, with reserve cell hyperplasia. H & E

Microglandular Hyperplasia of the Endocervix

With increasing potency of the gestagen used, endocervical glandular proliferation is more likely to develop into microalveolar changes with disappearance of the intervening stroma. (Figs. 61–63). The low cuboidal, undifferentiated, glandular epithelial cells can hardly be distinguished from the surrounding hyperplastic reserve cells. Occasionally a solid sheetlike proliferation of reserve cells, signet-ring cells or hobnail cells may be observed. These changes, too, may be misdiagnosed as invasive adenocarcinoma or clear cell carcinoma (Taylor et al. 1967; Candy and Abell 1968; Kyriakos et al. 1968; Talbert and Shery 1969; Helmerhorst et al. 1984; Wells and Brown 1986; Young and Scully 1989).

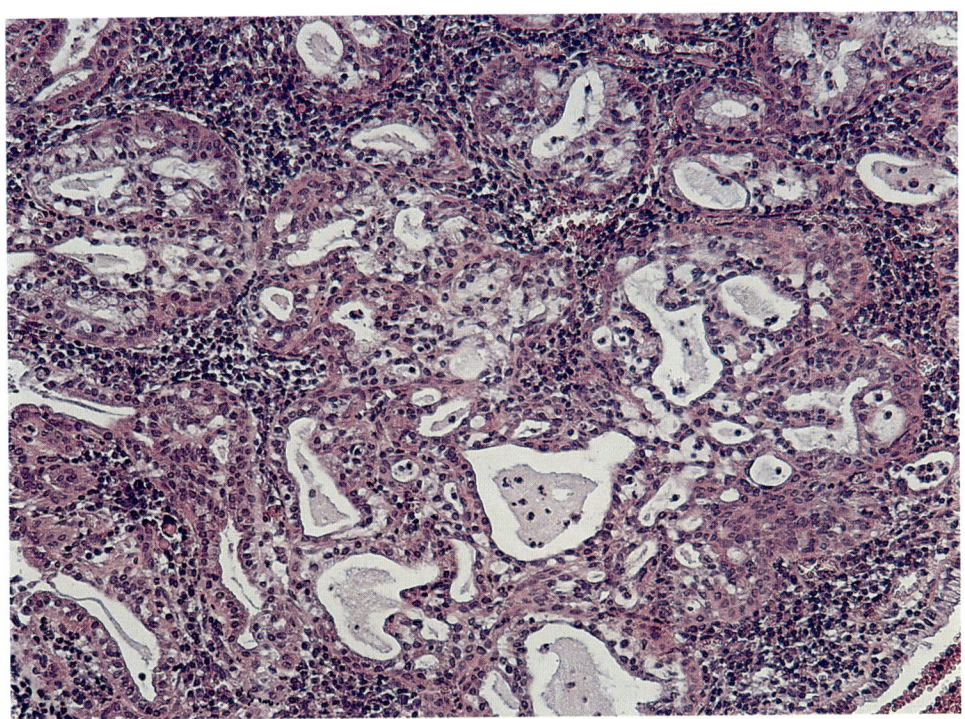

Fig. 63. Microglandular hyperplasia of endocervix. H & E, higher magnification

Differential Diagnosis. Several features may help to differentiate a microglandular hyperplasia from an invasive carcinoma. The cells of microglandular hyperplasia show less nuclear atypia; their cytoplasm contains mucin, not glycogen. In contrast to invasive adenocarcinoma, microglandular hyperplasia reacts negatively for CEA.

Glandular Papillary Ectropium
(Fig. 64)

As a result of excessive proliferation and growth pressure the endocervical mucosa frequently protrudes onto the ectocervical surface (Fig. 64). Under gestagenic stimulation, epidermization of such an ectropium is usually initiated by reserve cell hyperplasia ("Descending Repair," p. 18).

Polyps of the Ecto- and Endocervix (Figs. 65-67)

Focal proliferation of the endocervical mucosa leads to polyp formation. Depending upon their glands, they may be either cystic (Fig. 65), adenomatous, or microglandular; depending upon their stromal content either fibrous, angiomatous (Fig. 66), edematous (Fig. 65), or cellular (Fig. 66). Their surface may be papillary (Fig. 65) or smooth (Fig. 66). When these polyps protrude through the external os, the surface epithelium may be replaced by reserve cell hyperplasia (Fig. 66), which can differentiate to squamous metaplasia and finally to mature stratified squamous epithelium. When such polyps are completely overgrown by squamous epithelium, they are then classified as ectocervical polyps (Fig. 67).

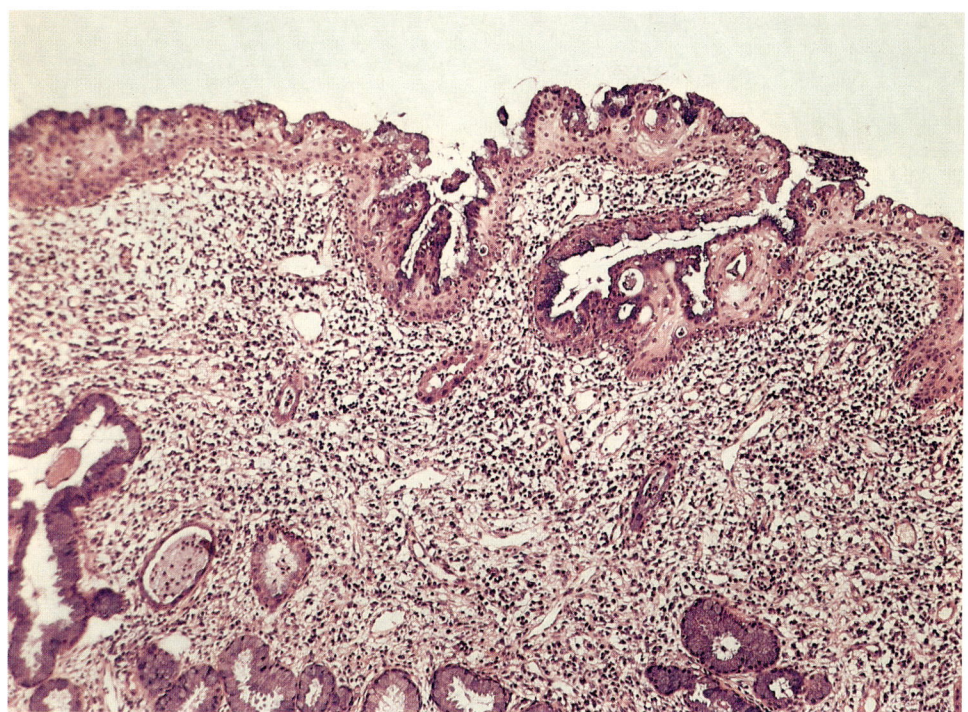

Fig. 64. Protrusion of hyperplastic endocervical mucosa onto the ectocervical surface with epidermization (descending repair). H & E

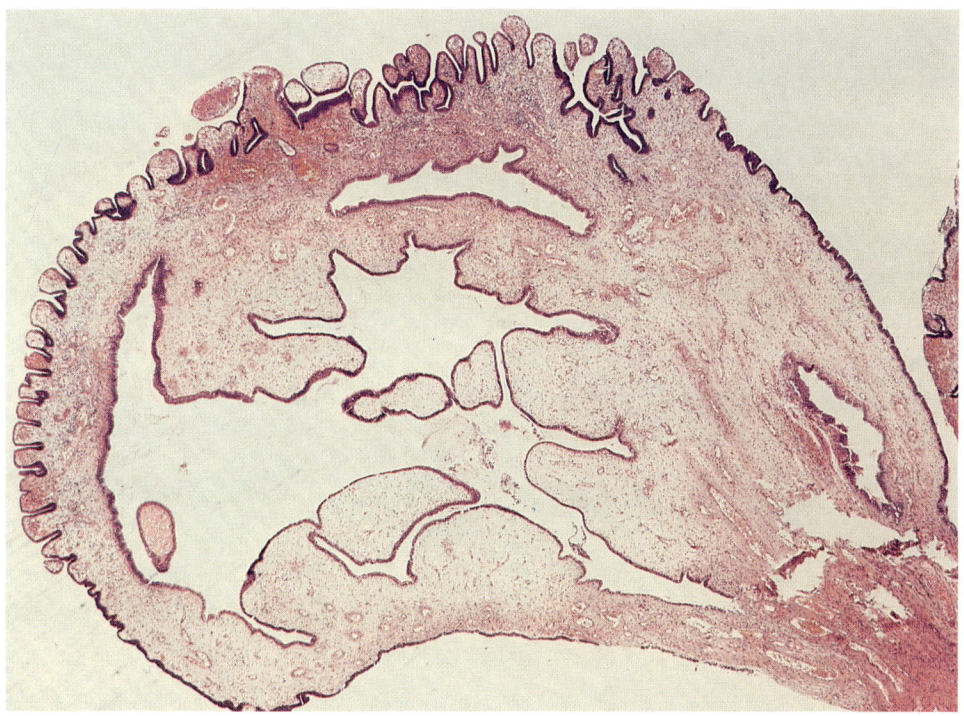

Fig. 65. Papillary, cystic endocervical polyp. H & E

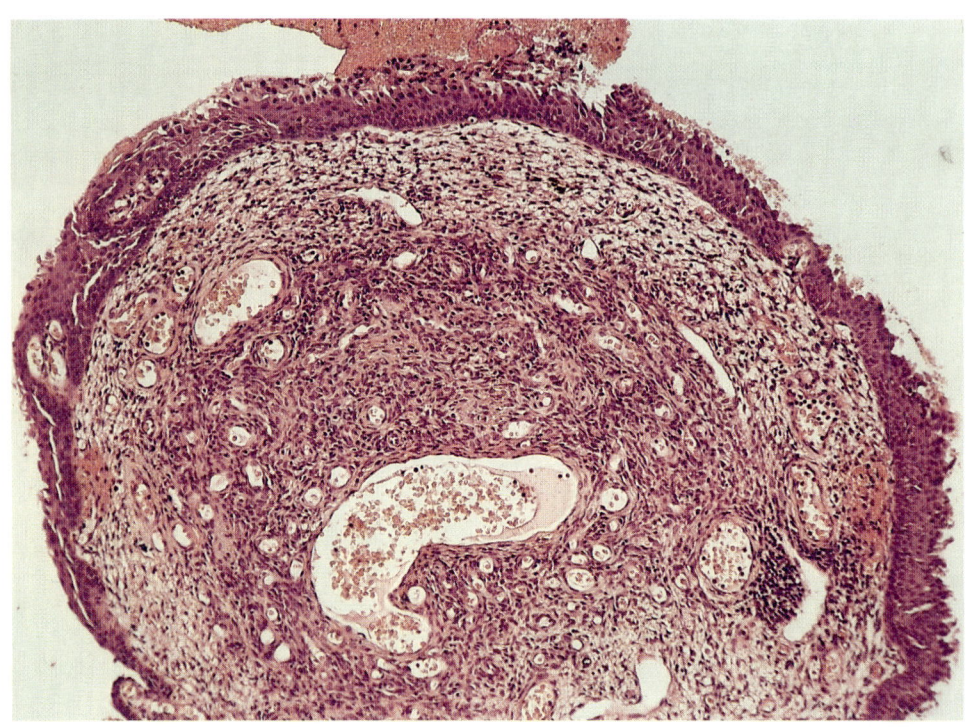

Fig. 66. Endocervical polyp with angiomatous, cellular stroma, covered by reserve cell hyperplasia. H & E

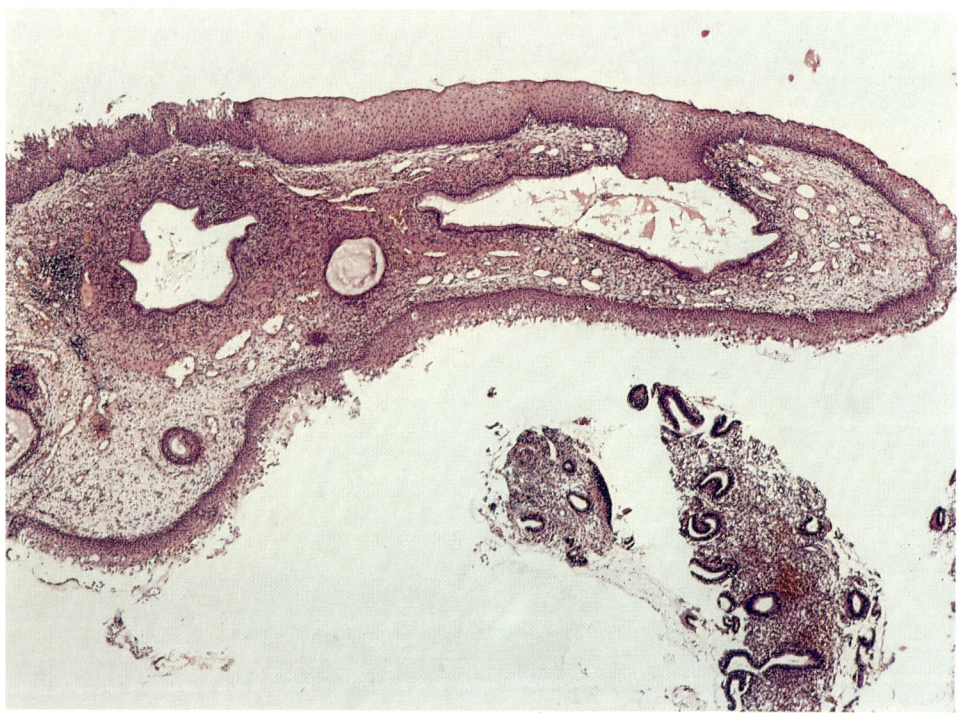

Fig. 67. Ectocervical polyp. H & E

Inflammatory Lesions

Nonspecific Ecto- and Endocervicitis (Figs. 68–73)

Nonspecific cervicitis may be chemically induced or caused by trauma in the presence of a "locus minoris resistentiae," such as postmenopausal atrophy of the ectocervical epithelium, or eversion of the vulnerable endocervical mucosa onto the ectocervix (ectropium) during the reproductive age.
Acute and subacute ectocervicitis (Figs. 68, 69) is characterized by vascular congestion, edema, and infiltration of inflammatory cells, mainly neutrophilic granulocytes. When the inflammation is mild, the overlying epithelium remains intact (Fig. 68). With more severe inflammation the epithelium is destroyed, sloughed off, leading to an erosive or ulcerative ectocervicitis (Fig. 69).
Acute and subacute endocervicitis (Figs. 70–72) presents similar signs of inflammation (Figs. 70, 71) and occasionally ulceration (Fig. 72).

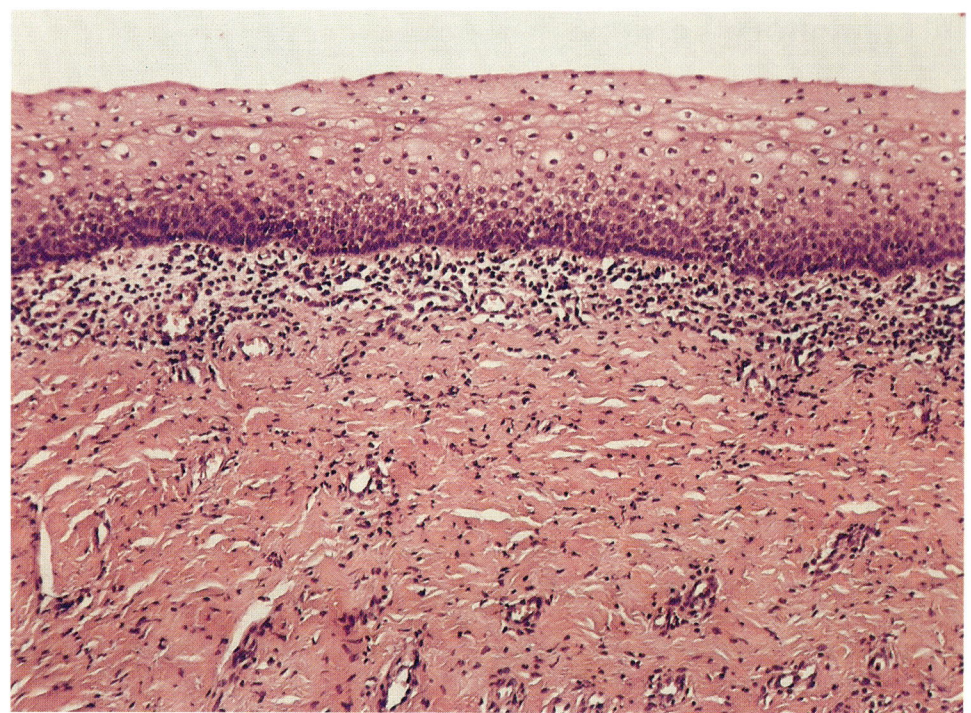

Fig. 68. Subacute ectocervicitis, mild. H & E

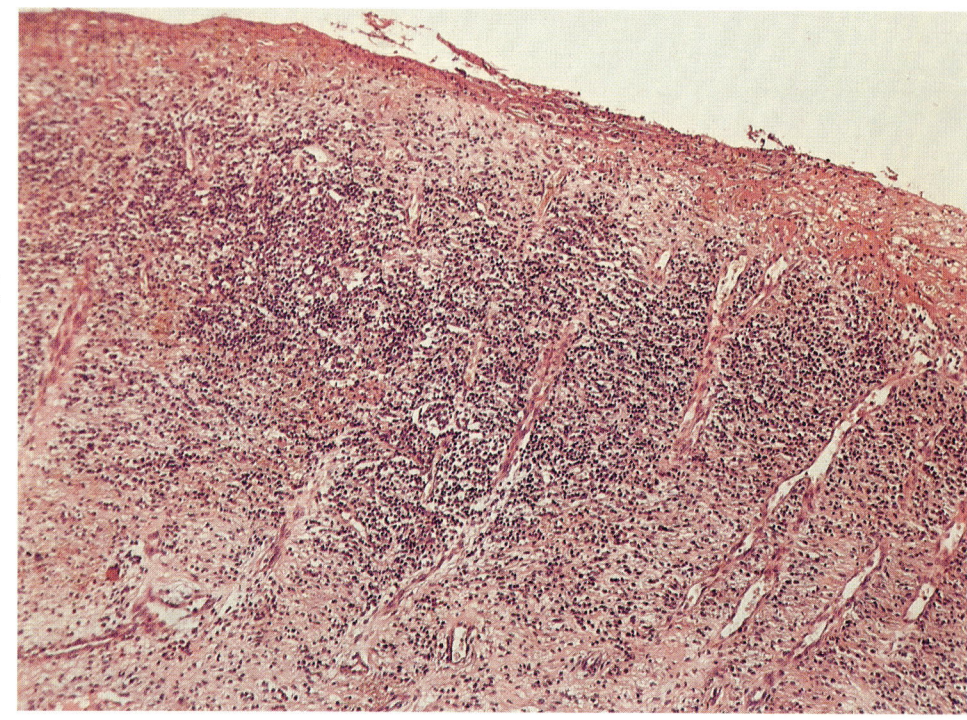

Fig. 69. Subacute ulcerative ectocervicitis. H & E

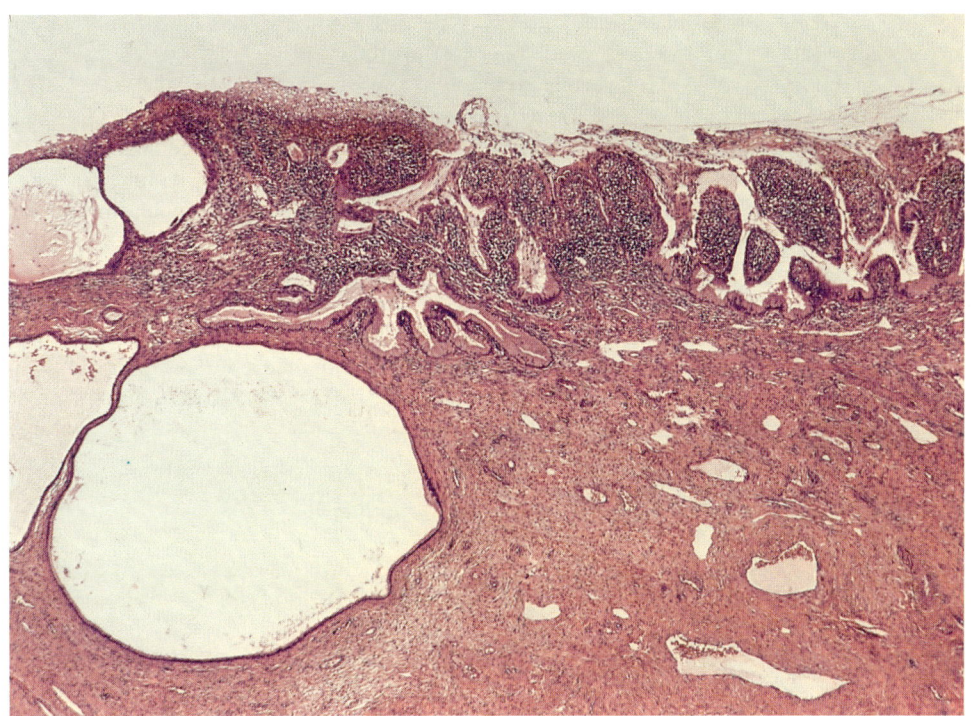

Fig. 70. Subacute endocervicitis. H & E

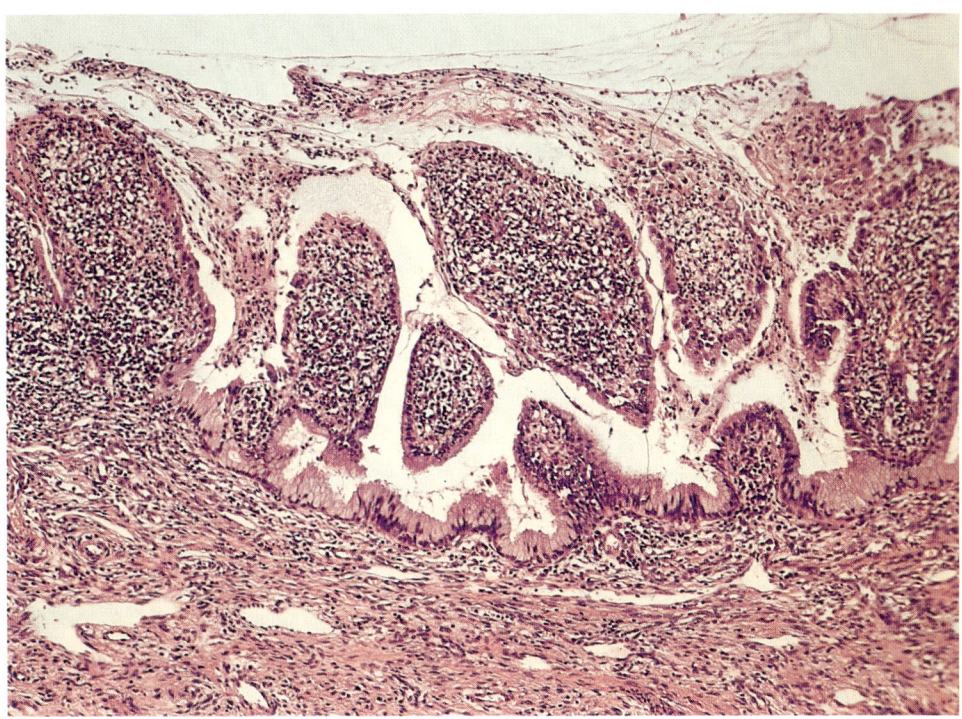

Fig. 71. Subacute endocervicitis. H & E, higher magnification

In *chronic ecto- and endocervicitis* rather dense subepithelial infiltrates of predominantly lymphocytes and plasma cells are found, often accompanied by proliferating capillaries and fibroblasts. The overlying epithelium is usually intact. In prolonged or severe chronic endocervicitis lymphoid follicles may develop, *(follicular endocervicitis,* Fig. 73), and the overlying columnar epithelium may show polymorphic, hyperchromatic, and depolarized nuclei. When detected in cervical smears, such reactive nuclear changes may be misinterpreted by the screening cytologist and lead to false-positive readings.

Differential Diagnosis. Severe subacute and chronic follicular and ulcerative cervicitis may be misdiagnosed as lymphoma when large lymphoid cells, immunoblasts, and mitoses are found. However, surface ulceration and a polymorphic inflammatory infiltrate with neutrophils and plasma cells are rarely seen in lymphomas, which show instead an extensive, monomorphic infiltrate of lymphoid cells (Fig. 208; Young et al. 1985).

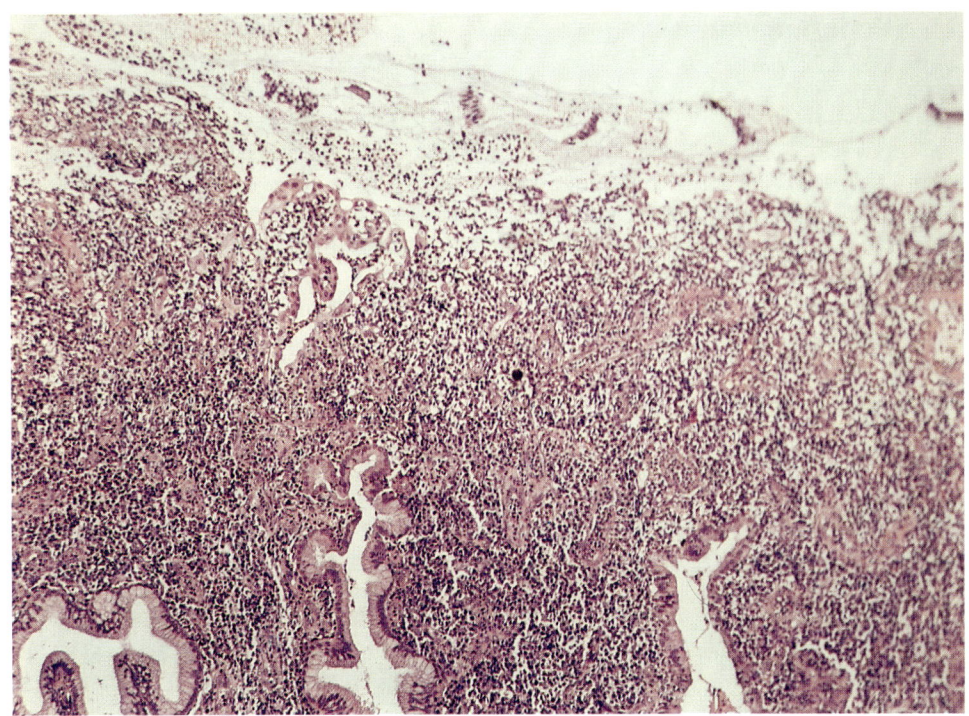

Fig. 72. Subacute ulcerative endocervicitis. H & E

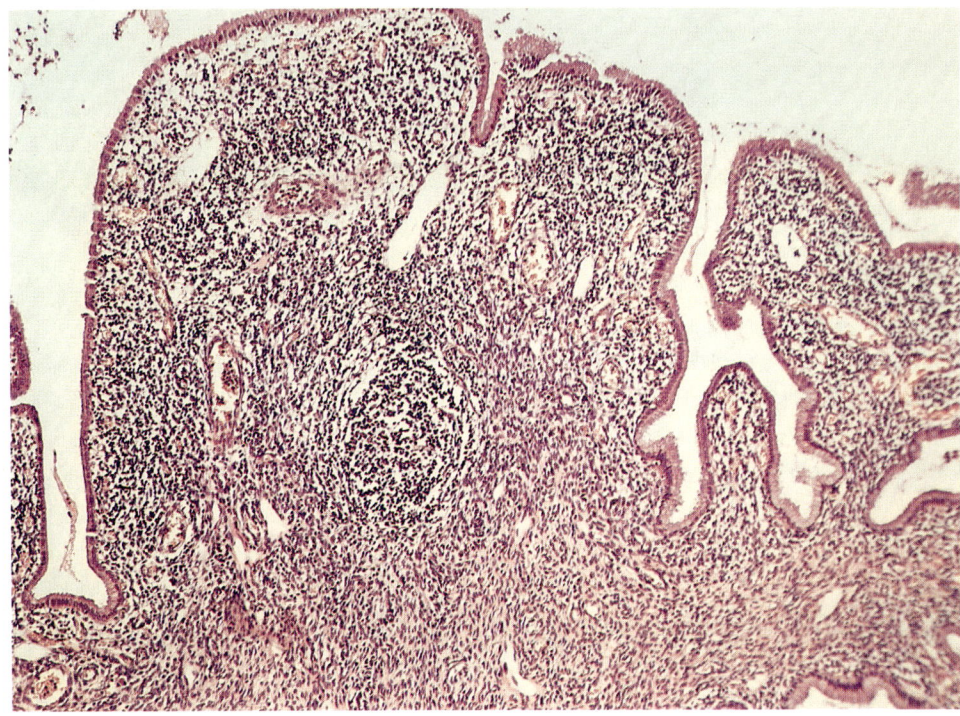

Fig. 73. Follicular endocervicitis. H & E

Specific Inflammations (Figs. 74–85)

Viral Infections

Viral infections of the ecto- and endocervix cause often characteristic nuclear changes, by which they can be recognized. The accompanying inflammatory infiltrate may be scant (as with HPV infection) or extensive (as with herpes virus infection).

Infection with *papilloma virus* induces koilocytosis of the ectocervical (Fig. 74) and endocervical epithelia. In addition, other changes may occur, such as: acanthosis, papillomatosis, giant nuclei, multinucleated cells, monocellular keratinization, hypergranulation, and superficial orto- and/or parakeratosis.

A *koilocyte* can be defined as a dyskaryotic epithelial cell with a deformed, often angulated, hyperchromatic nucleus surrounded by a swollen cytoplasm, which shows a clear perinuclear halo and a thickened cytoplasmic membrane (Fig. 75 a). Both signs, the atypical degenerating nucleus and the clear, blown-up cytoplasm must be present before one can call a cell a koilocyte. By strictly adhering to the above criteria it is possible to differentiate nonspecific koilocyte-like cellular changes caused by other agents. For example, clear cells with ballooned cytoplasm and a normal nucleus may be seen after a gestagen-predominant hormonal stimulation, whereby glycogen accumulates in the cytoplasm (Fig. 75 b). In contrast, the cytoplasm of koilocytes is devoid of glycogen. A degenerative vacuolation of the cytoplasm may occur in nonspecific inflammation. Nuclear atypicality alone develops in all types of dyskaryosis and may be caused by a variety of carcinogens or cocarcinogens, independent of HPV infection. Koilocytes can also be observed in columnar epithelial cells (Fig. 110) of the endocervix.

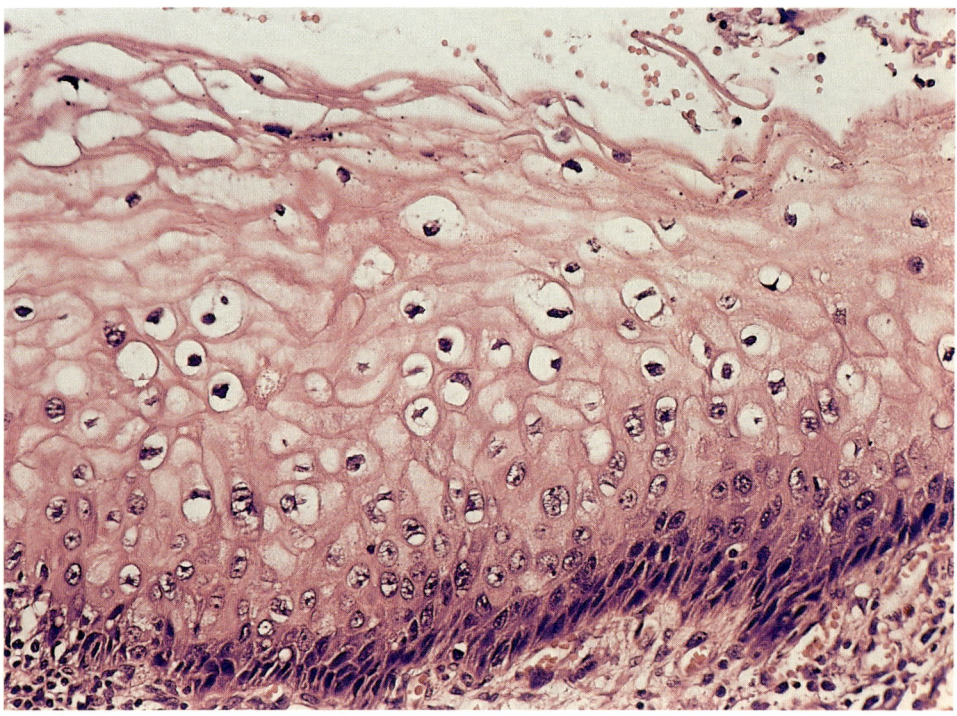

Fig. 74. Infection of ectocervical epithelium with papilloma virus. H & E

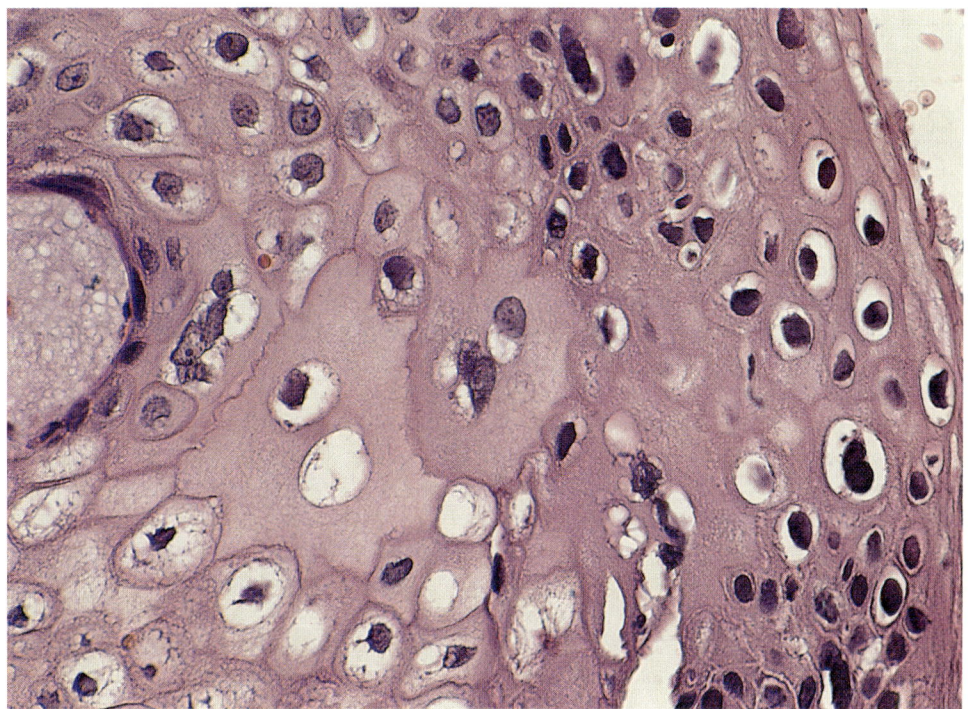

Fig. 75a. Dysplastic squamous epithelium with true koilocytes. H & E

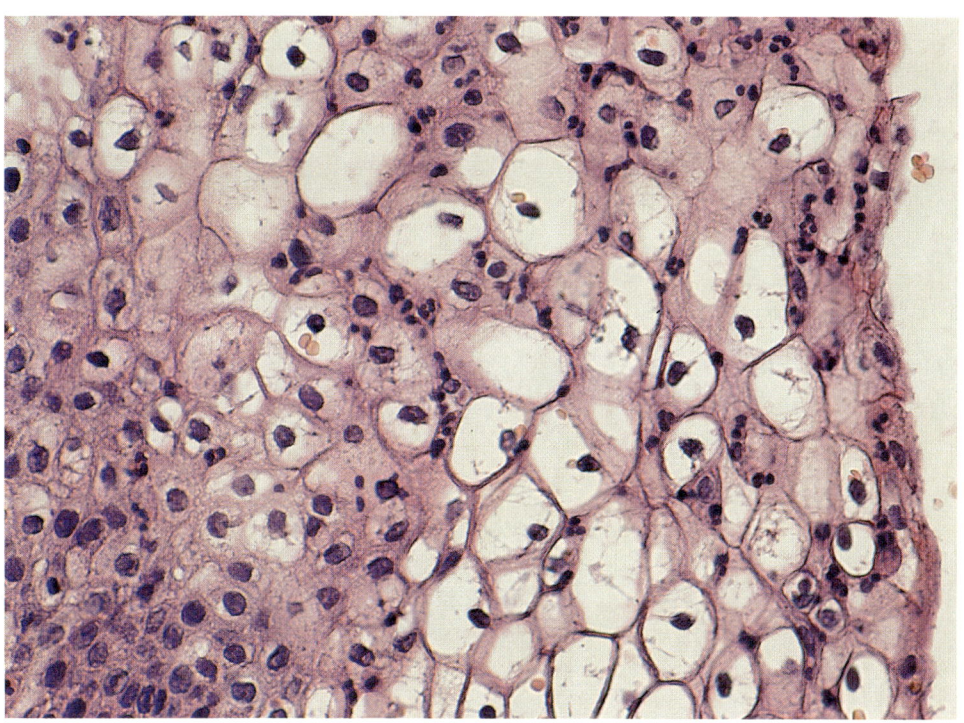

Fig. 75b. Squamous epithelium with "false" koilocytes. H & E

In the early, nondysplastic stage of infection, the perinuclear halo of the koilocyte caused by the virus is the first cellular change that can be detected. Depending on the type of the virus, the change may regress slowly or, at a later stage, the virus may induce atypical proliferation by its interaction with the nuclear DNA, often resulting in carcinogenesis. HPV infection is discussed therefore at greater length in "Premalignant Lesions."

A HPV-induced koilocytic or even an occult nonkoilocytic infection (Nuovo et al. 1988) of the cervical epithelium is often chronic or latent and involves the entire ecto- and endocervical mucosa, persisting at the margins even after total removal of a koilocytic dysplasia. Hence, these infected areas may give rise later to recurrent precancerous lesions (Bistoletti et al. 1988; see also Fletcher 1983; Koss 1987).

Infection with *herpesvirus* (Figs. 76-79) involves chiefly herpes simplex virus (HSV) type 2, a DNA-containing virus that replicates within the nuclei of the epithelial cells by synthesizing viral protein (Wagner 1974). In the acute stage, the infection can be easily recognized cytologically by the large multinucleated epithelial cells with characteristic intranuclear, ground-glass, viral inclusions (Fig. 76). On histological examination, small or larger vesicles may be found within the ectocervical epithelium containing such giant cells with intranuclear viral inclusions (Fig. 77). These vesicles ultimately burst, forming confluent ulcers surrounded by cellular debris and dense inflammatory infiltrates (Figs. 78, 79). Identification of herpesvirus infection is important since it may, like the papilloma viruses, be involved in cervical carcinogenesis (Fenoglio et al. 1981). During pregnancy, infection of the fetus or placenta may cause spontaneous abortion (Corey 1984).

Differential Diagnosis. Intraepithelial vesicles (bullae) may be seen in the ectocervix in patients with generalized pemphigus vulgaris, or as isolated small cysts (see below). These, however, lack the characteristic intranuclear viral inclusions of Herpes. An ulcerative and necrotizing infection of the cervix may occasionally be caused by *Chlamydia trachomatis,* or by protozoa, like *Trichomonas vaginalis,* or rarely by *Entamoeba histolytica.* Identification of the causative agent is essential for a definitive diagnosis. The cytoplasmic chlamydial inclusions can best be detected immunohistochemically (see below). The motile protozoa are most readily identified in fresh native smears under phase contrast microscopy.

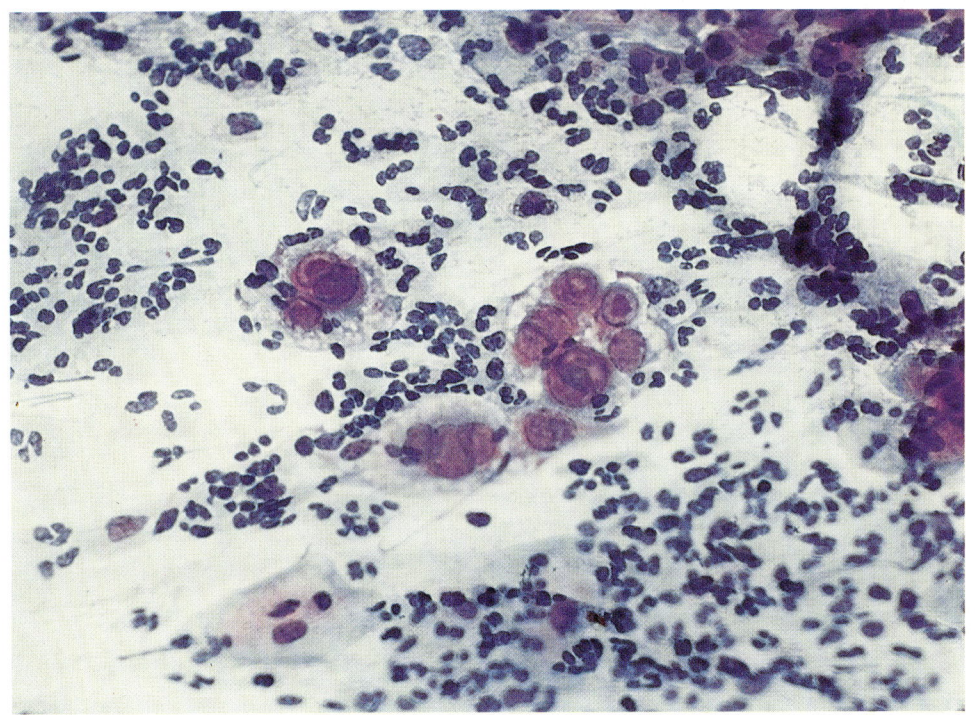

Fig. 76. Vaginal cytological smear with intranuclear inclusions of herpesvirus. Papanicolaou

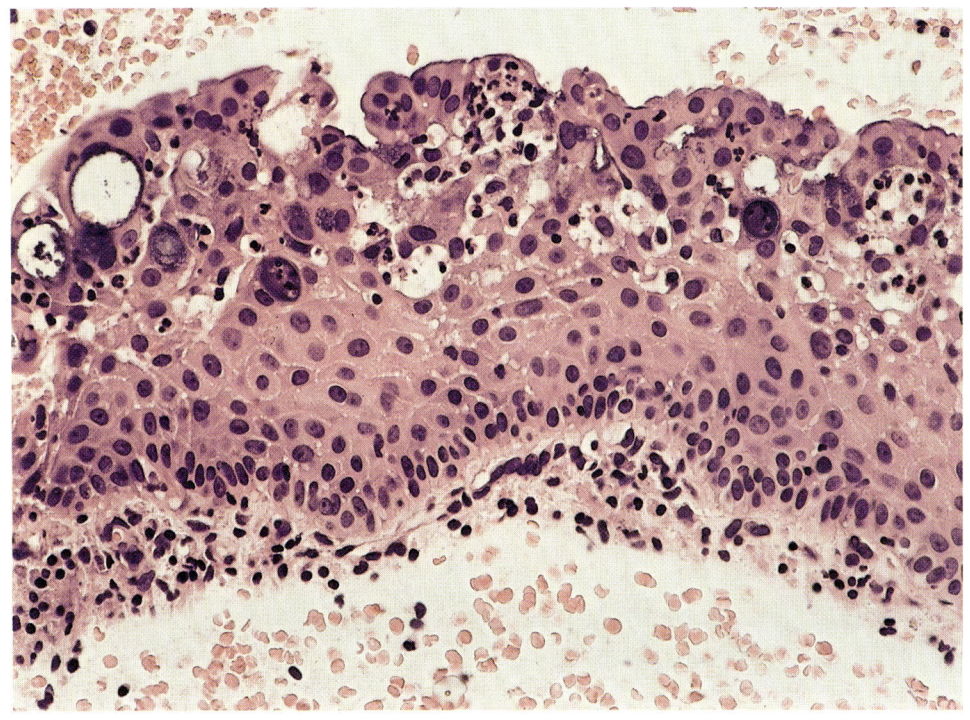

Fig. 77. Ectocervical epithelium with intranuclear inclusions of herpesvirus. H & E

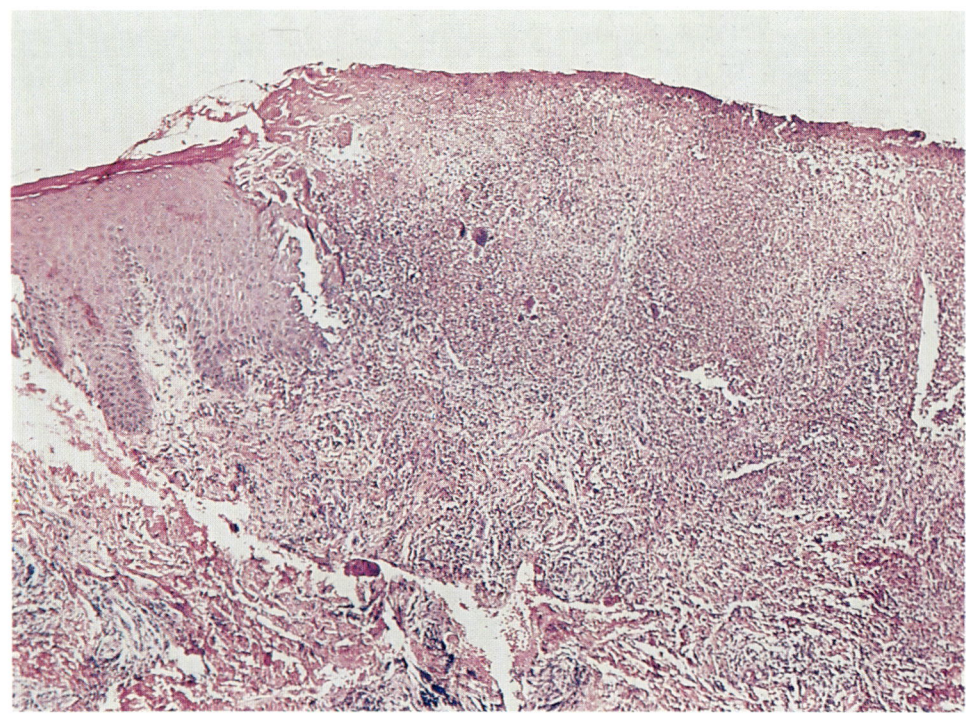

Fig. 78. Florid ulcerative ectocervicitis caused by herpesvirus. H & E

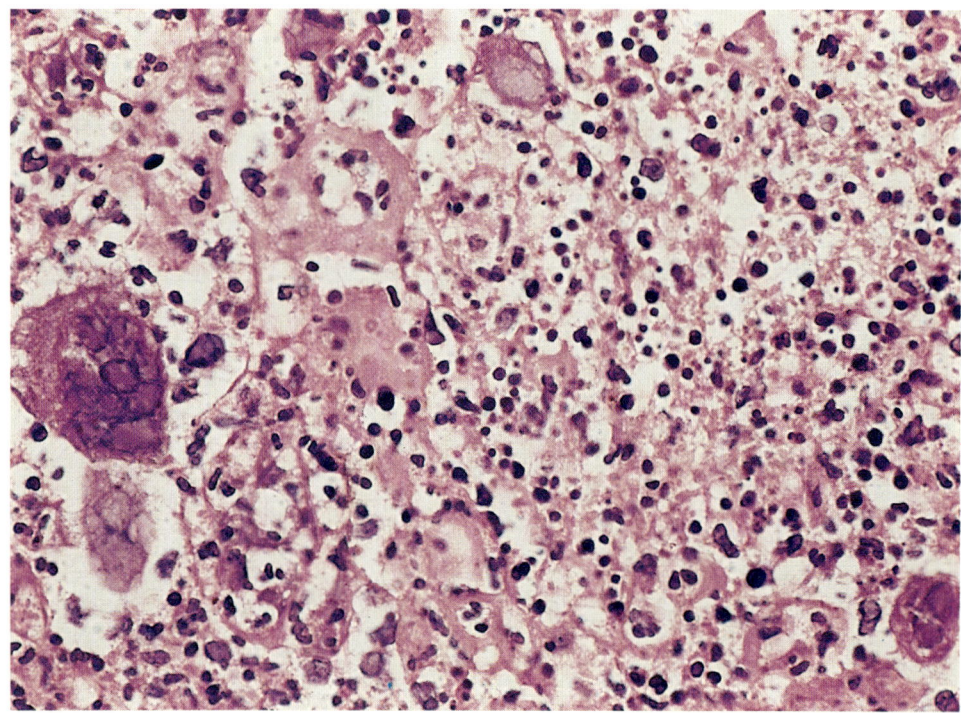

Fig. 79. Florid ulcerative ectocervicitis caused by herpesvirus. H & E, higher magnification

Bacterial Infections

Tuberculous cervicitis (Fig. 80) almost always develops from an infection descending from tuberculous salpingitis or endometritis. The tuberculous granulomas can be recognized by aggregates of epitheloid cells and Langhans giant cells surrounded by lymphocytes. Caseation is rare in the cervix. Since similar granulomatous lesions of other causes may occur here, and some of them are even more common, the diagnosis of tuberculosis has to be verified by the demonstration of acid-fast mycobacteria (tuberculosis), with the Ziehl-Neelsen stain, or a modification of it.

Differential Diagnosis. Under low microscopic magnification foreign body granulomas may appear very similar. They can often be distinguished from tuberculous granulomas by identifying intracytoplasmic inclusions of foreign material in multinucleated giant cells under polarized light. Most of these inclusions are double refractile under polarized light (such as talcum crystals or suture material). Infectious granulomas such as *lues, lymphogranuloma venereum, granuloma inguinale, schistosomiasis,* and *sarcoidosis* must be distinguished from tuberculosis by using special stains or bacteriological and immunological methods, since individual morphological features are often lacking.

Chlamydial cervicitis is being observed with increasing frequency (Winkler and Crum 1986) and is now the most common sexually transmitted infection in the Western world (Stamm and Holmes, 1984). The causative agent, chlamydia trachomatis, is sexually transmitted and has an affinity for cervical columnar cells or basal (reserve) cells. Concomitant infection of other tissues leads to urethritis, endometritis, salpingitis, and proctitis, which are common. Other infections, such as gonorrhoea, often occur at the same time.

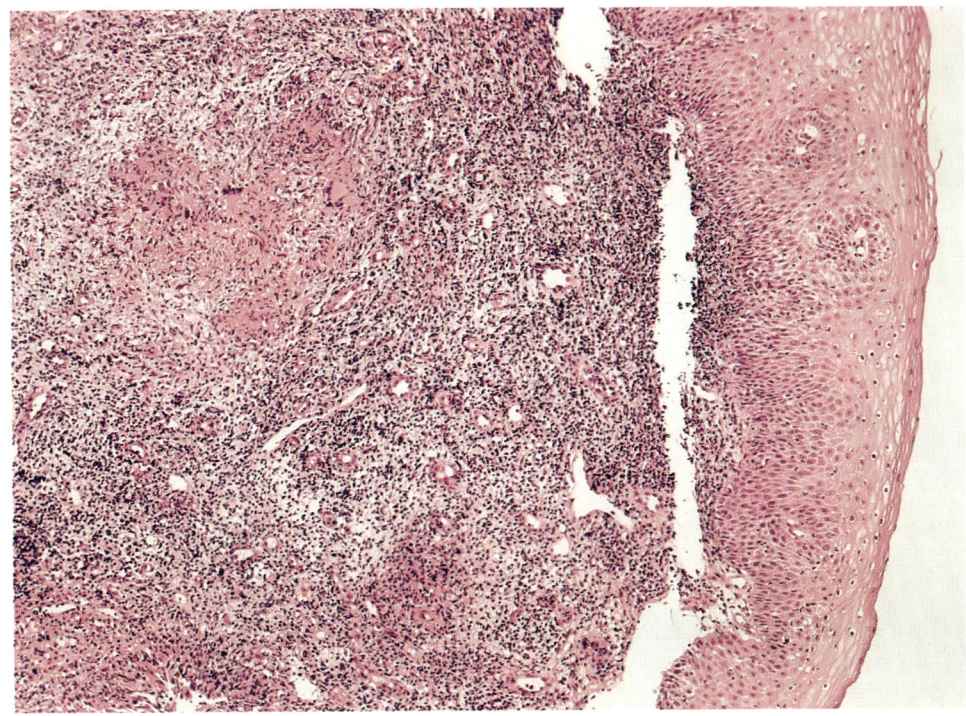

Fig. 80. Tuberculous cervicitis. H & E

Histologically, severe nonspecific inflammation is typical, but in some cases chronic follicular endocervicitis is observed (Winkler and Crum, 1986). Slight atypia of both columnar and metaplastic cells has been described. Only in a small number of cases can cytoplasmic inclusions, comprising aggregates of chlamydia trachomatis organisms, be found in columnar or metaplastic basal cells of smears or sections (Fig. 81a). Recognition in vaginal PAP smears is difficult, since many degenerative cytoplasmic inclusions occurring in metaplastic epithelial cells closely resemble the various developmental stages of chlamydial inclusions. These consist of cytoplasmic vacuoles containing few or numerous tiny particles. The microorganisms can best be detected by immunohistochemistry (Tam et al. 1984; Fig. 81b) or culture (Crum et al. 1984). It is important to treat the patients as well as their male partners since chlamydial urethritis may be asymptomatic.

Differential Diagnosis. Distinction from severe subacute or chronic nonspecific cervicitis is virtually impossible on histological grounds alone. Many of these so-called nonspecific infections actually are unrecognized chlamydial cervicitis, as Paavonen et al. (1982) could show for follicular endocervicitis. Distinction from gonorrhea is possible bacteriologically, from trichomonal infection by vital cytology under phase contrast microscopy (see below).

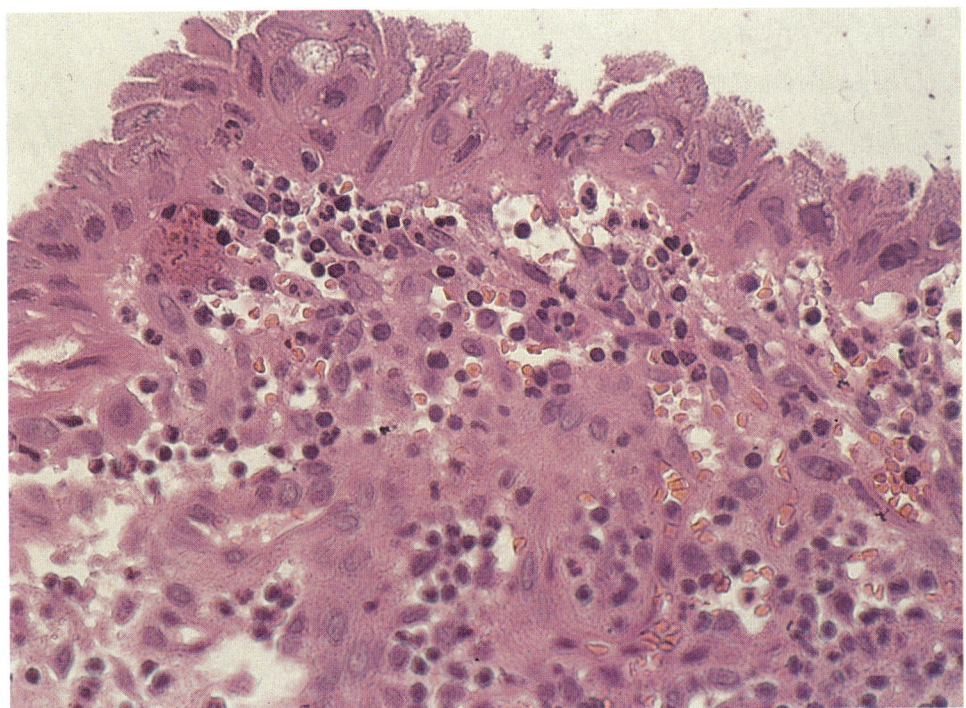

Fig. 81a. Subacute endocervicitis with intracytoplasmic inclusions of *Chlamydia* trachomatis in metaplastic epithelial cells. H & E

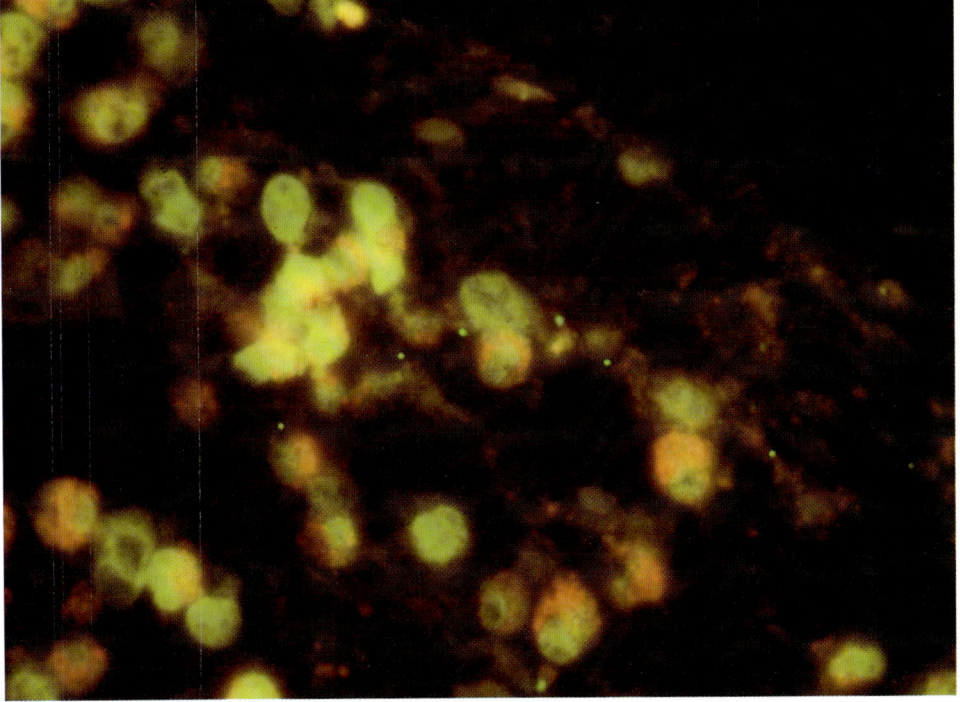

Fig. 81b. Intracytoplasmic inclusions of *Chlamydia trachomatis* showing uniform green flourescence. Immunhistochemistry with specific antibodies

Parasitic Infections

Trichomonas cervicitis (Fig. 82) is caused by an ascending infection with *Trichomonas vaginalis,* a flagellated protozoan most easily recognized in a fresh vaginal smear under phase contrast microscopy (Stoll 1969). In histological preparations an inflammatory infiltrate is seen, whereby the desquamating epithelial cells reveal nuclear swelling and chromatin clumping.

Differential Diagnosis. Nonspecific acute and subacute purulent cervicitis, follicular (chlamydial) cervicitis, granuloma inguinale, lymphogranuloma can be distinguished by detecting the causing agent. Rare parasitic infections involving the cervix are: schistosomiasis (endemic in Africa), echinococcosis, and infections with *Entamoeba histolytica.*

Fungal Infections

Actinomycosis of the cervix (Fig. 83) may result from infectious trauma from an IUD or surgical procedures (Burkman and Damewood 1985). Microscopically, a dense inflammatory infiltrate with abscess formation is seen, consisting mainly of neutrophils and histiocytes. Characteristic gram-positive rods arranged in a radial fashion, and located in the center of the abscess, are diagnostic.

Differential Diagnosis. Inspissated mucus or groups of autolytic, swollen, endocervical epithelial cells arranged in a radial position may have a very similar appearance. Distinction is possible by immunohistochemical detection of actinomyces organisms (Pine et al. 1985).

Infection with candida albicans rarely involves the cervix and is secondary to involvement of vulva and vagina.

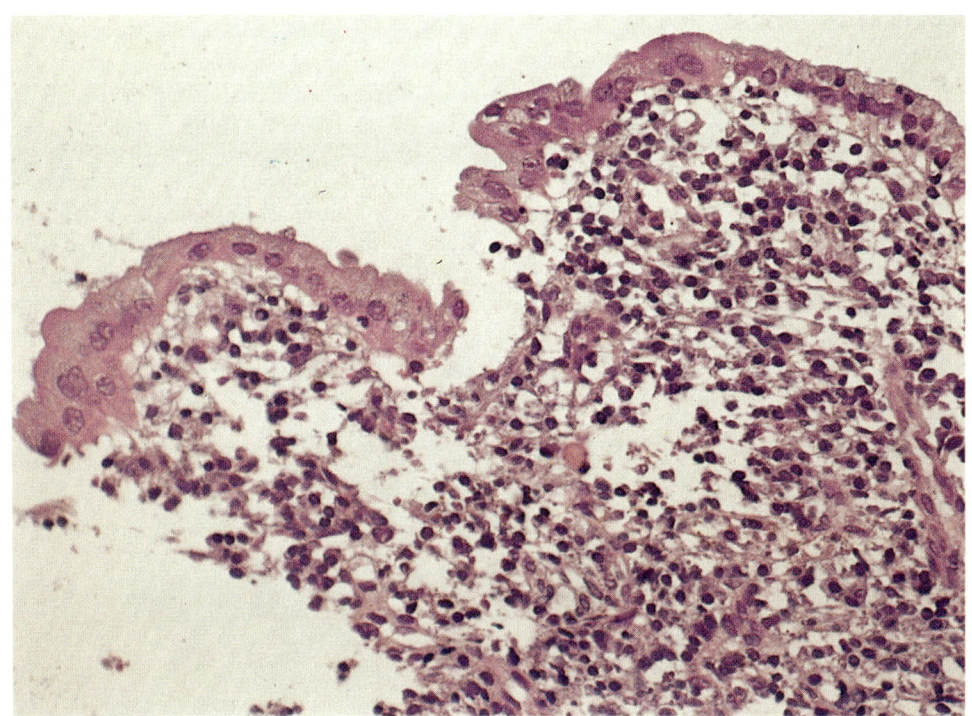

Fig. 82. Endocervicitis caused by ascending infection with *Trichomonas vaginalis*. H & E

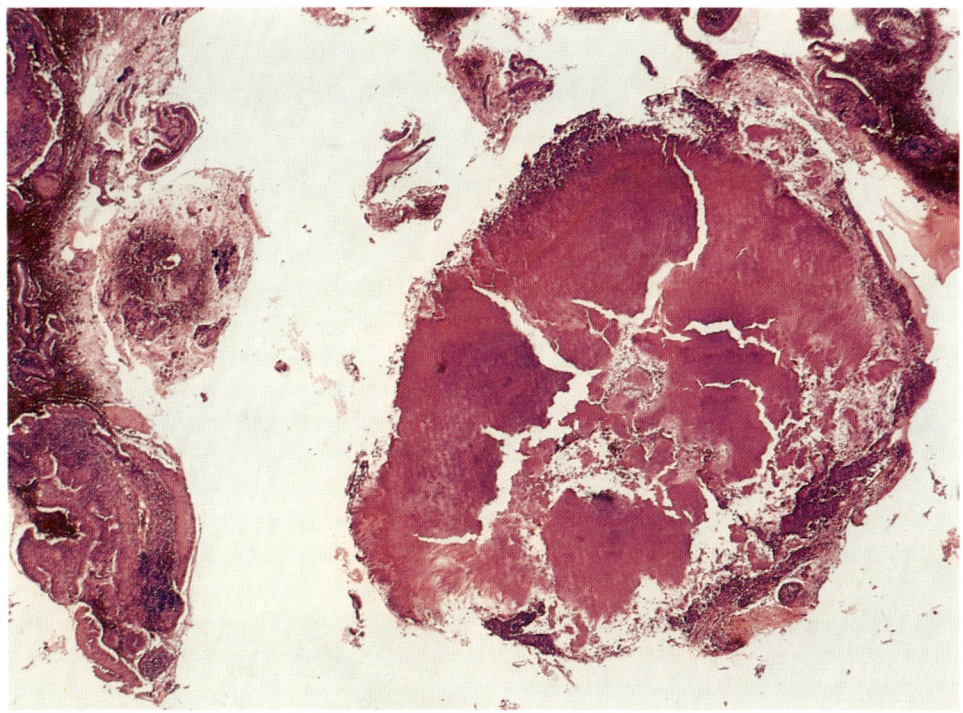

Fig. 83. Aktinomycosis of the cervix. H & E

Infections of Unknown Etiology

In *cervicitis emphysematosa* subepithelial cysts are found as dilated, empty spaces in the connective tissue without epithelial lining. The etiology is unknown. Intraepithelial cysts are occasionally observed (Fig. 84), which may have a similar cause.

Polyarteriitis nodosa (Fig. 85) can involve the cervix only, or appear as part of a generalized (autoimmune) disease.

Irradiation Changes (Fig. 86)

After irradiation therapy, preexisting glandular patterns become distorted (Fig. 86). The muclei of the glandular epithelial cells are pleomorphic, hyperchromatic and enlarged due to replication of DNA without cell division. In the cytoplasm, damage of various organelles and destruction of lysosomal membranes may result in vacuolation. Similar cellular changes may be observed in the ectocervical epithelium resulting in postirradiation dysplasia.

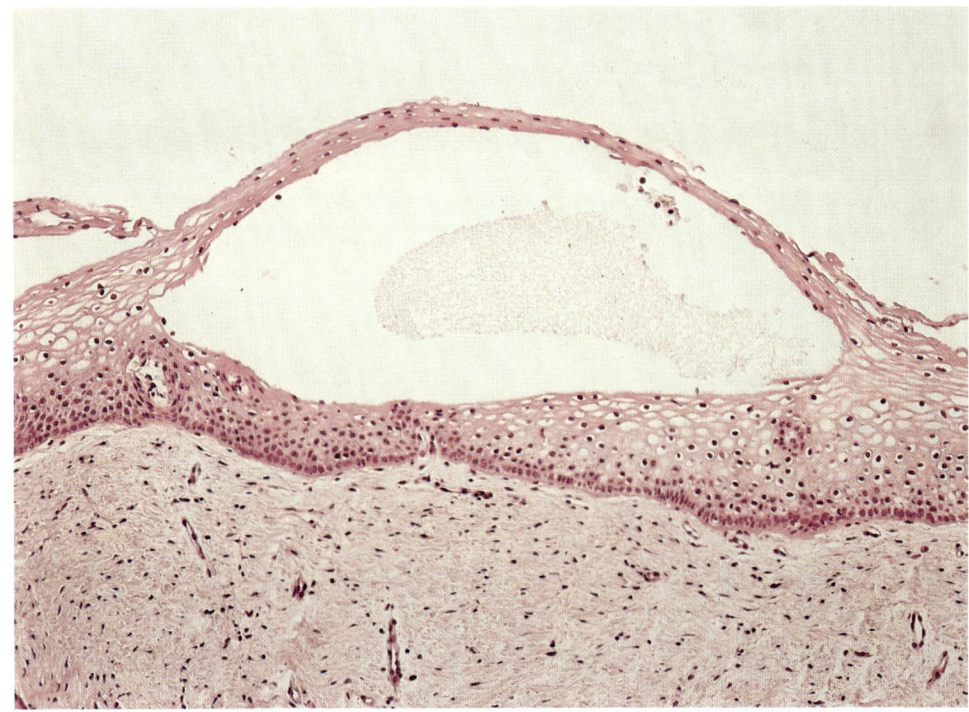

Fig. 84. Cervicitis emphysematosa. H & E

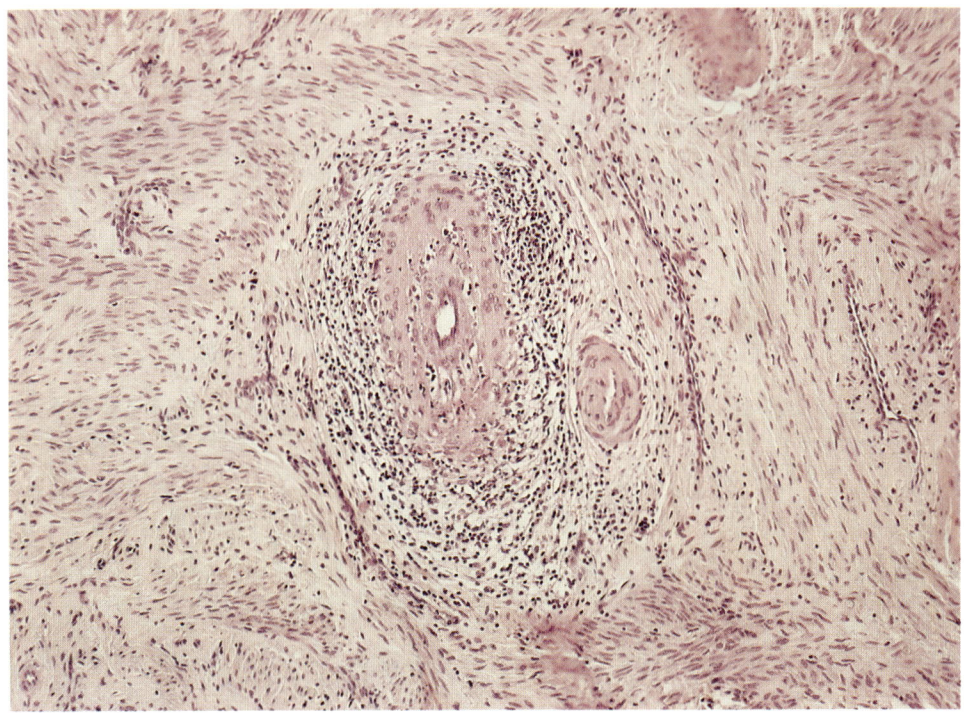

Fig. 85. Polyarteriitis nodosa of the cervix. H & E

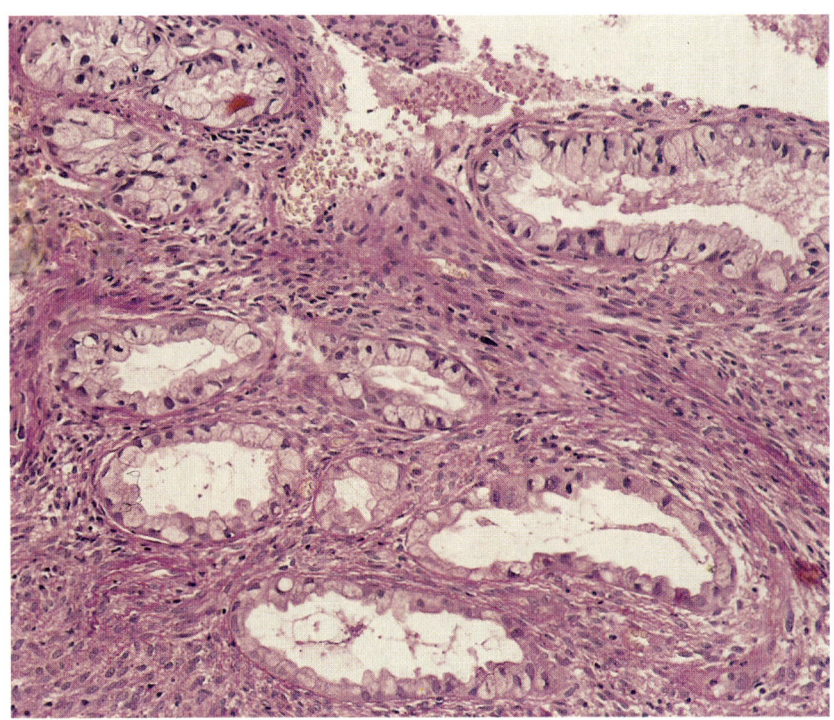

Fig. 86a. Endocervical glands after irradiation therapy with periglandular fibrosis. H & E

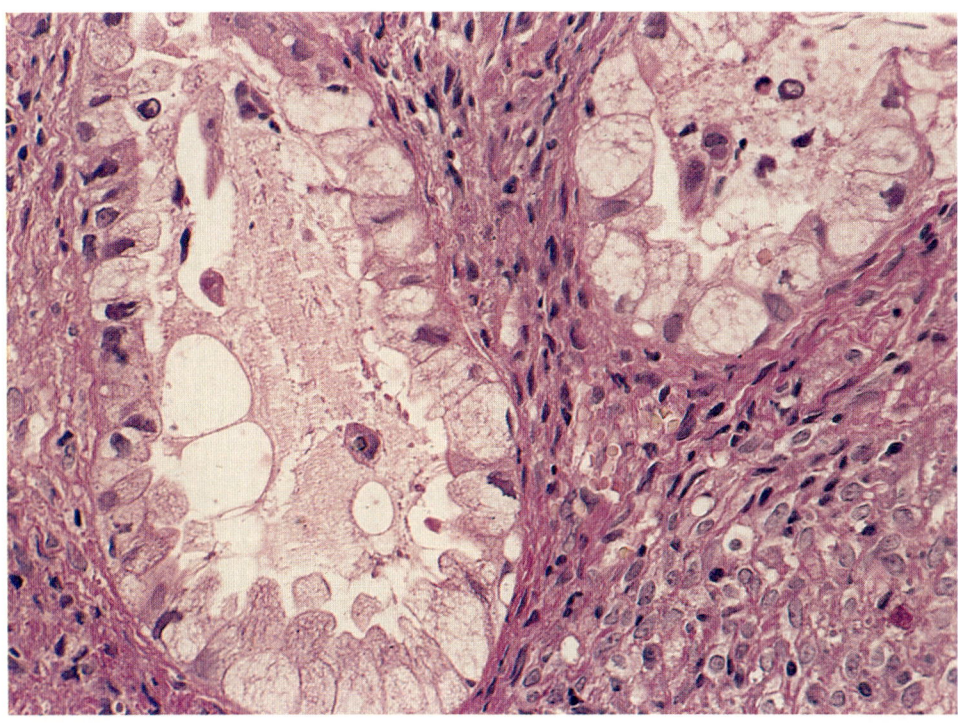

Fig. 86b. Same as Fig. 86a. Pleomorphic nuclei and vacuolated cytoplasm of glandular epithelium. H & E

Benign Tumors

Epithelial Tumors (Figs. 87–89)

Papillomas of the ectocervix (Figs. 86–89) occur predominantly in young women and are mainly caused by HPV infection 6 and 11. Some may be inverted, hence their surfaces are flat. Histologically they consist of thick layers of stratified squamous epithelium with elongated rete pegs that extend deeply into the lamina propria (Fig. 87). The basal membrane is intact, the epithelial layers are well differentiated, and acanthosis is usually pronounced. More advanced lesions may also contain koilocytes in the upper layers. Mitoses are rare. Besides the flat, inverted type of papilloma, others may be quite condylomatous and closely resemble the condylomata of the vulva and vagina (Fig. 88) or form verrucae covered by parakeratosis or hyperkeratosis (Fig. 89). These papillomas may be sessile or pedunculated.

Differential Diagnosis. On gross examination the condylomatous papillomas may resemble an invasive carcinoma. Histologically, they can be distinguished by their lack of cellular atypicality, absence of mitoses, and the intact basal membranes. The previously introduced term "flat condyloma" for inverted papilloma should be avoided, as it may mislead the clinician. Ectocervical papilloma, depending on the type of HPV causing it, may later become malignant, whereas condylomas of the vulva and vagina almost invariably remain benign (Willett et al. 1989).

Besides diffuse or focal adenomatous hyperplasia (see p. 42) circumscribed benign *adenomas* may rarely develop from metaplastic foci. A *villous adenoma* derived from intestinal metaplasia of the endocervical epithelium has recently been described (Michael et al. 1986).

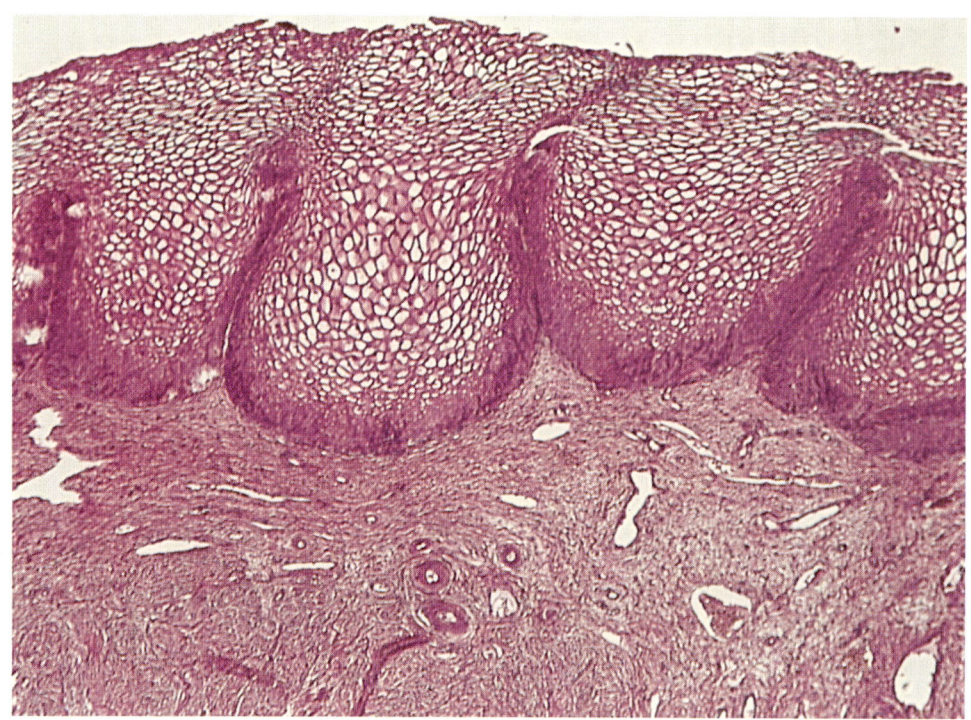

Fig. 87a. Papilloma of the ectocervix, early stage. H & E

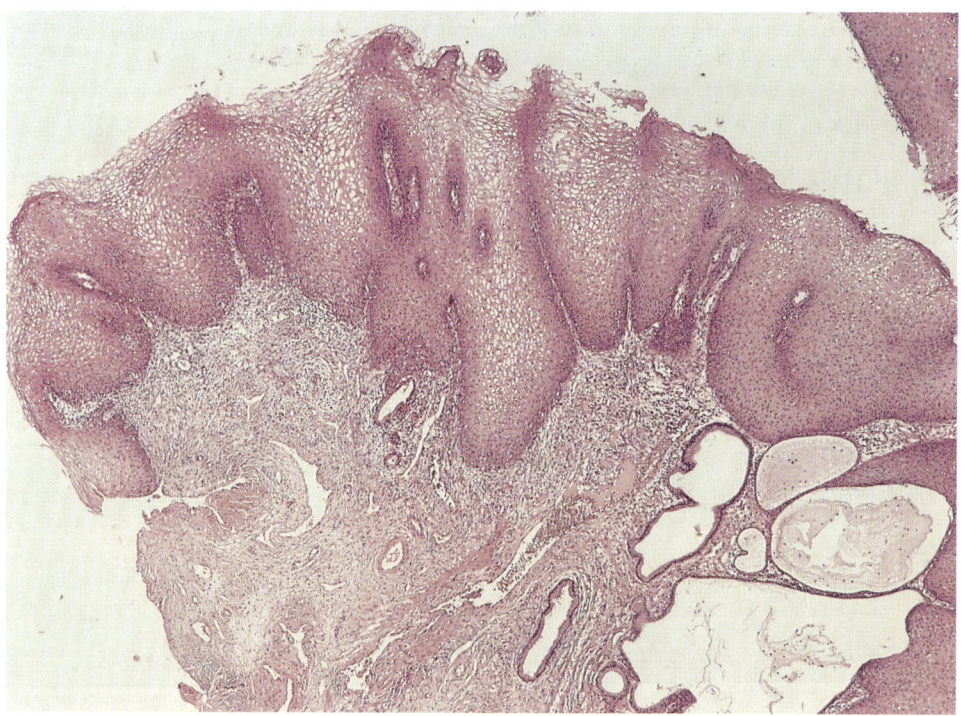

Fig. 87b. Papilloma of the ectocervix, advanced stage. H & E

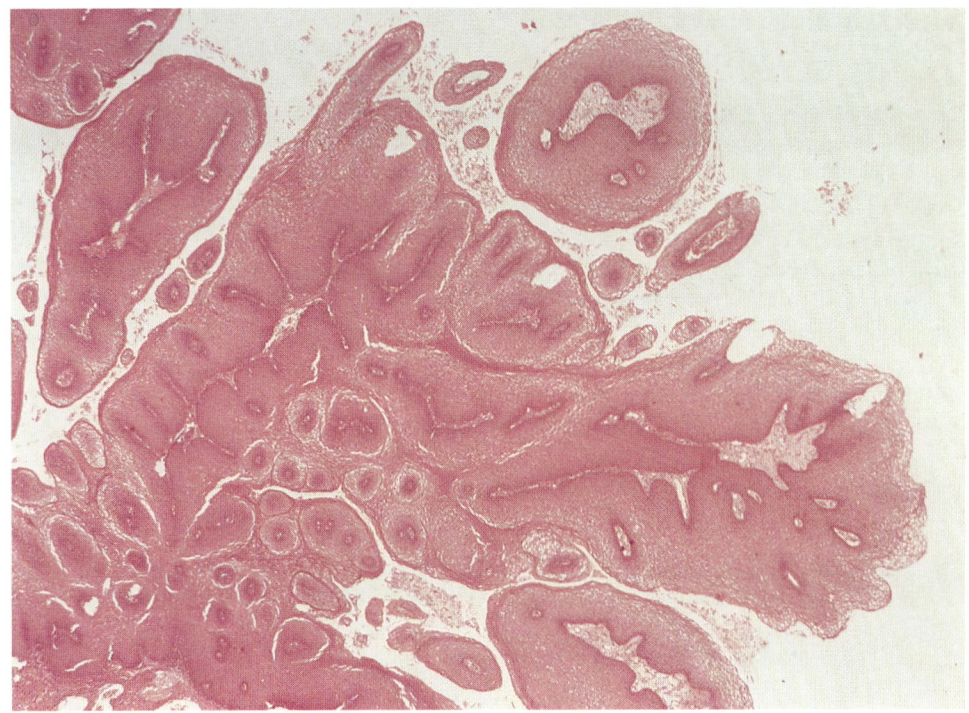

Fig. 88. Papilloma of the ectocervix, condylomatous. H & E

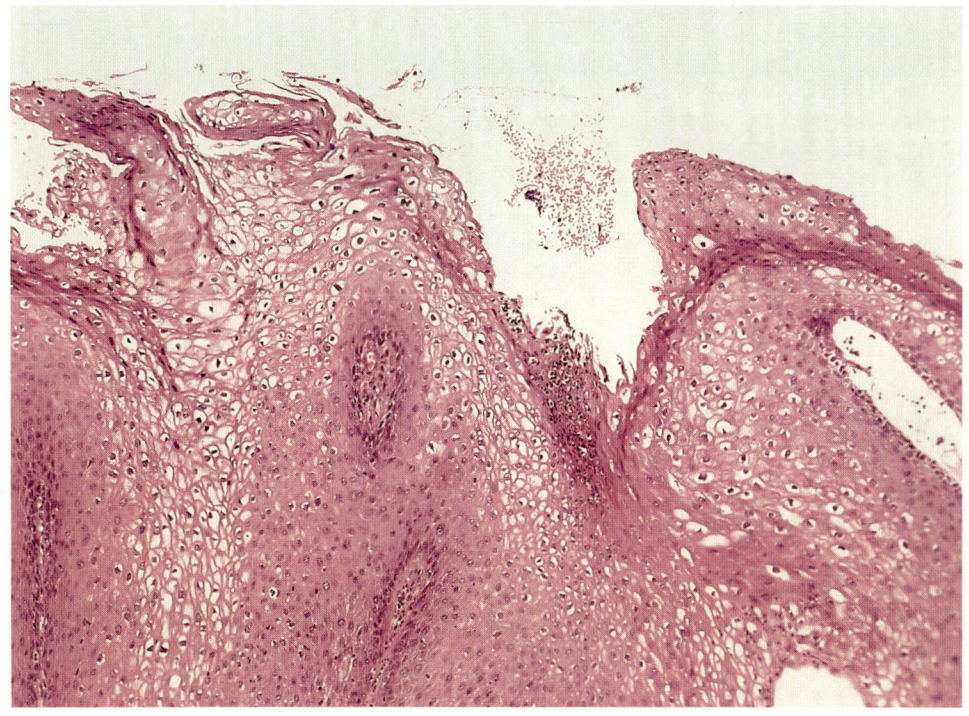

Fig. 89. Papilloma of the ectocervix, verrucous surface. H & E

Mesenchymal Tumors (Fig. 90-92)

Leiomyomas (Fig. 90) consist of smooth muscle cells more or less intermingled with fibroblasts and abundant blood vessels of various sizes. These leiomyomas resemble in most respects those of the myometrium.

Hemangiomas (Fig. 91) of the cervix are rare (Gusdon 1965). They consist of compact tangles of venules (Fig. 91) or capillaries that through their growth often cause a bulging of the surface.

Blue Nevi (Fig. 92) very rarely occur in the endocervix (Patel and Bhagavan 1985). They are composed of slender, wavy dermal melanocytes with long dendritic processes. These cells, either grouped or dispersed among variable numbers of melanophages, fibroblasts, and collagenous fibers, are usually laden with fine granules of melanin.

Other benign mesenchymal tumors, such as neurinoma, neurofibroma, and lipoma are rare, compared with their counterparts in other tissues.

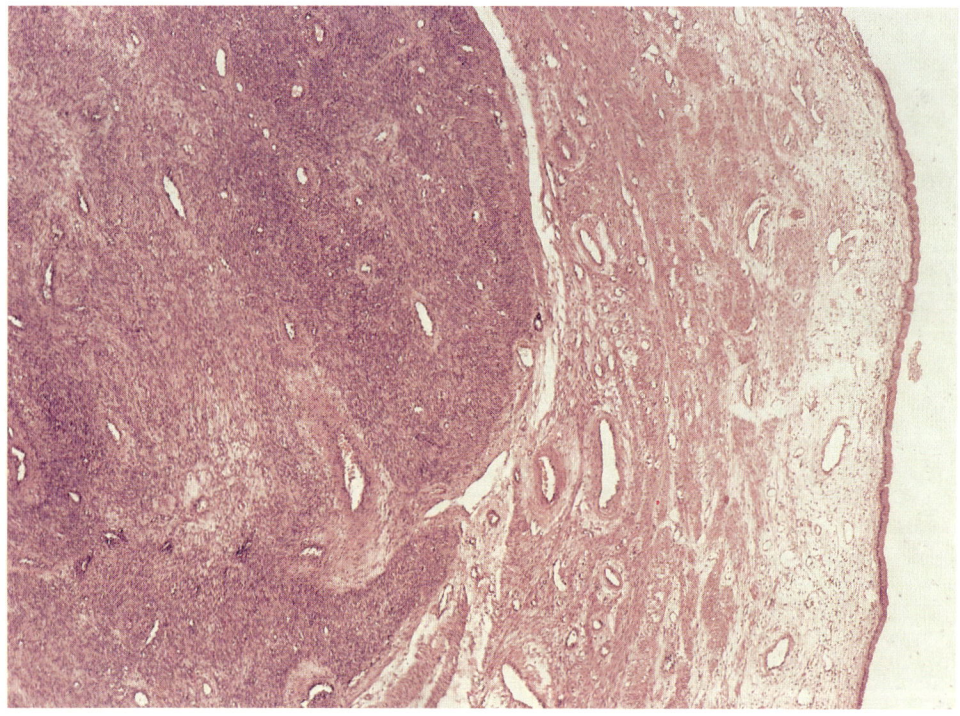

Fig. 90. Leiomyoma of the cervix. H & E

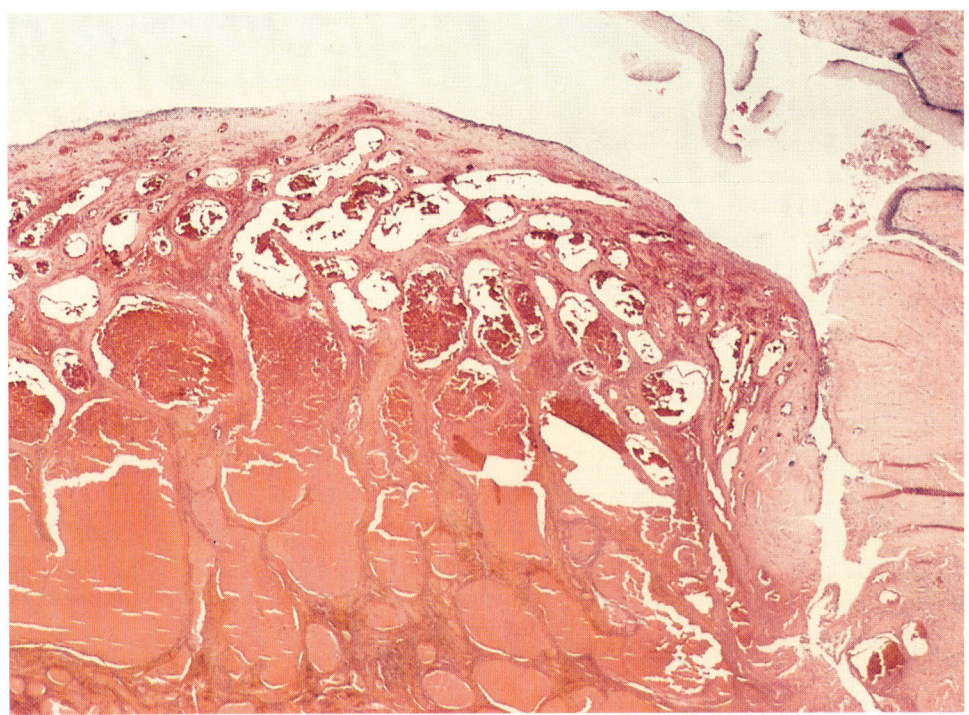

Fig. 91. Hemangioma of the cervix. H & E

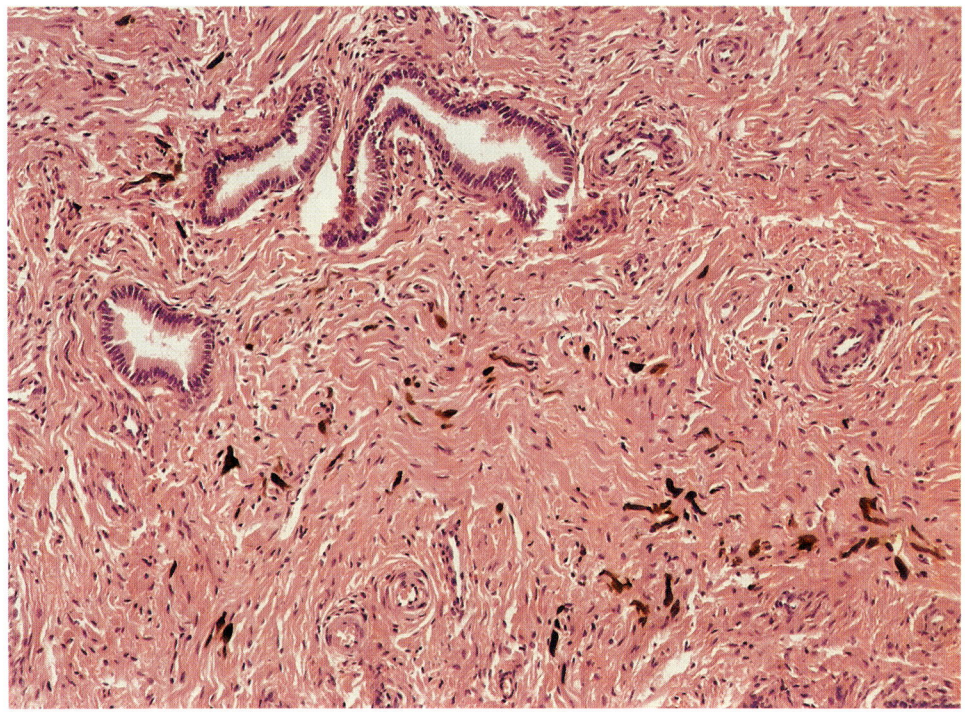

Fig. 92. Blue nevus of the cervix. H & E

Mixed Tumors (Figs. 93 and 94)

Papillary adenofibromas (Figs. 93, 94) are shaped like large endocervical polyps with fingerlike projections at their surface. The covering epithelium is of the endocervical type, single layered, and inconspicuous. Their stroma is very cellular and dense, consisting of fibroblasts, occasionally intermingled with leiomyoblasts. Mitoses are rare (Abell 1971). These tumors are seen almost exclusively in postmenopausal women. They recur frequently, and after several recurrences, their stroma may undergo malignant change to become an adenosarcoma (see Figs. 215, 216).

Differential Diagnosis. Endocervical polyps can be distinguished by their either loose, edematous or fibrous, acellular stroma. Adenosarcomas are recognized by their high mitotic activity, their periglandular cuffs, and the polymorphism of their stromal cell-nuclei.

Adenomyomas rarely arise within the cervix. Polypoid adenomyomas of the endometrium may occasionally prolapse and protude from the endocervical canal, giving the impression they have arisen there.

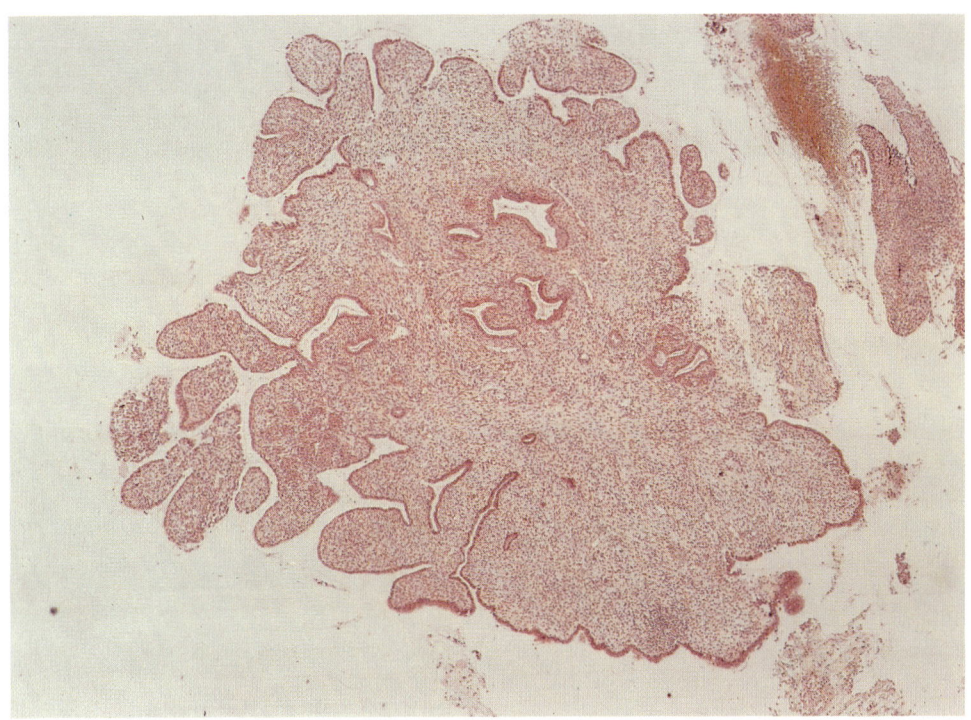

Fig. 93. Papillary adenofibroma of the endocervix. H & E

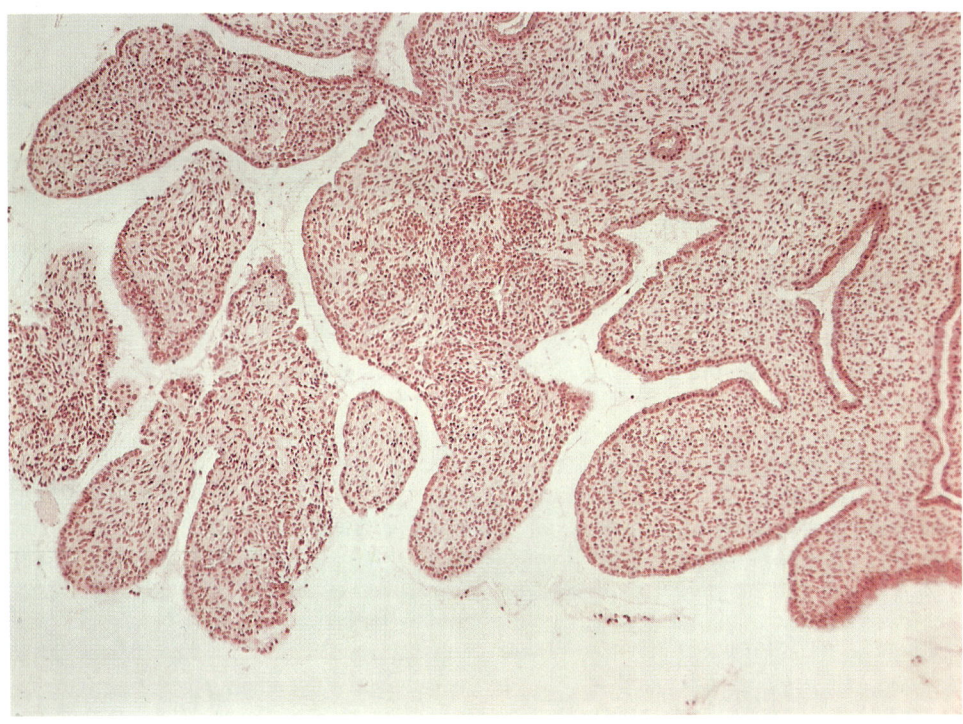

Fig. 94. Papillary adenofibroma of the endocervix. H & E, higher magnification

Premalignant Lesions

Introduction

Dysplasia and carcinoma in situ are common lesions; most pathology laboratories receive several cases weekly. It is important to have well-defined terms and criteria for each type of these lesions, thereby promoting correct diagnoses and proper treatment. Unfortunately, as the literature shows us, there is confusion about how to interpret these lesions, in part, because of disagreement about how best to name them (e. g., dysplasia and carcinoma in situ versus cervical intraepithelial neoplasia, CIN), but also because the various lesions form a broad spectrum of biological and cytological changes with no sharp and precise limits. We have chosen to use the terms dysplasia and carcinoma in situ instead of CIN, because these are the original names recommended by the WHO and most widely used. The differences between the two nomenclatures are, however, small. The WHO classification is a 4-step division, the CIN a 3-step. CIN I corresponds in general to mild dysplasia, CIN II to moderate dysplasia, and CIN III covers both severe dysplasia and carcinoma in situ.

The spectrum reaches from the mildest dysplasia to carcinoma in situ, changes that may be found in very small regions of the cervix, but virtually always in the transformation zone. They may involve the whole circumference of the cervical orifice to include smaller or larger parts of the endocervical mucosa. The dysplastic or anaplastic epithelium lies not only on the surface, but may also extend down into the endocervical glands.

It must be emphasized that often varying degrees of dysplasia and carcinoma in situ are found together in the same cervix. The prime diagnosis is made from the most advanced and severe change.

Dysplasia and adenocarcinoma in situ of the endocervical glandular epithelium are much less common. Nonetheless, they seem to be associated with dysplasia and carcinoma in situ of the squamous and reserve cell epithelium.

Etiology and Pathogenesis

Precursors of cervical cancer may develop from regenerating ectocervical squamous epithelium, from proliferating columnar epithelial cells of the endocervical glands, or, most frequently, from hyperplastic reserve cells beneath the endocervical glandular epithelium. Since proliferative activity with high mitotic rates is known to be a prerequisite of cancerogenesis, those cells undergoing proliferation will be most vulnerable to carcinogenic agents. In addition to mechanical or chemical irritation, cellular proliferation is largely initiated by excessive (mainly exogenous) hormonal stimulation of target cells (see page 42). Among the oncogenic factors affecting prestimulated, rapidly proliferating cells, DNA-containing viruses, especially human papilloma viruses (HPV) are most frequent. To a lesser extent, herpes simplex virus II and cytomegaly virus may be considered as potential carcinogens (Fenoglio and Ferenczy 1982). Specific subtypes of HPV predominate in certain kinds of premalignant lesions and invasive carcinomas (Table 2). Of the more than 60 subtypes of

Table 2. Types of human papilloma virus (HPV) found in premalignant lesions and invasive carcinomas of the cervix

	HPV		
	6, 11	16	18
Squamous epithelium			
Ectocervix			
Papilloma	+	+	
Mild koilocytic dysplasia	+	+	
Severe koilocytic dysplasia		+	
Carcinoma in situ		+	
Invasive carcinoma		+	
Reserve cell			
Endocervix			
Mild koilocytic dysplasia		+++	+
Severe koilocytic dysplasia		+++	+
Carcinoma in situ		+++	+
Invasive carcinoma		+++	+
Clear cell carcinoma		+	++
Adenosquamous carcinoma		+	++
Adenocarcinoma		+	++
Glandular epithelium			
Endocervix			
Adenocarcinoma in situ		+	++
Adenocarcinoma		+	++
Adenosquamous carcinoma		+	++

HPV identified to date, mainly subtypes 16 and 18, but also subtypes 31, 33, 35, 39, and rarely a few in the 40s and 50s are associated with cervical carcinogenesis (Richart 1987).

During the acute (productive) phase of infection, the virus replicates in superficial (degenerating) epithelial cells with low or arrested DNA synthesis, resulting in koilocytosis with subsequent cell death. If viral DNA fragments become integrated into the nuclear DNA, as in rapidly replicating cells of the basal or reserve cell layer or in regenerative epithelium, immortalization and finally malignant transformation may occur. This development is thought to be a multistep event, in which not only cell proliferation, but also malignant transformation is strongly enhanced by steroid hormones. A direct influence of the hormone-receptor complex on the viral genome has also been discussed (Pater et al. 1988). The progesterone receptor in particular, which is mainly increased under oral contraceptive use, appears to be a determinant risk factor. It has also been shown that HPV enhances hydroxylation of estradiol, and the resulting metabolite enhances virus expression. Besides steroid hormones, additional inductive factors may be postulated, such as immune deficiency, e. g., that following immunosuppressive therapy for renal transplantation (Schneider et al. 1983). Other risk factors may be smoking, promiscuity, and alcohol.

The infection with HPV is not always accompanied by koilocytosis (Fuchs et al. 1988) or a precancerous lesion: The cells of 10% of women between 15 and 50 years of age with normal cytologic smears expressed DNA of HPV, 6.9% of which were subtypes 16 and 18 (de Villiers er al. 1987). This appears explainable in view of the multistep development requiring additional cocarcinogenic factors for malignant transformation.

The viruses can best be detected in biopsy samples with the Southern blot hybridization technique (Southern 1975) or in paraffin sections by in situ hybridization with DNA probes (Nagai et al. 1987). With these techniques it was shown that the great majority (up to 90%) of carcinomas in situ and invasive cervical carcinomas contain genomically integrated HPV. Of these, roughly 50% were subtype 16 and 20% subtype 18; the remaining 20% were associated with various other subtypes (Gissmann 1984; and cited by Richart 1987). Whereas virus subtype 16 predominates in the reserve cell carcinoma in situ (up to 77%; Franquemont et al. 1989) and invasive squamous cell carcinomas, subtype 18 is mainly observed in adenocarcinoma in situ and invasive adenocarcinomas of the endocervix (Tase et al. 1988, 1989; Wilczynski et al. 1988; Farnsworth et al. 1989). Since these two kinds of carcinoma histogenetically derive from reserve cells (Christopherson et al. 1979; Boon et al. 1981), the virus apparently acts not only as an oncogen on the nuclear DNA, but in addition seems to influence cellular differentiation towards squamous or glandular epithelial cells. When endocervical adenocarcinoma is associated with carcinoma in situ of the reserve cell type, the same subtype 18 virus is often found in both lesions. In these cases, a bidirectional differentiation of the affected reserve cells is postulated, giving rise to both types of carcinoma.

The virus subtypes 6 and 11, which are most frequently found in condylomas of the vulva and vagina, rarely affect the cervix (Willett et al. 1989). If they do, the resulting koilocytic lesion nearly always regresses and almost never progresses beyond the stage of mild or moderate dysplasia since these viruses remain episomal and are not integrated into the cellular genome. On the contrary, up to 85% of mild dysplastic lesions progressing to preinvasive or invasive carcinoma contained virus subtype 16, as could be shown in a prospective study (Campion et al. 1986). Hence, it is of paramount clinical importance to determine what subtype of HPV has caused the lesion.

Histopathology and Immunohistochemistry

Dysplasia and Carcinoma In Situ
(CIN I-III; Figs. 95-127)

The development of dysplasia and carcinoma in situ is a continuum, extending from slight to severe cytological atypia with a gradual loss of epithelial stratification, an increase in nuclear changes, and an increase in the number of atypical mitoses. Because the changes merge into one another, it may be difficult in some instances to differentiate between mild and moderate dysplasia, moderate and severe dyplasia, or severe dyplasia and carcinoma in situ. On the other hand, the distinction between a mild dysplasia and an irregular regenerative or reparative epithelium should not prove difficult: The nuclei of regenerative epithelium may be enlarged, slightly irregular, yet the chromatin pattern normal. The epithelial stratification may be barely altered. On the other hand, the nuclei of dysplastic epithelium are dyskaryotic from the beginning, enlarged, and irregular with chromatin clumping. In addition, abnormal mitotic figures, loss of basal polarity and multinucleated cells may be present. Depending upon the cell of origin, structural variations can be observed between squamous cell and reserve cell intraepithelial neoplasias.

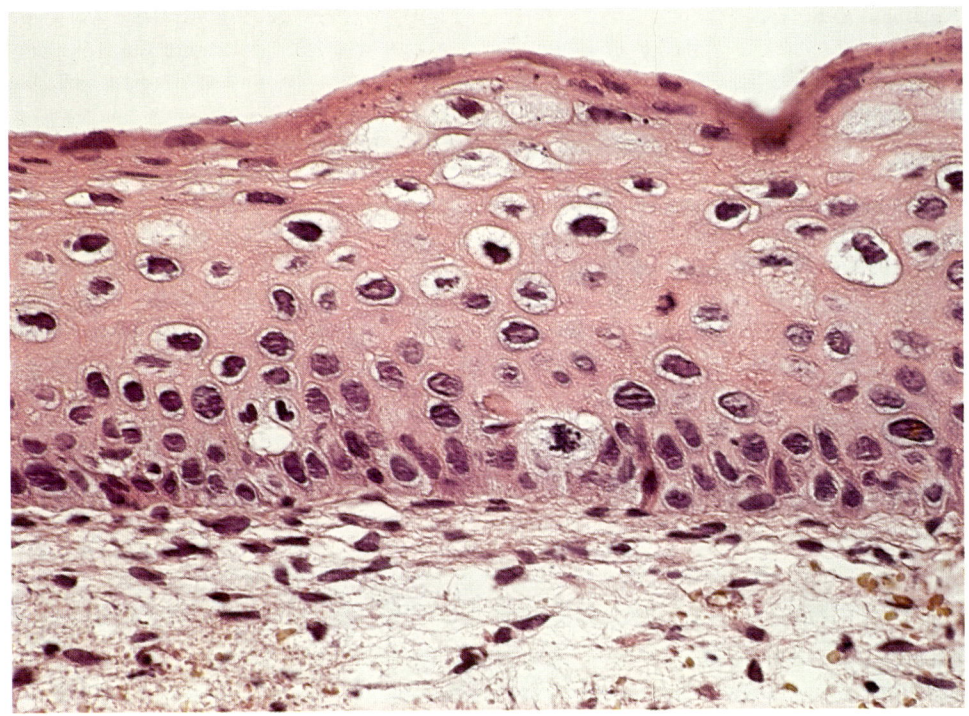

Fig. 95. Mild dysplasia, squamous cell type, koilocytic. H & E

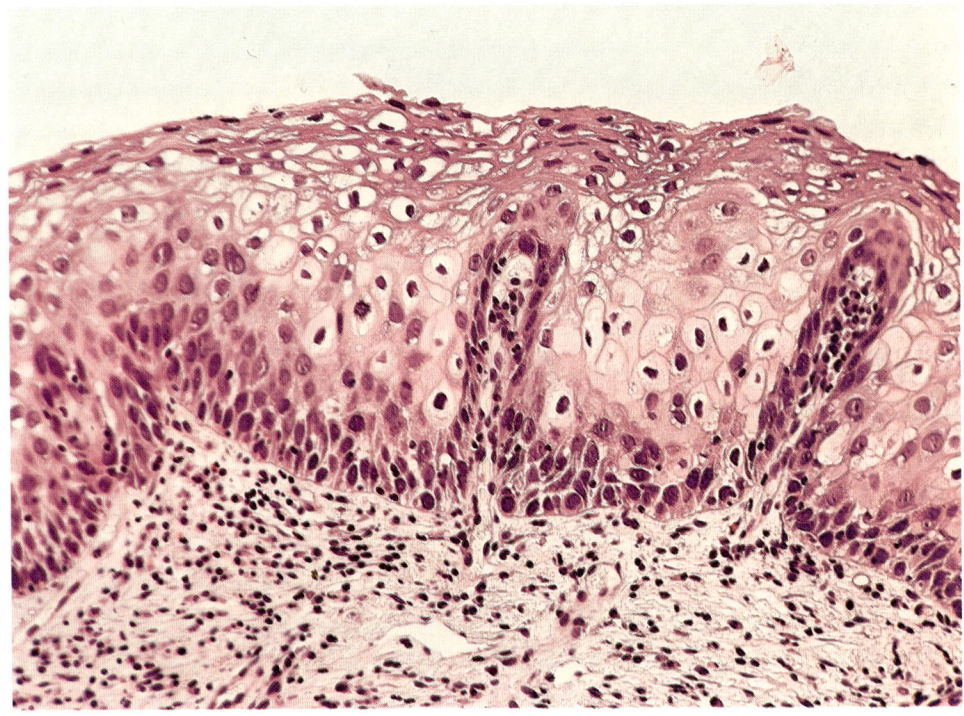

Fig. 96. Mild dysplasia, squamous cell type, slightly papillomatous. H & E

Squamous Cell Type

In mild and moderate dysplasia of squamous cell type (Figs. 95–100), epithelial stratification is only partly lost, with an increasing basal hyperplasia and a general thickening (Figs. 95, 98) or slightly papillomatous change (Figs. 96, 97) of the epithelial layer. Basal polarity and cellular orientation are gradually lost. The nuclei become irregular, hyperchromatic with an abnormal, coarsely granular chromatin pattern. Mitoses increase in number, primarily in the basal and middle epithelial layers. Depending on the causative agent, the upper epithelial layers may (Fig. 99) or may not (Fig. 98) show koilocytosia, as a result of viral replication following HPV infection. In mild or moderate dysplasia, the presence of koilocytes may indicate replication of papilloma viruses subtypes 6 or 11, which will remain episomal; such a dysplasia is virtually always reversible. If, however, the infection is with virus subtypes 16 or 18, the viral DNA will most likely become integrated into the cellular genome and initiate malignant change. The dysplastic change starts at the squamocolumnar junction and is usually located there.

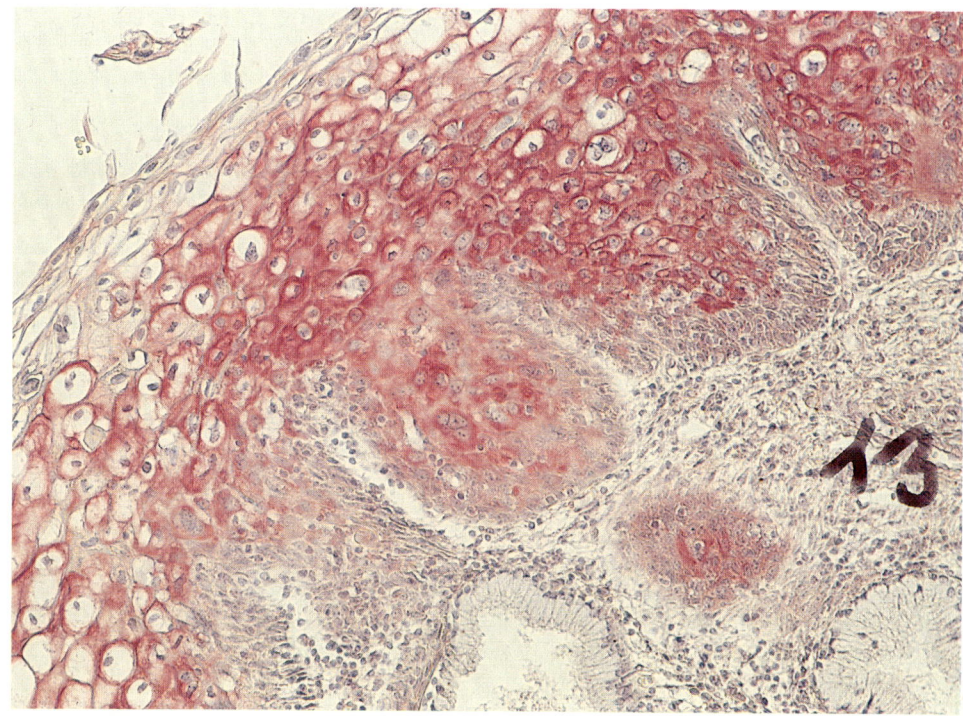

Fig. 97. Mild dysplasia, squamous cell type. Immunohistochemical reaction with anticytokeratin 13

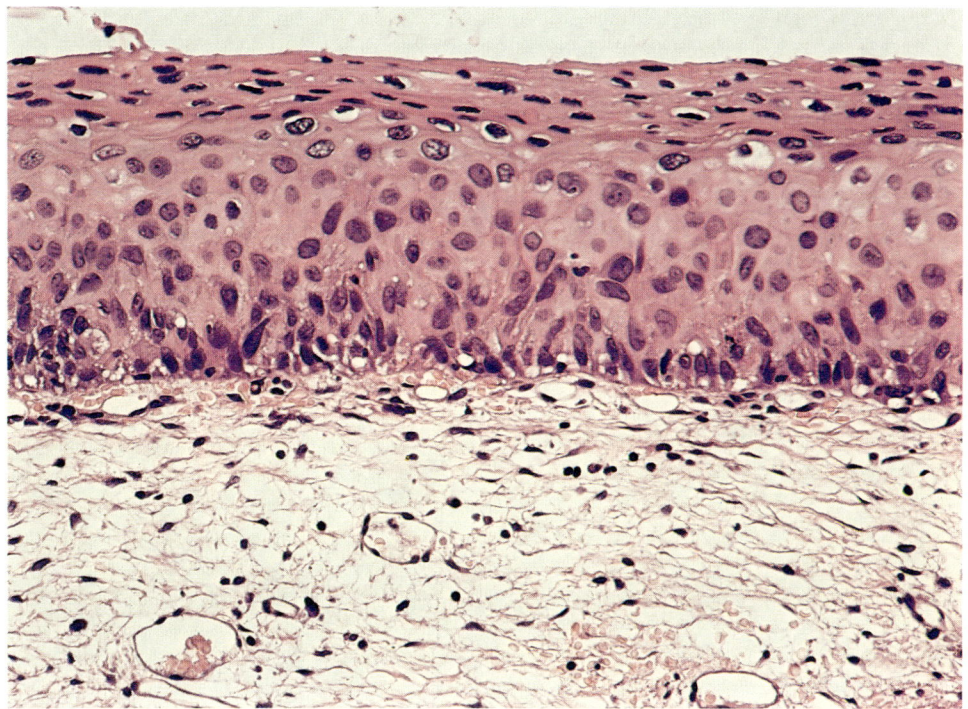

Fig. 98. Moderate dysplasia, squamous cell type, nonkoilocytic. H & E

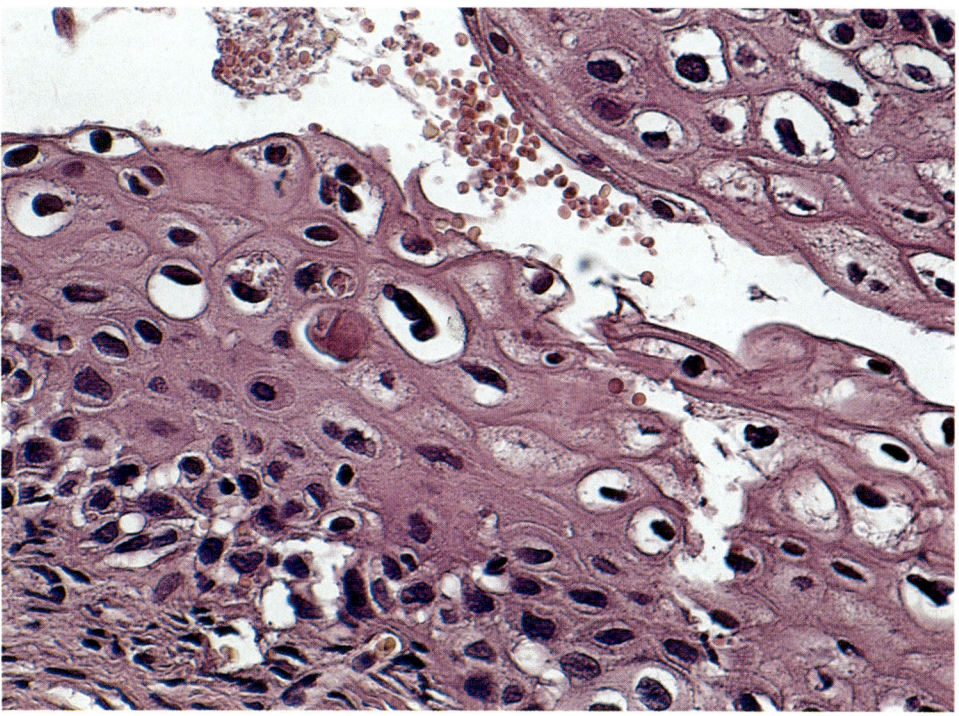

Fig. 99. Moderate dysplasia, squamous cell type, koilocytic. H & E

Differential Diagnosis. It is possible to distinguish between reversible and irreversible koilocytic dysplasia at this early stage by Southern blot or in situ hybridization with DNA probes to identify the type of infective virus (Figs. 100 a–c). If that is not possible, histological (Winkler et al. 1984; Crum et al. 1985) or immunohistochemical (Dallenbach-Hellweg and Lang 1990) distinction should be attempted: Dysplasias infected with HPV 6 or 11 have dyskaryotic polyploid nuclei but normal mitoses and express cytokeratin 13 only. Those infected with HPV 16 or 18 have aneuploid nuclei and atypical mitoses and in most instances show a coexpression of cytokeratins 13, 8, 18, and CEA. Such coexpression of intermediate filaments and CEA may indicate that the dysplasia is most likely of reserve cell type (see below). The distinction is clinically important for deciding how to treat the patient further.

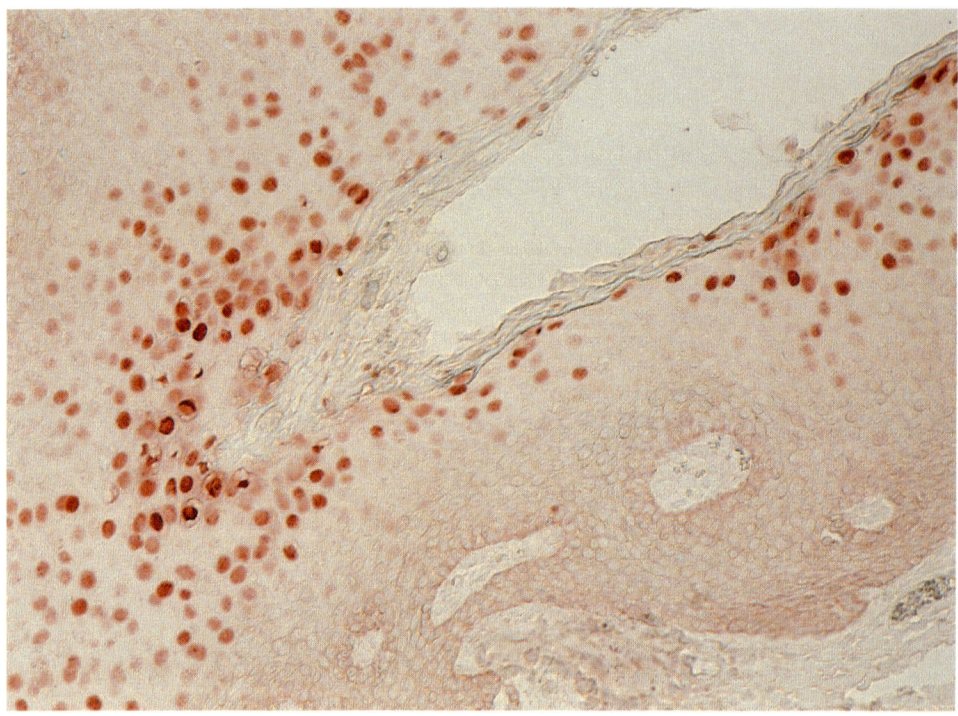

Fig. 100a. Mild to moderate dysplasia, squamous cell type. In situ hybridization with DNA probe for HPV 6 and 11

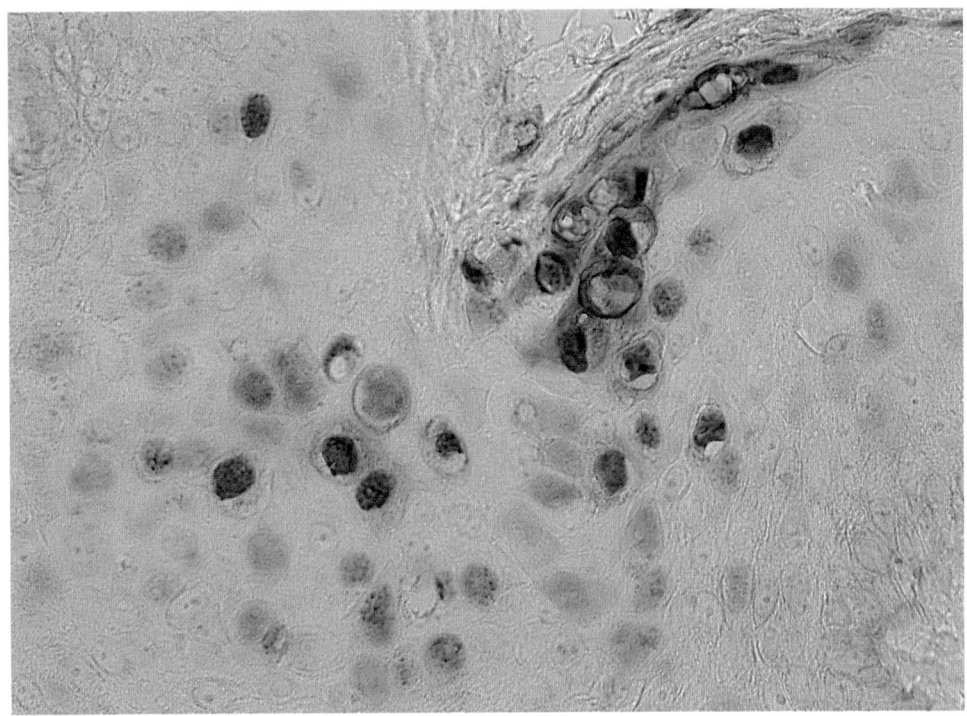

Fig. 100b. Same as Fig. 100a. Higher magnification. Positive nuclear reaction of superficial epithelial cells

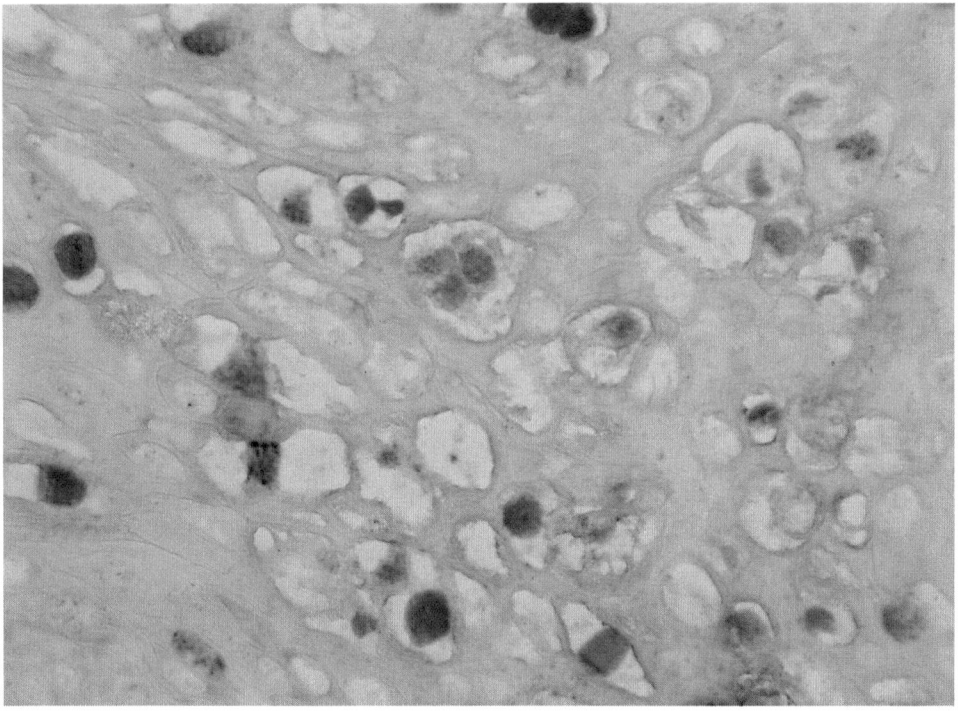

Fig. 100c. Same as Fig. 100b. Positive nuclear signals in koilocytes located in intermediate cellular layers

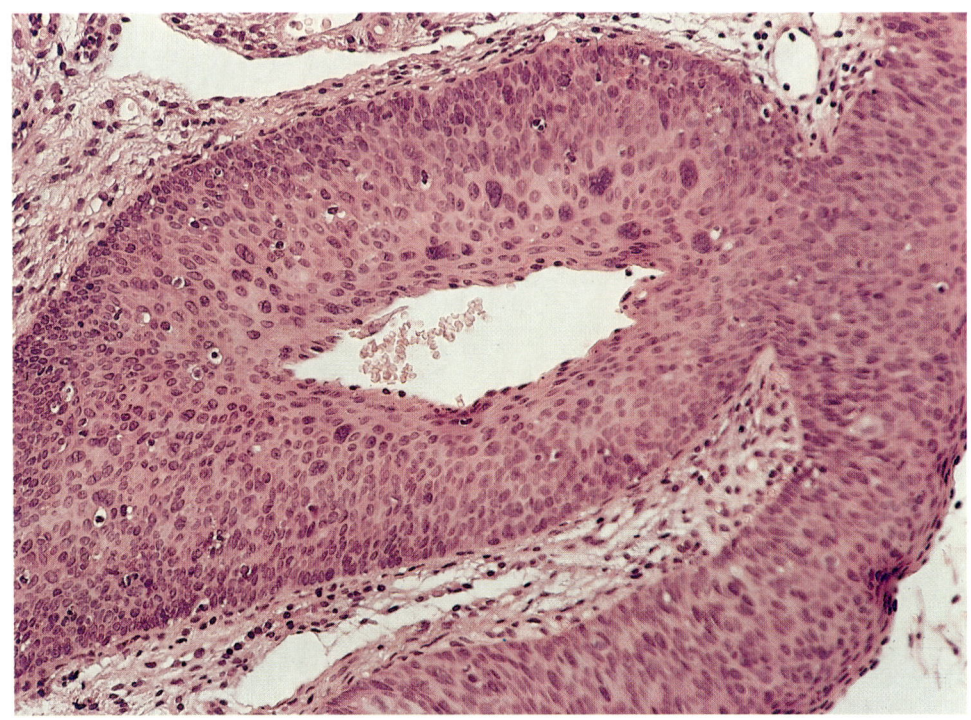

Fig. 101. Severe dysplasia, nonkoilocytic. H & E

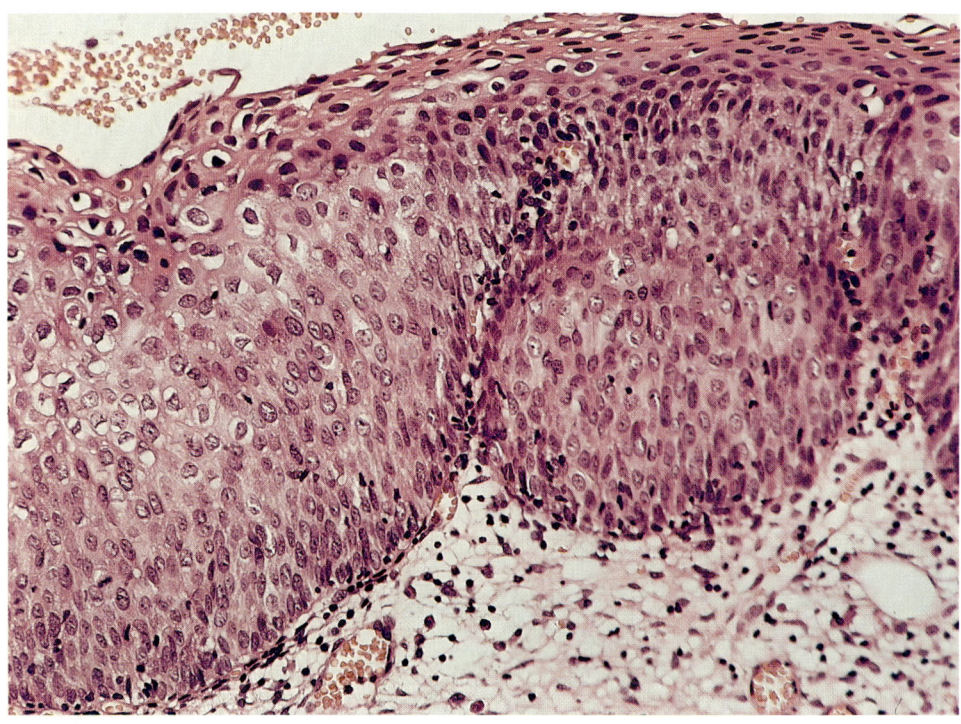

Fig. 102. Severe dysplasia, koilocytic, H & E. Histogenetic type in Figs. 101, 102 cannot be determined without special stains

In *severe dysplasia of squamous cell type* (Figs. 101–103), loss of epithelial stratification is almost complete. Nuclear changes (enlargement, chromatin clumping, polymorphism, hyperchromasia) and the number of mitoses are considerably increased. Since koilocytes can only develop in maturing cells, they will be less numerous than in mild or moderate dysplasia. They are rarely present at all in the squamous cell type of severe dysplasia, which often develops independent of an HPV infection. If koilocytes are present in severe dysplasia, then they almost always indicate infection with HPV 16 or 18 and mean that the dysplasia is most likely not of squamous, but of reserve cell origin (see below). The dysplastic epithelium is usually quite high, may be covered by a thick layer of parakeratosis (Fig. 103), and may form broad papillae that extend downwards into the underlying stroma (Fig. 102) or into the mouths of endocervical glands (Fig. 101).

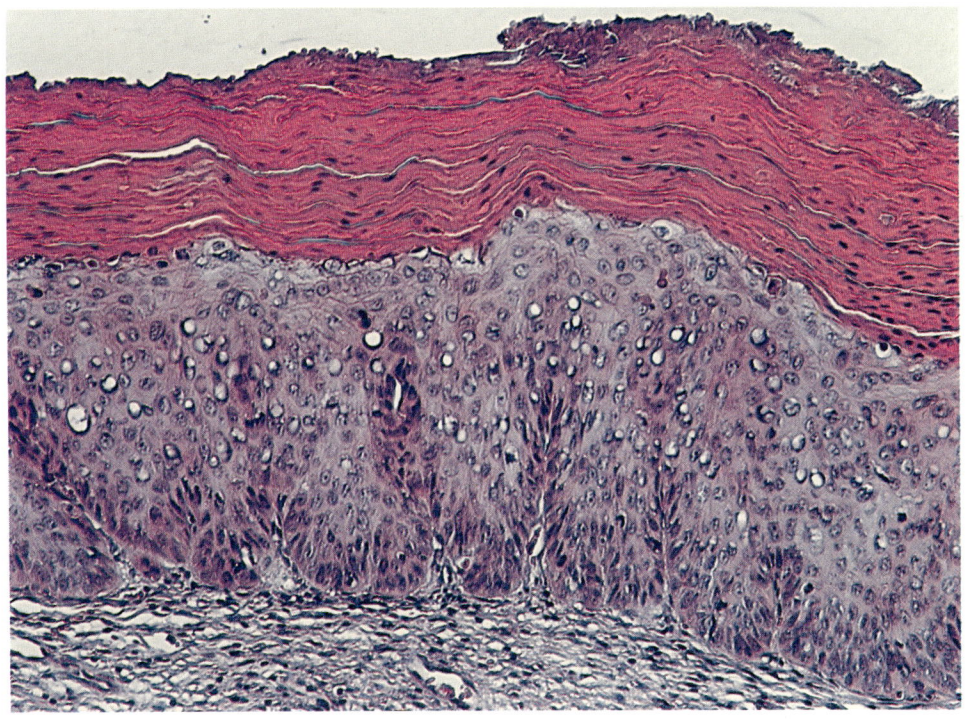

Fig. 103. Severe dysplasia, squamous cell type, covered by a broad layer of parakeratosis. H & E

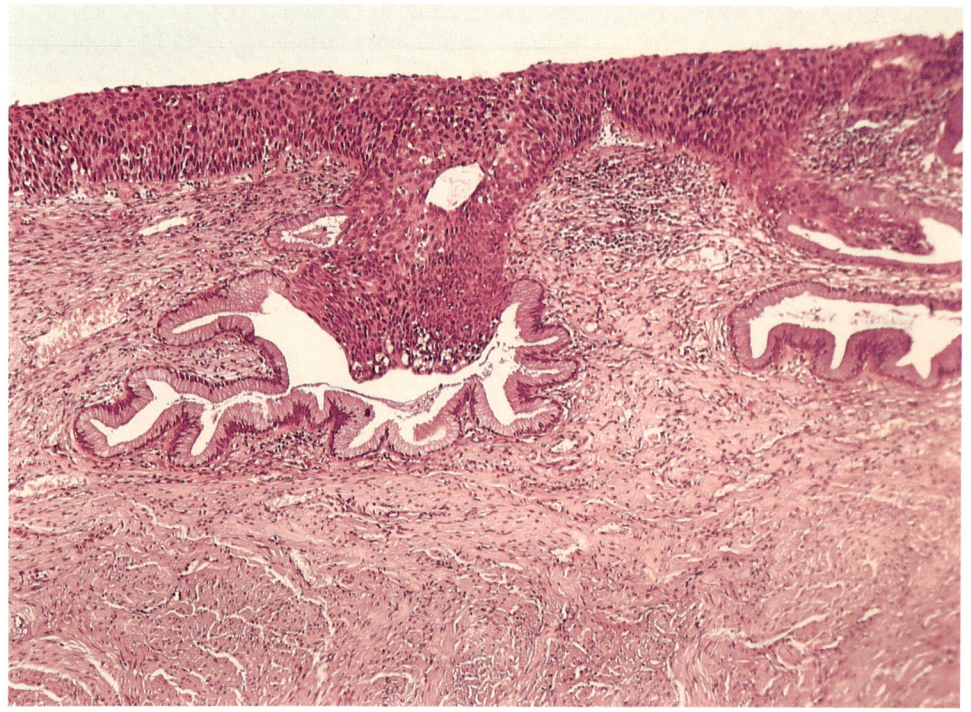

Fig. 104. Carcinoma in situ, squamous cell type. H & E

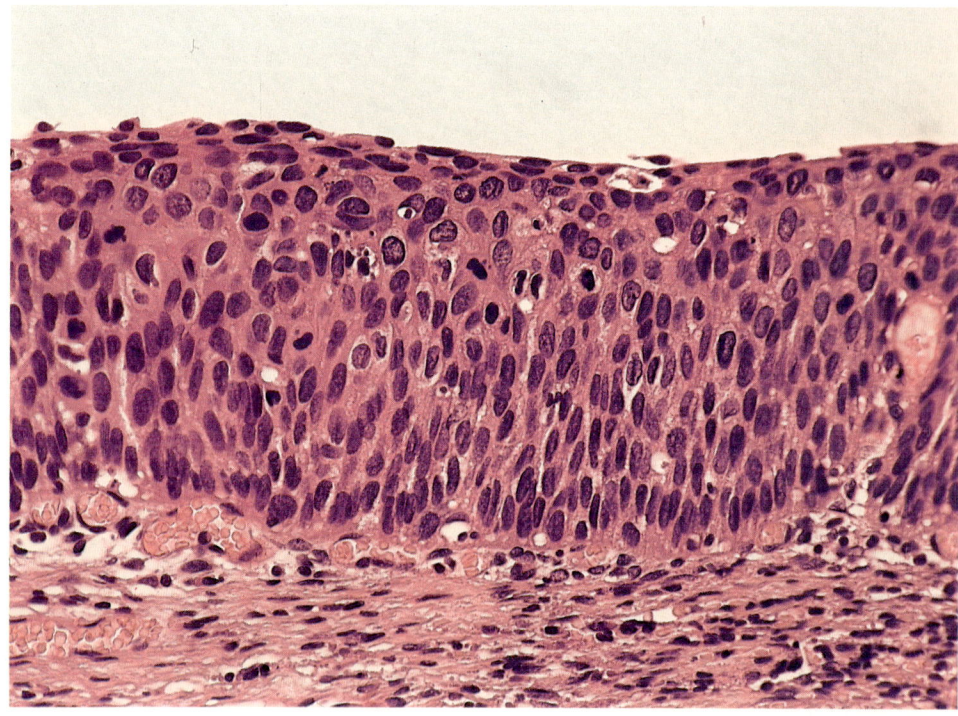

Fig. 105. Carcinoma in situ, squamous cell type. H & E, higher magnification

Carcinoma in situ of the squamous cell type (Figs. 104–106) shows a complete loss of stratification. The entire epithelium consists of poorly differentiated neoplastic cells, which contain disorganized, large, atypical, hyperchromatic nuclei surrounded by little cytoplasm. Atypical mitoses are frequent in all layers; koilocytes are not present. This neoplastic epithelium originates at the squamocolumnar junction and from there may grow out to replace large areas of the ecto- and endocervical surface epithelium. It is usually covered by a layer of atypical parakeratosis. Its spread into glands is much less pronounced than that of the reserve cell type of carcinoma in situ.

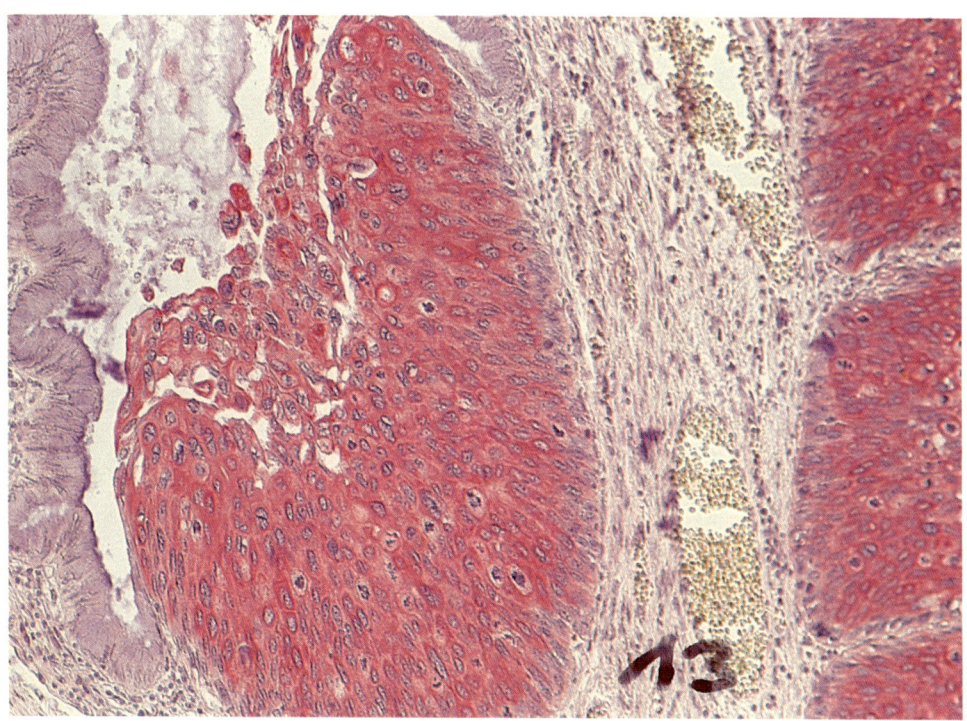

Fig. 106. Carcinoma in situ, squamous cell type. Immunohistochemical reaction with anticytokeratin 13

Reserve Cell Type

Mild, moderate or severe dysplasia of reserve cell type (Figs. 107-120) develops from the reserve cell layer of the endocervical epithelium and is usually preceded by a reserve cell hyperplasia. The gradual increase in cytological and nuclear atypicality corresponds closely to the various degrees of squamous dysplasia. Because the reserve cells are bipotential, irregular maturation towards mucin formation, often monocellular (Fig. 111; mucoid dysplasia), clear cell change (Fig. 112), or maturation towards keratinization (see Fig. 127) may be seen. Koilocytosis is often present and nearly always caused by infection with HPV 16 or 18 (Fig. 114), whereas types 6 and 11 are almost exclusively found in squamous epithelium. Topographically, reserve cell dysplasia is not always concentrated at, but rather above the squamocolumnar junction, and may also arise anywhere within the endocervical mucosa (surface epithelium and glands; Figs. 108, 109).

In rare instances a rather mild type of reserve cell dysplasia may form papillary structures resembling a pedunculated papilloma of the ectocervix (Figs. 117, 118). Since an invasive carcinoma may develop at their base, the papillomatous growths should be excised in total and examined carefully (see page 94; Randall et al. 1986).

At the stage of severe dysplasia, it is important to distinguish the rapidly progressing koilocytic type (HPV 16 or 18) from the non-koilocytic type. That, again, is best done using hybridization techniques (Fig. 114).

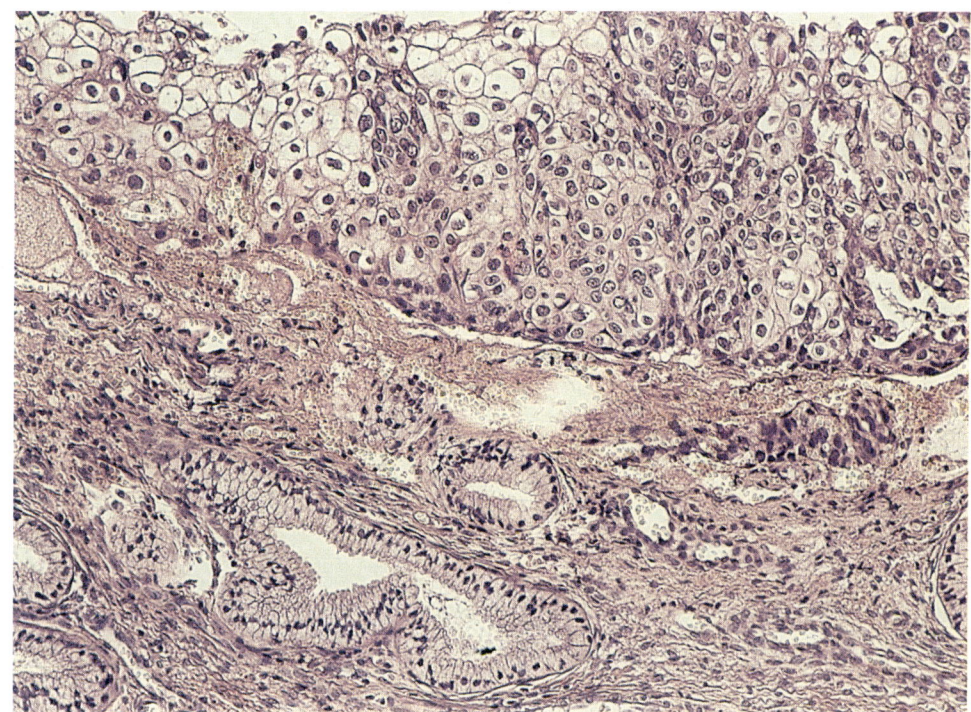

Fig. 107. Mild dysplasia, reserve cell type with koilocytes. H & E

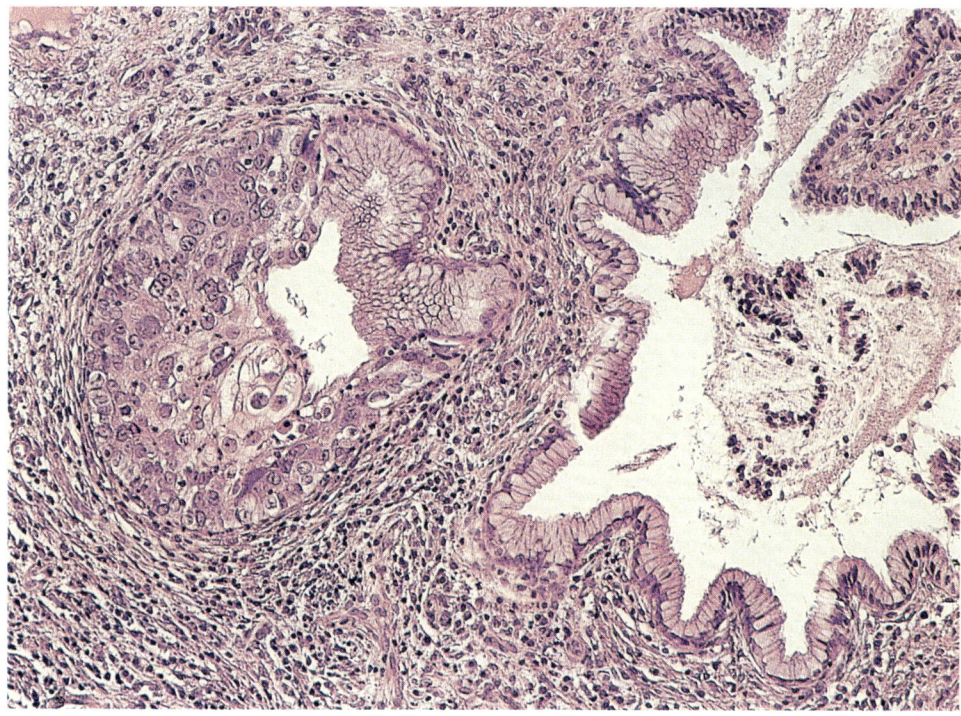

Fig. 108. Mild dysplasia, reserve cell type with koilocytes in endocervical gland. H & E

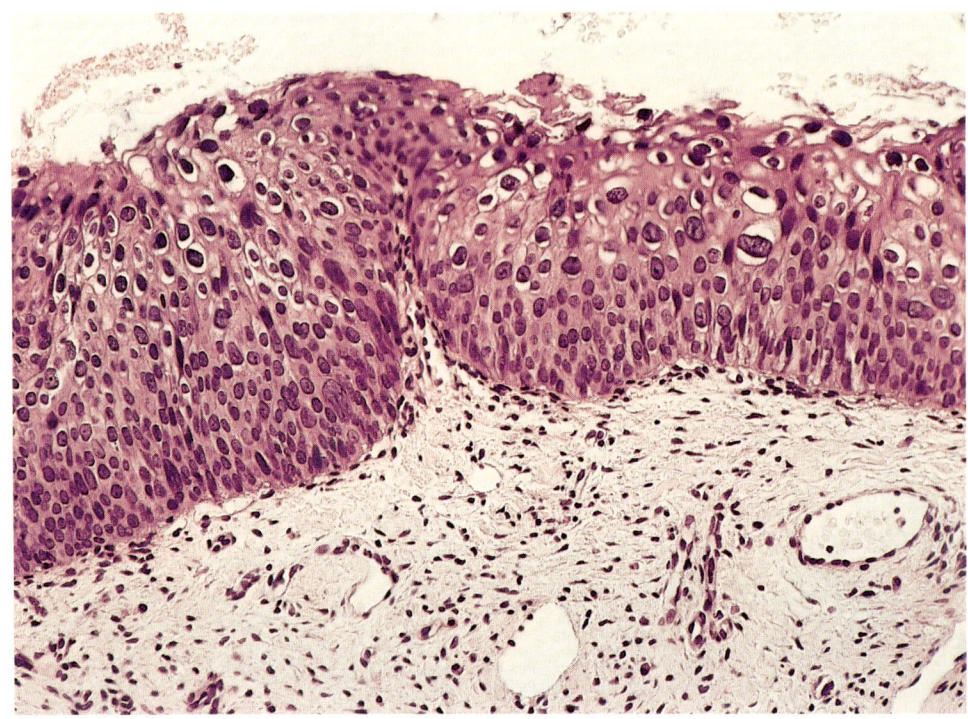

Fig. 109. Moderate dysplasia, reserve cell type, with koilocytes. H & E

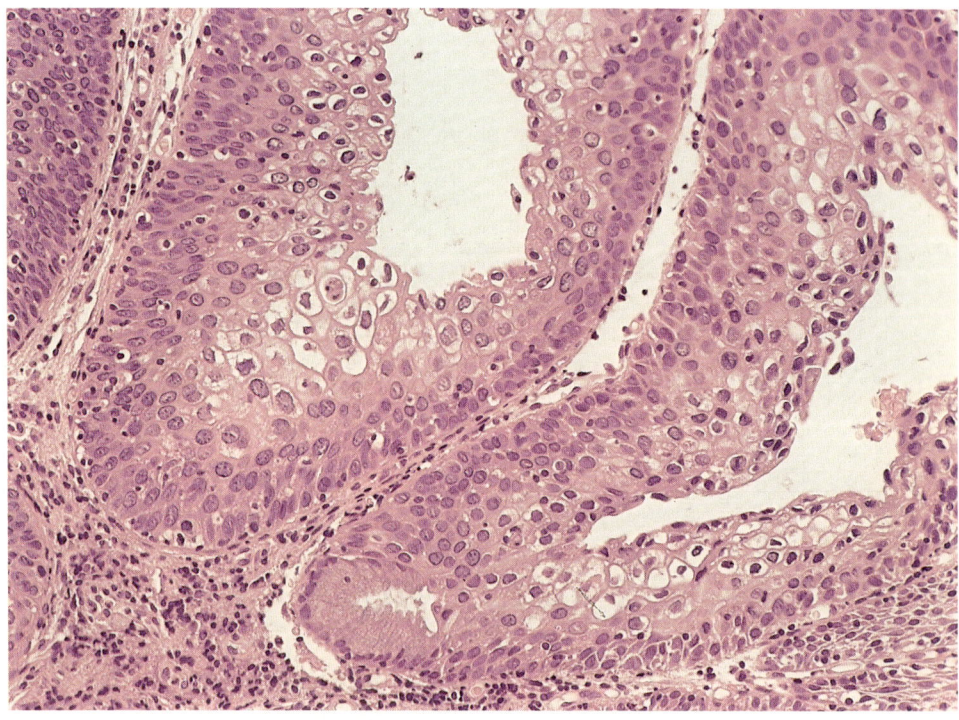

Fig. 110. Moderate koilocytic dysplasia, reserve cell type, in endocervical glands. H & E

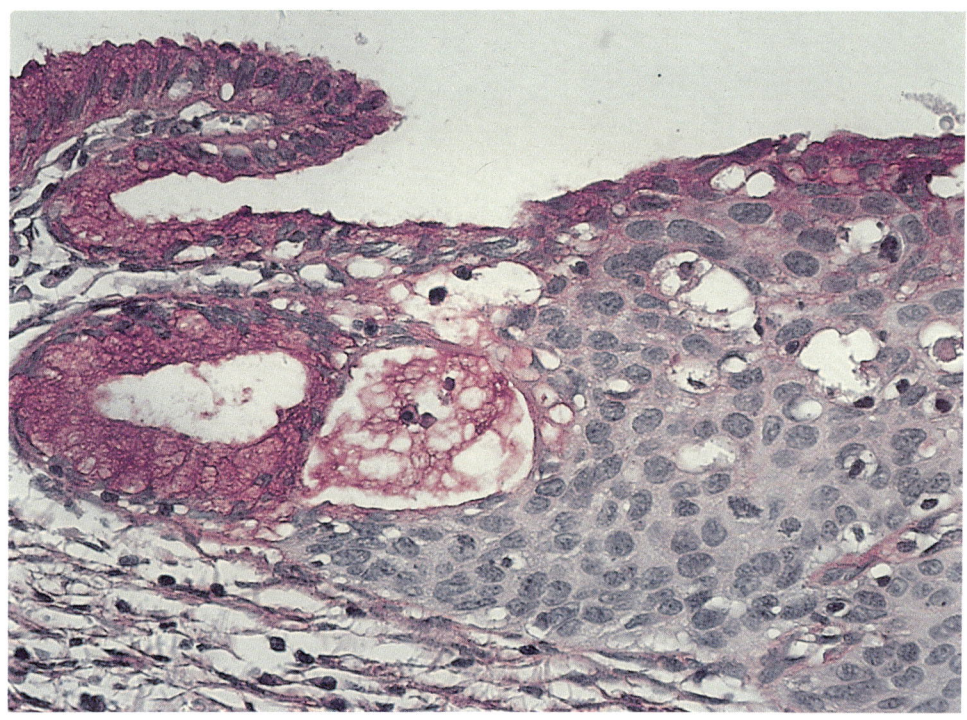

Fig. 111. Mucoid dysplasia, reserve cell type with monocellular mucin formation. PAS reaction

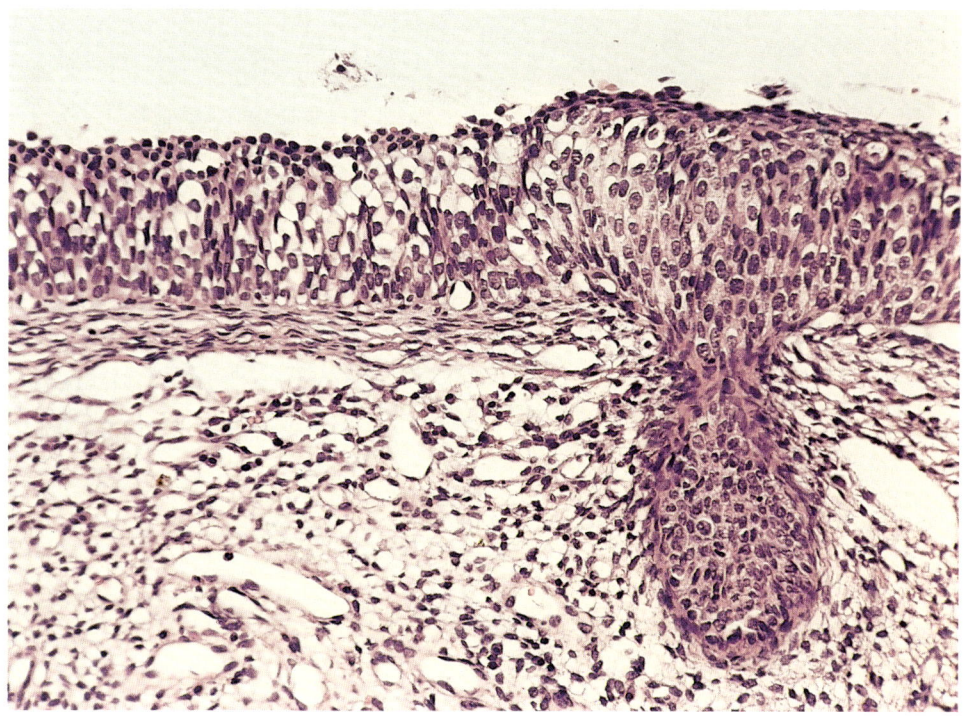

Fig. 112. Severe dysplasia, reserve cell type, with clear cell change and with protrusion towards stroma. H & E

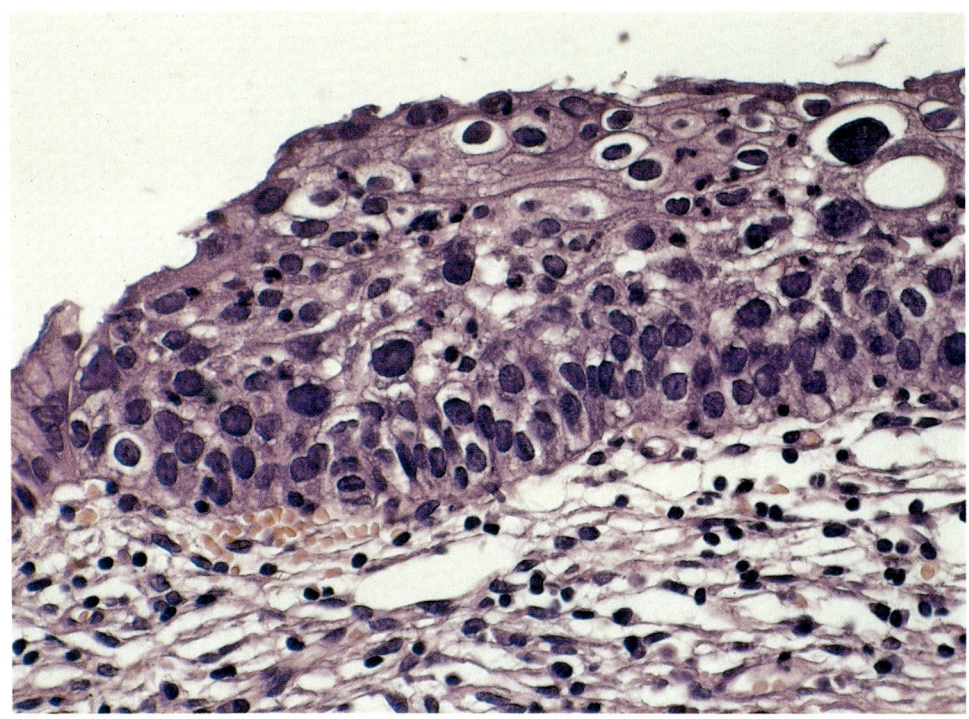

Fig. 113. Moderate dysplasia, reserve cell type, with koilocytes. H & E

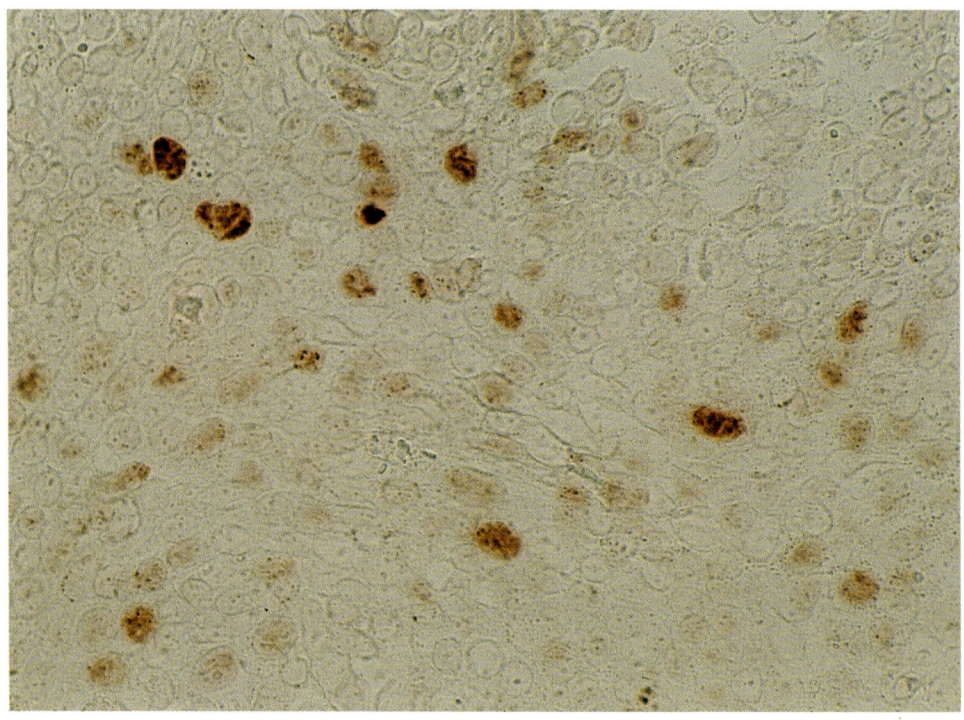

Fig. 114. Koilocytic dysplasia, reserve cell type. In situ hybridization with DNA probe for HPV 16 and 18

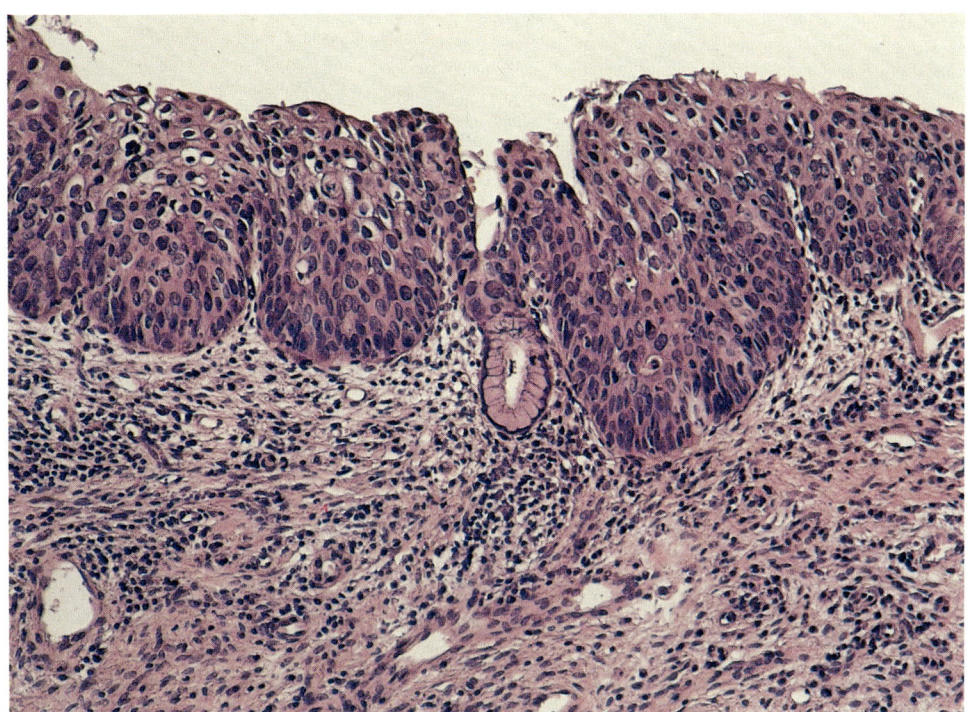

Fig. 115. Severe dysplasia, reserve cell type, almost complete loss of stratification. H & E

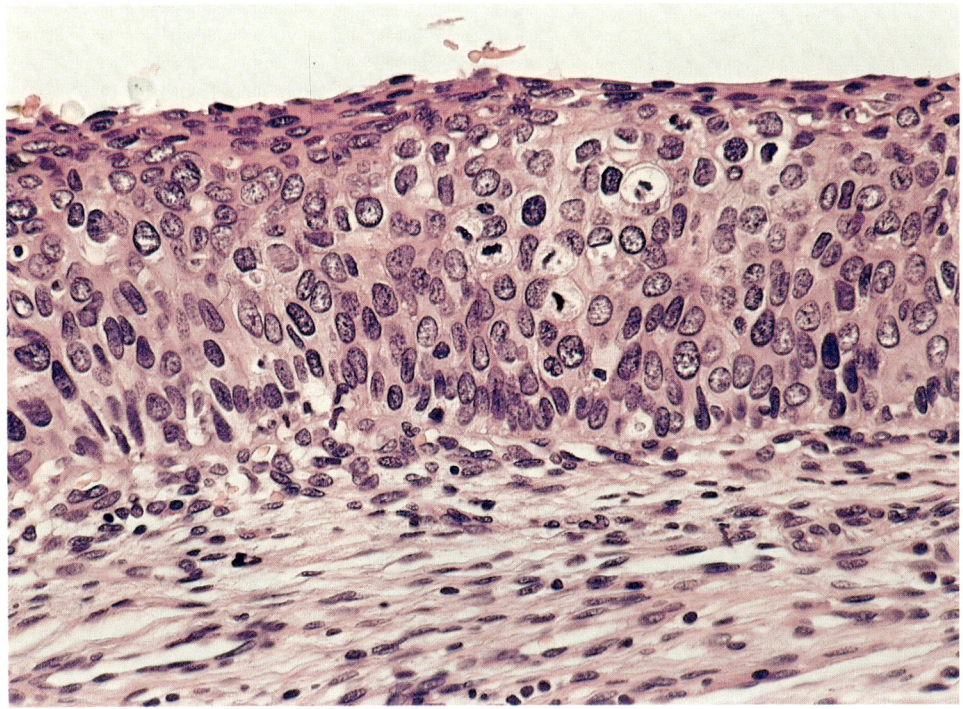

Fig. 116. Severe dysplasia, reserve cell type with frequent mitoses. H & E

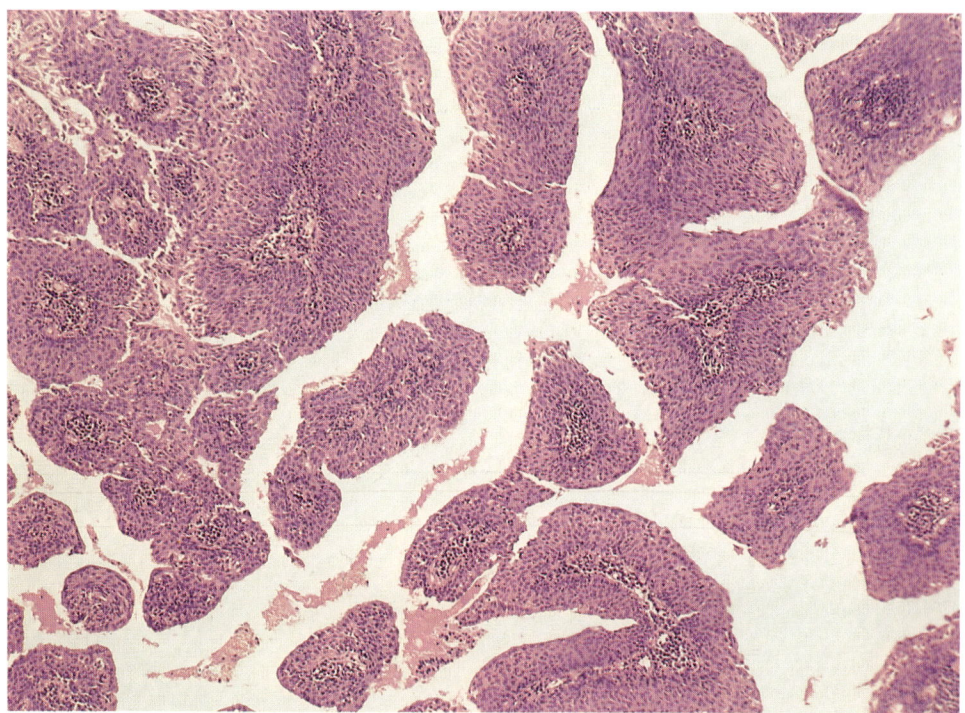

Fig. 117. Papillary type of reserve cell dysplasia. H & E

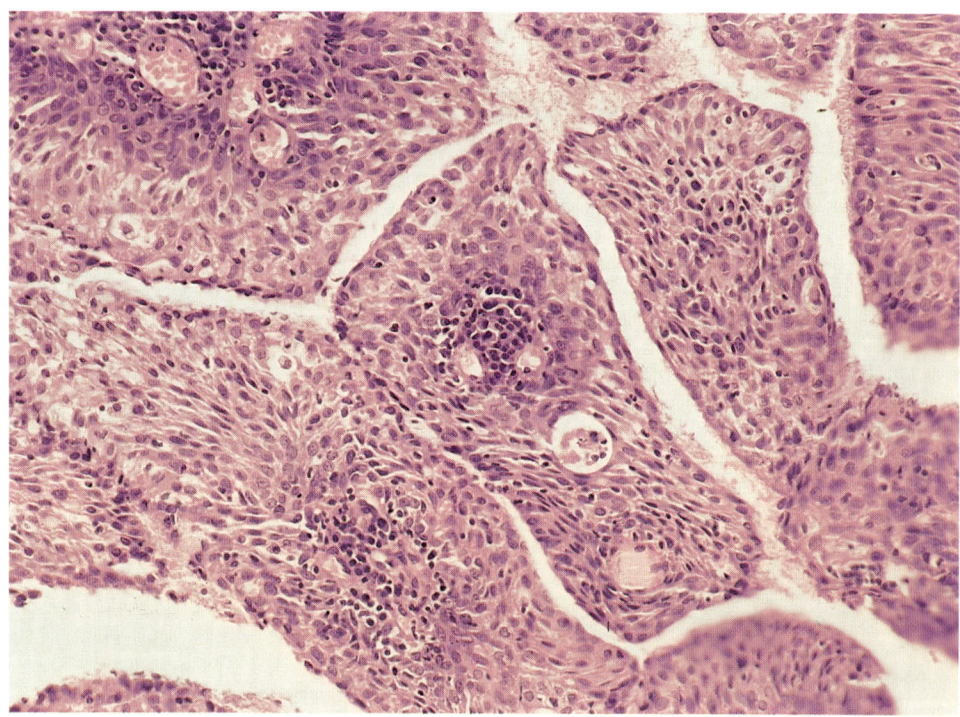

Fig. 118. Papillary type of reserve cell dysplasia. H & E, higher magnification

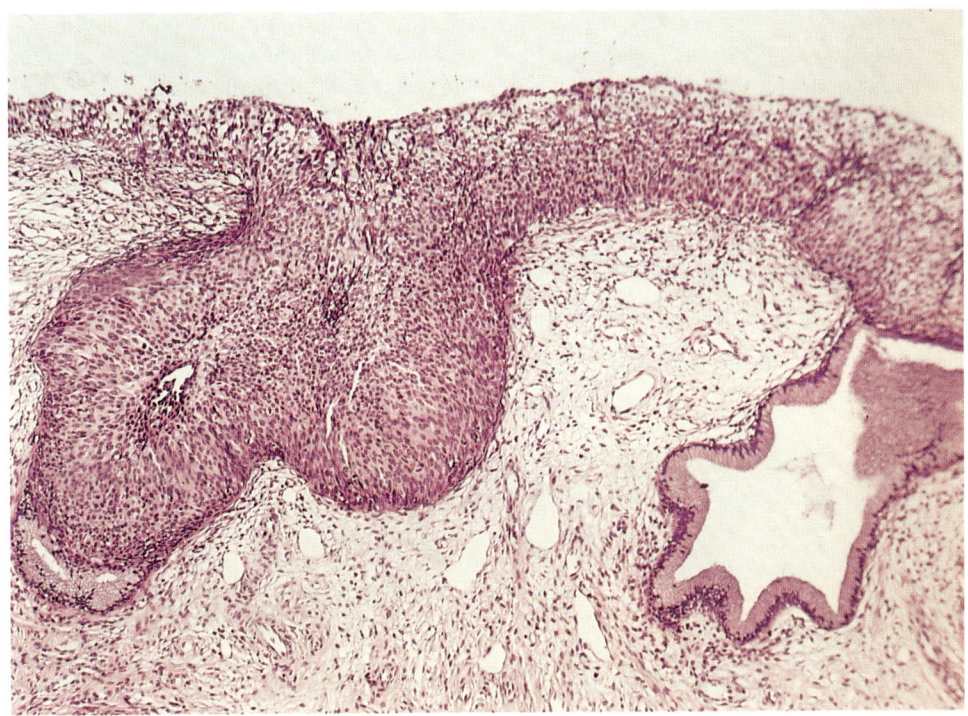

Fig. 119. Severe dysplasia, reserve cell type, with transition to carcinoma in situ. H & E

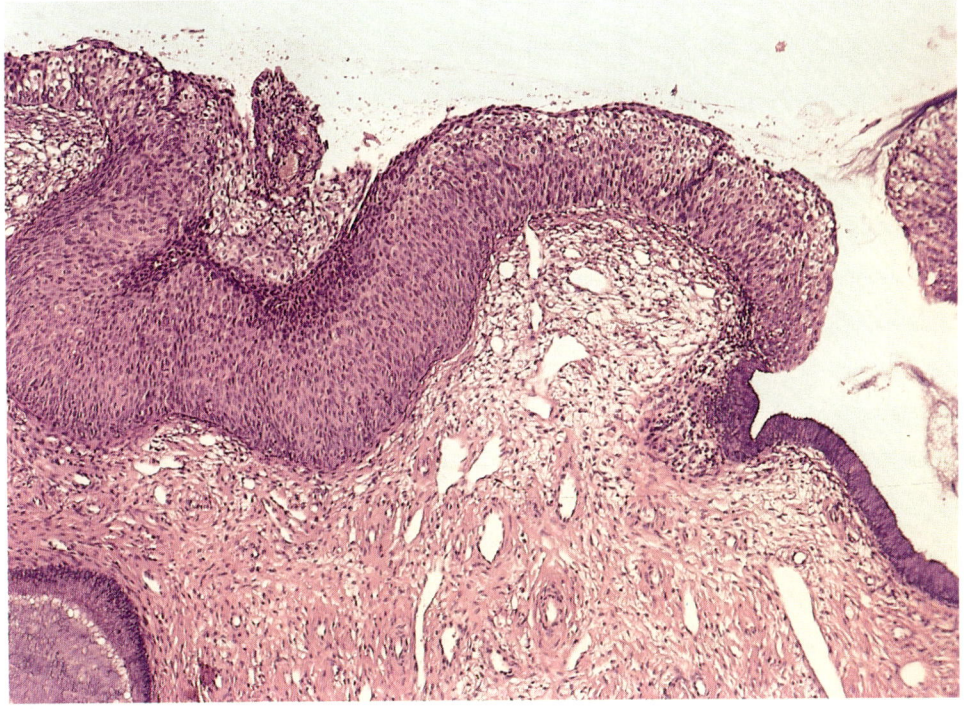

Fig. 120. Severe dysplasia, reserve cell type, with transition to carcinoma in situ. H & E

The *carcinoma in situ of reserve cell type* (Figs. 121–127) also presents a complete loss of stratification with densely arranged atypical nuclei. These are generally elongated and usually smaller than those of the squamous type. Atypical mitotic figures such as three-group metaphases are frequently observed (Fig. 124). Koilocytes are not seen, because no mature cells are present in the upper layers. The very sparse cytoplasm of the tumor cells may show incomplete differentiation in some areas, forming either keratin or mucin or clearing (Fig. 125). In contrast to that of the squamous type, carcinoma in situ of the reserve cell type often grows into glands, and in the noninvasive stage may even spread out over large areas of the endocervical mucosa (Fig. 126).

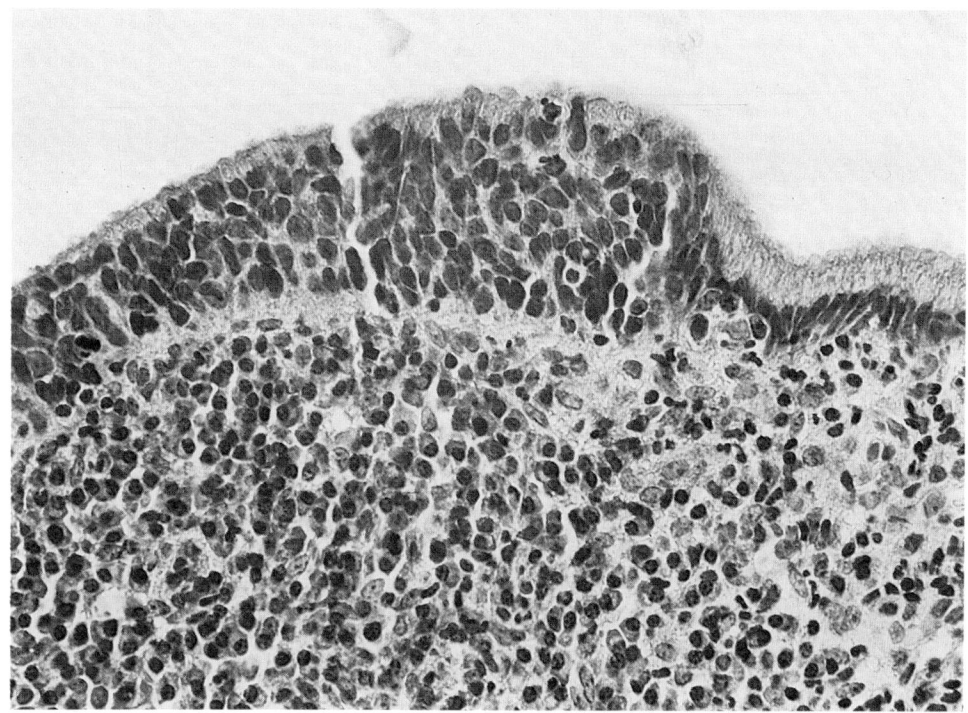

Fig. 121. Carcinoma in situ, reserve cell type, early change. H & E

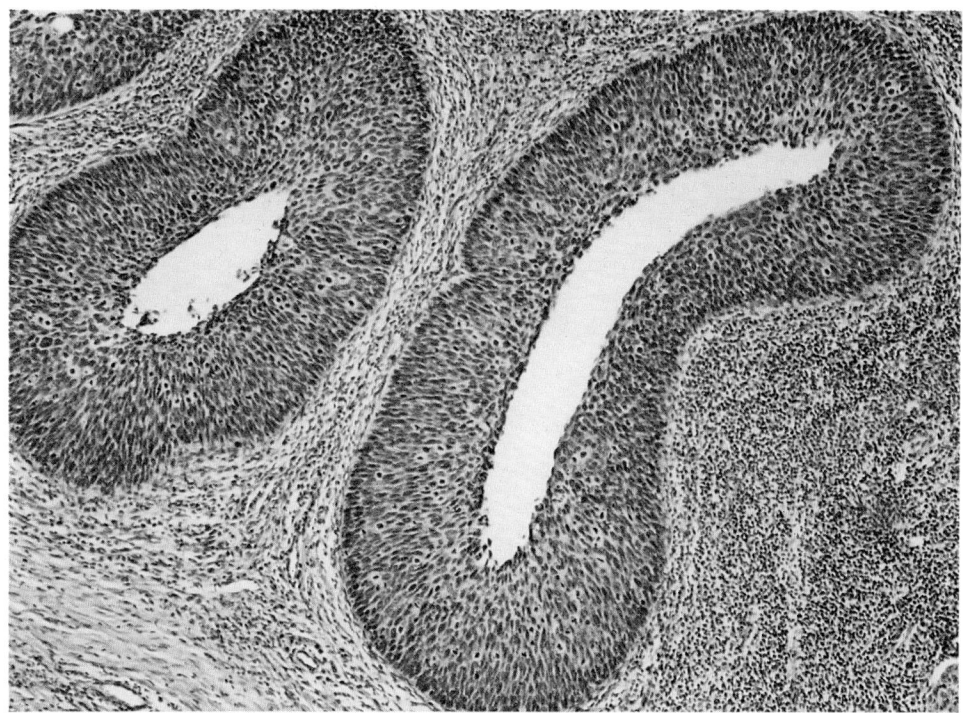

Fig. 122. Carcinoma in situ, reserve cell type, intraglandular spread. H & E

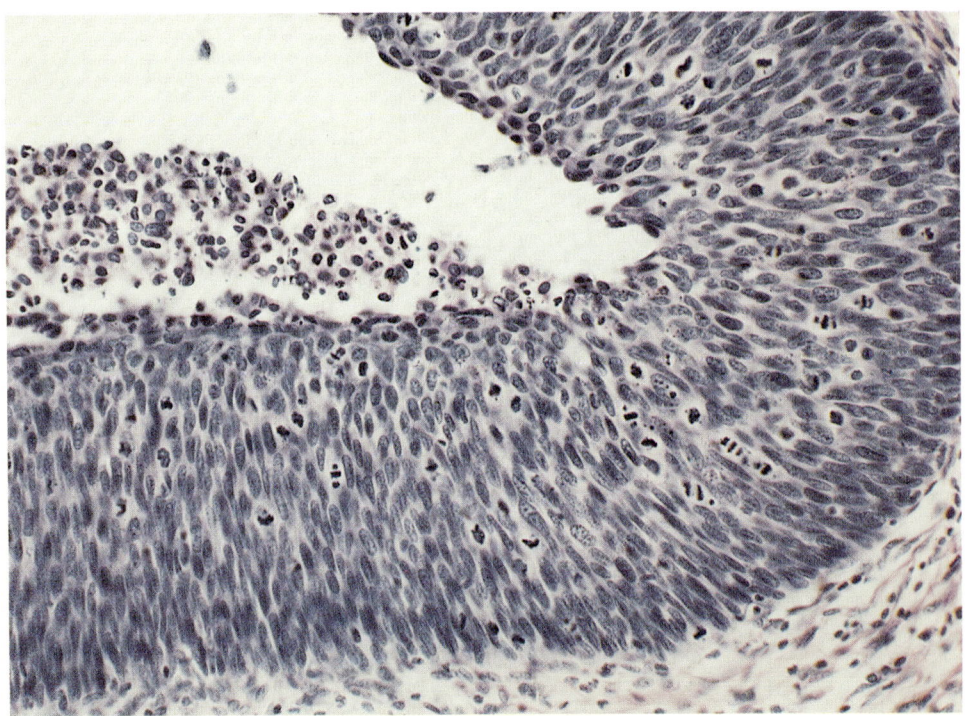

Fig. 123. Carcinoma in situ, reserve cell type, higher magnification. H & E

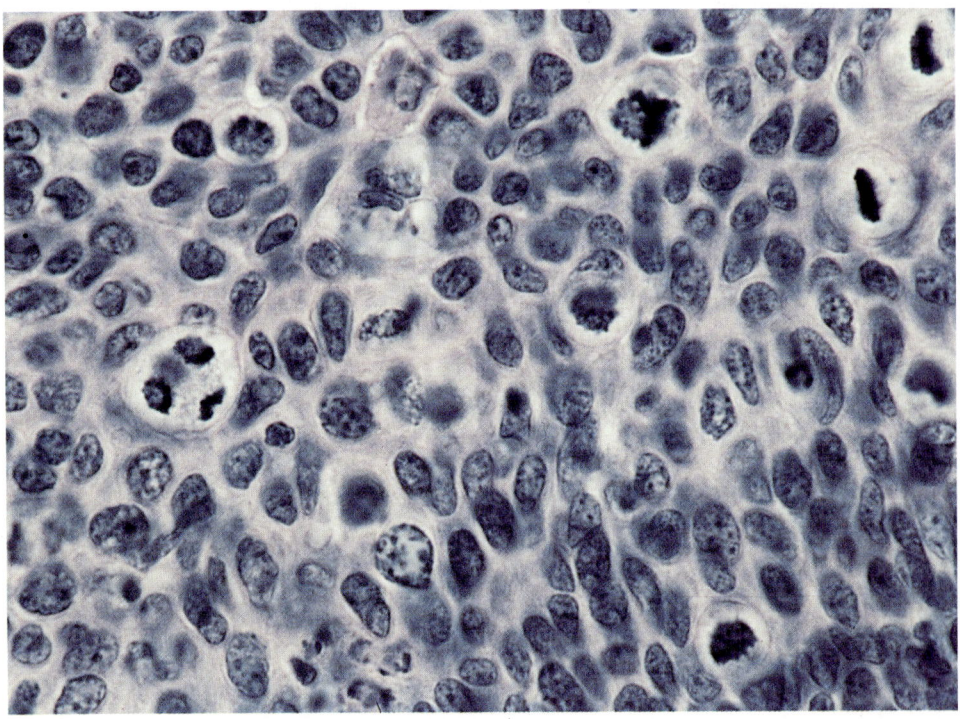

Fig. 124. Carcinoma in situ, reserve cell type, three group metaphases. H & E

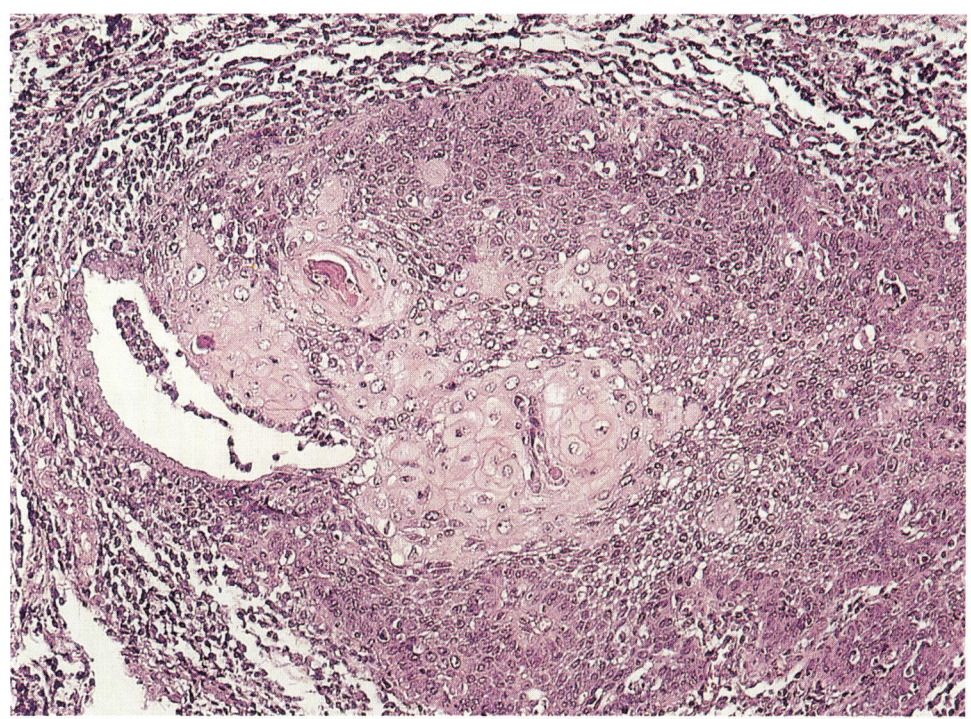

Fig. 125. Carcinoma in situ, reserve cell type, with metaplastic squamous differentiation. H & E

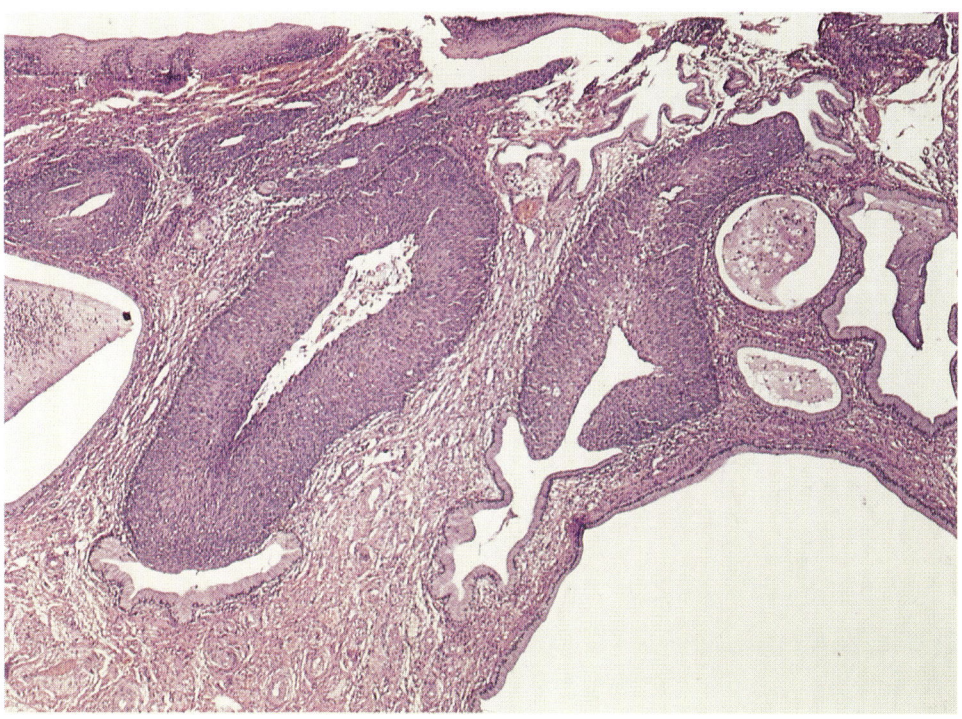

Fig. 126. Carcinoma in situ, reserve cell type, intraglandular spread with deep extension. H & E

Differental Diagnosis. The two types of carcinoma in situ can be distinguished in most cases by their topographical localization and spread (pattern of growth), and by the variation in their nuclear structure, as pointed out above. In rare instances, both types of carcinoma in situ develop simultaneously in neighboring areas. There are, however, intermediate lesions in which it is difficult to make a distinction. In those instances immunohistochemistry will be of considerable help, since both types have different compositions of intermediate filaments in their cytoplasm: the carcinoma in situ of the squamous cell type reacts positively with anticytokeratin 13 (Fig. 106), but negatively with anticytokeratin 8 and 18 and with anti-CEA. The carcinoma in situ of the reserve cell type, on the contrary, shows a coexpression of cytokeratin13, 8 and 18 and is also positive with anti-CEA (Fig. 127). The distinction between the two is clinically important, since the reserve cell type, which is the type most frequently observed in young women, is found in approximately 90% of the cases associated with HPV 16 (50%), HPV 18 (20%), or other subtypes (20%), whereas in the squamous cell type HPV tests are almost consistently negative. These differences are best explained by the fact that the cancerogenic virus subtypes 16 and 18 almost exclusively infect the stimulated vulnerable reserve cells, whereas squamous epithelia seem to be resistant to these viruses and more susceptible to virus types 6 and 11. Because the carcinomas in situ initiated by HPV 16 or 18 progress more rapidly and frequently recur later in the infected mucosa around the primary tumor, despite its complete removal by conization, they must be identified and differentiated from the carcinomas in situ not associated with HPV during all stages of development. Such recurrences are explained by the fact that normal epithelium around the carcinoma in situ may already be infected by HPV at the time of conization (Colgan et al. 1989). The differentiation is best achieved by histological appearance, immunohistochemistry, or in situ hybridization.

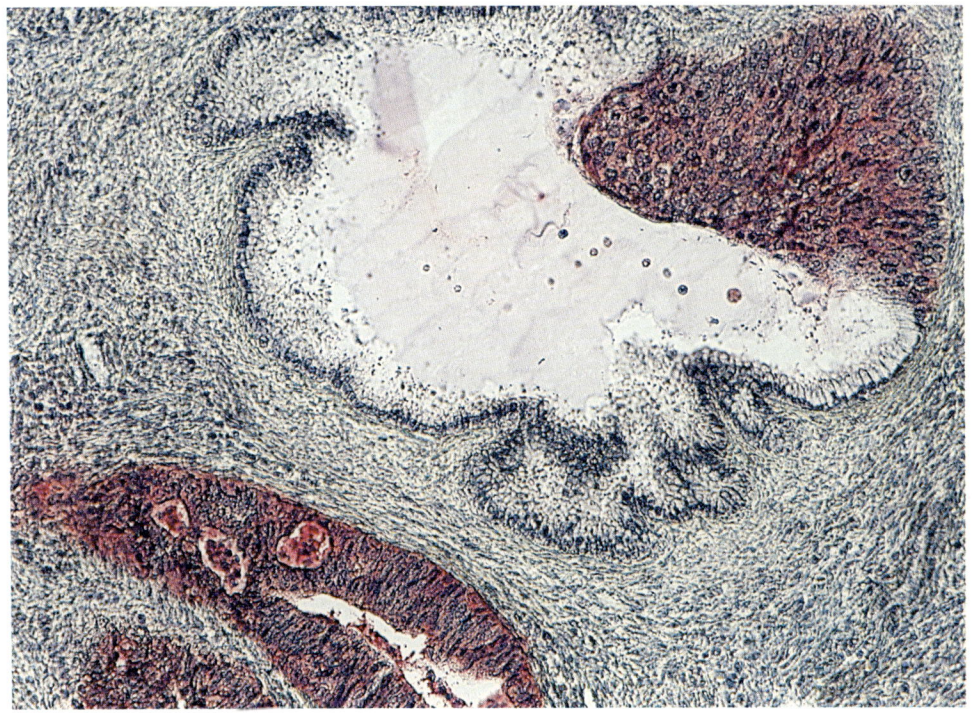

Fig. 127. Carcinoma in situ, reserve cell type. Positive immunohistochemical reaction with anti-CEA *(upper right corner)* and with coexisting adenocarcinoma in situ *(lower left corner)*

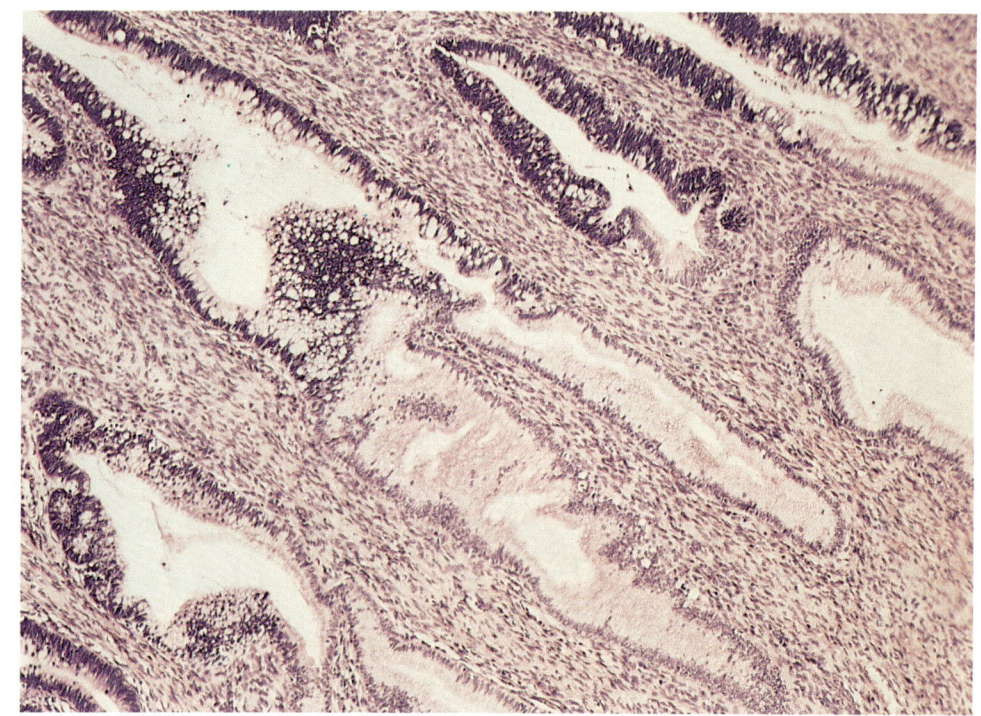

Fig. 128. Adenocarcinoma in situ, uniform type. H & E

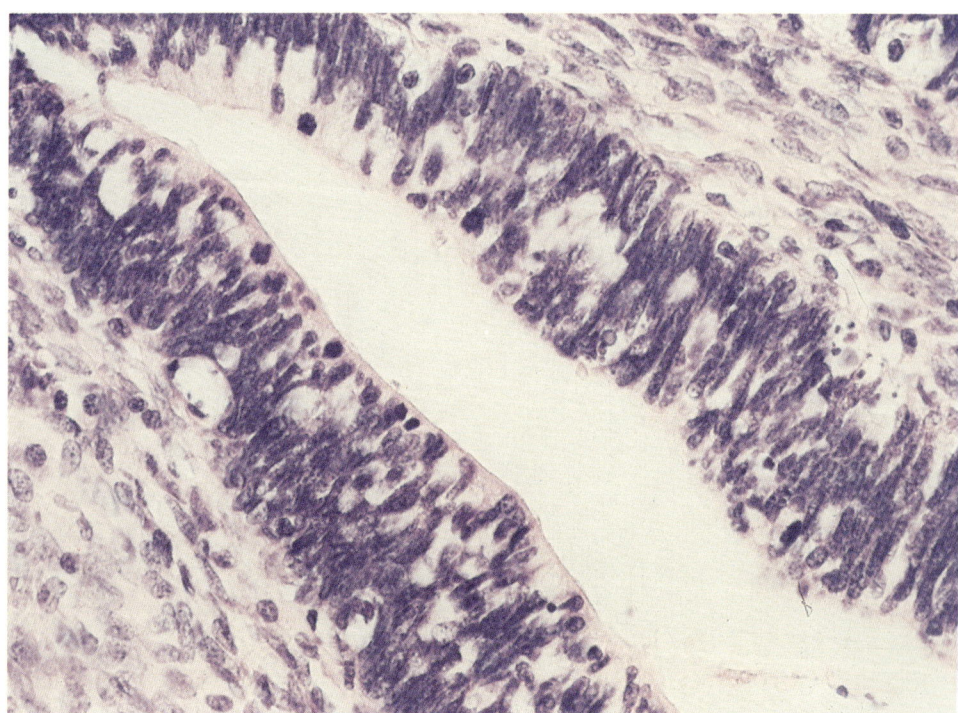

Fig. 129. Adenocarcinoma in situ, uniform type. H & E, higher magnification

Adenocarcinoma In Situ (Figs. 128–136)

In adenocarcinoma in situ the normal columnar epithelium of the endocervical glands may be replaced by two types of abnormal epithelial cells. In the first type, one sees a pseudostratified or even multilayered atypical glandular epithelium with enlarged, elongated, hyperchromatic nuclei surrounded by a sparse undifferentiated cytoplasm. Mitoses are frequent. Mucin formation is absent or minimal (uniform type of Gloor and Ruzicka 1982; Figs. 128, 129). The glandular lumina are preserved, but may show intraglandular budding or bridging (Fig. 130). This atypical change is usually focal and may be limited to only one part of the gland (Fig. 128). In the second type, seen less frequently, the glands may be lined by strikingly disorganized, irregular cells with enlarged depolarized, pleomorphic nuclei with disordered chromatin. The cytoplasm is clear, foamy, and PAS negative (pleomorphic type of Gloor and Ruzicka; Figs. 131, 132). These two types of adenocarcinoma in situ may replace smaller or larger portions of normal glandular epithelium of the endocervical mucosa. Occasionally, the surface epithelium of the endocervix may also be involved (Fig. 133).

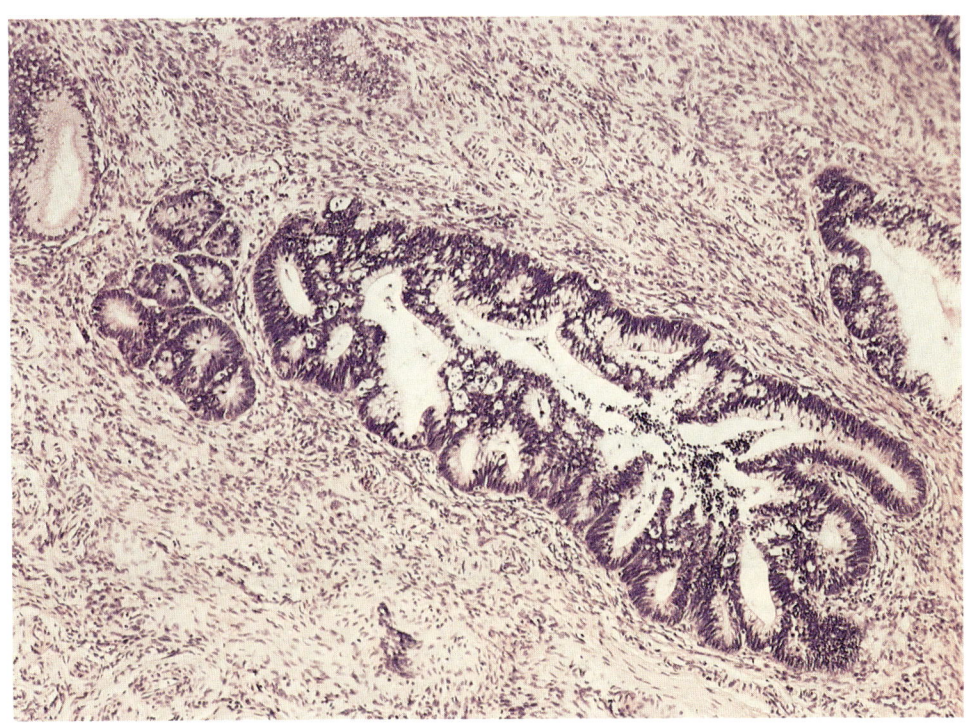

Fig. 130. Adenocarcinoma in situ, with intraglandular budding. H & E

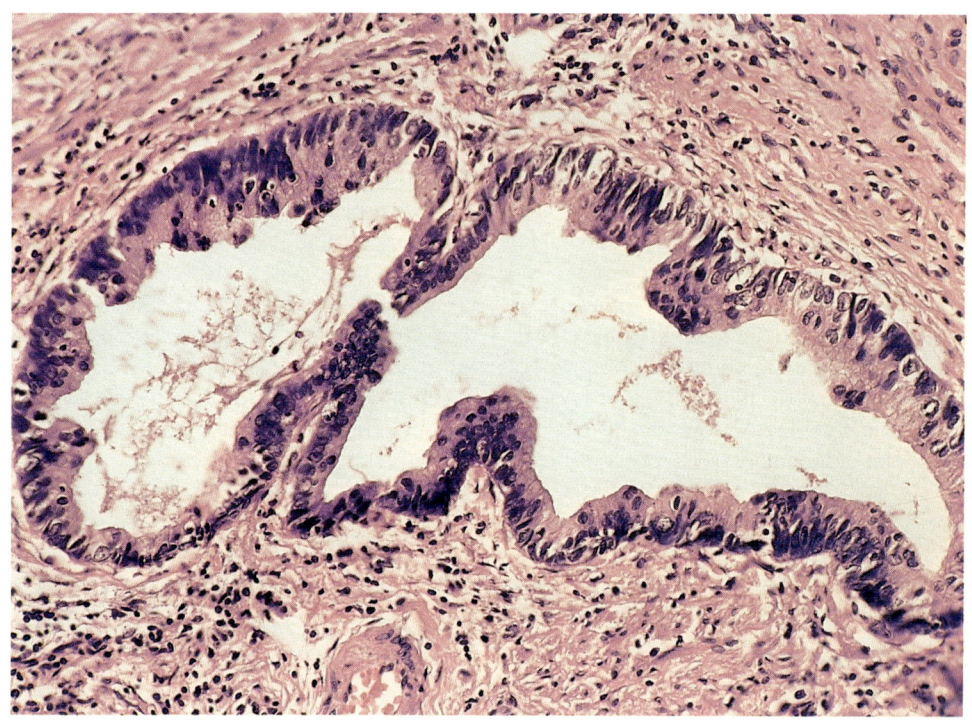

Fig. 131. Adenocarcinoma in situ, pleomorphic type. H & E

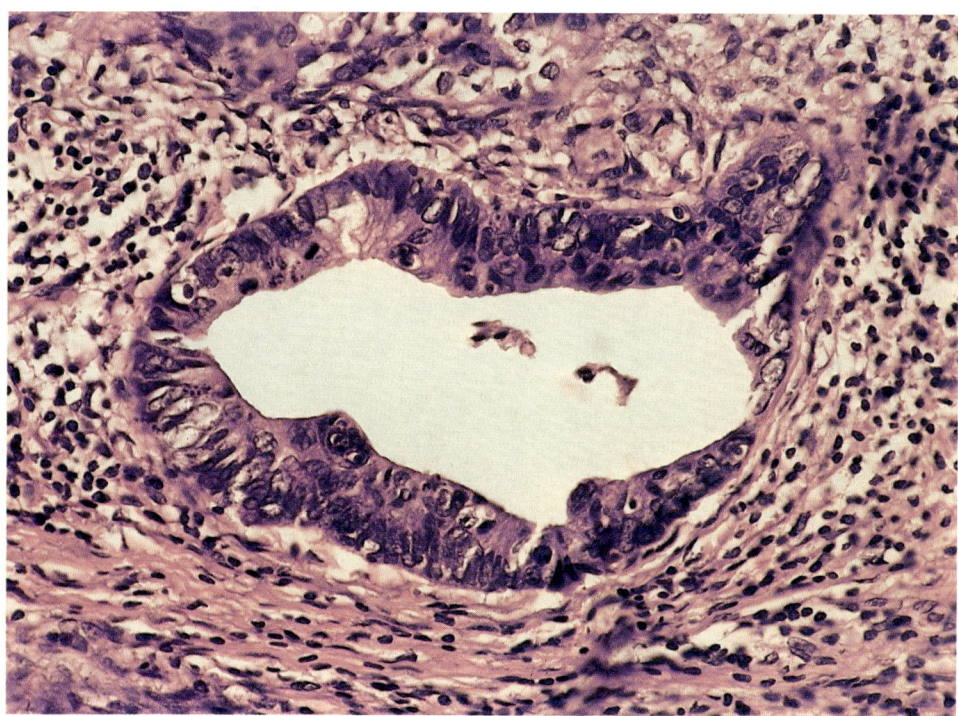

Fig. 132. Adenocarcinoma in situ, pleomorphic type. H & E

Adenocarcinoma in situ of the endocervix was once a rare lesion (Friedell and McKay 1953; Abell and Gosling 1962; Krimmenau 1966; Barter and Waters 1970; Sachs et al. 1975; Werner and Waidecker 1975), but has increased in frequency during past years (Jaworski et al. 1988). Since only a few glands may be affected and be focally distributed, they may be overlooked unless serial sections of a cone biopsy are examined. If the lesion is overlooked and incompletely excised, it will progress to invasive adenocarcinoma (Boon et al. 1981; Wells and Brown 1986). Since both glandular and squamous cells of the endocervix may originate from the subcolumnar reserve cell (Alva and Lauchlan 1975; Christopherson et al. 1979), their precancerous and neoplastic changes are often closely related. Consequently, they often show an identical or a very similar expression of intermediate filaments (Fig. 127). When dealing with a dysplasia or carcinoma in situ of the endocervix, it is essential to carefully search for a coexistent adenocarcinoma in situ.

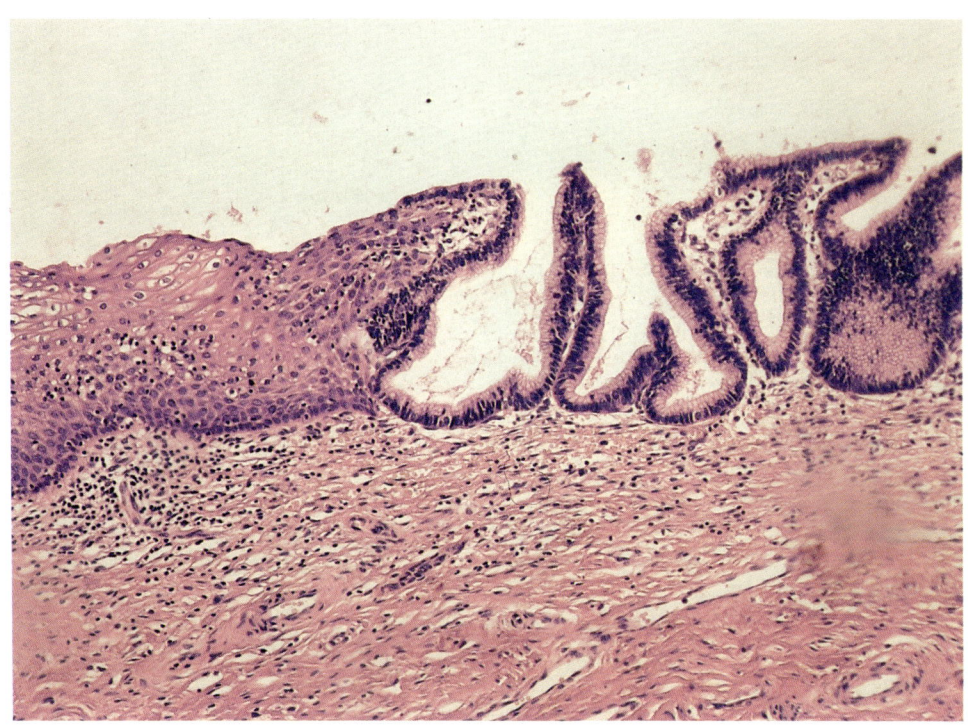

Fig. 133. Adenocarcinoma in situ, involving the surface epithelium. H & E

Differential Diagnosis. Adenocarcinoma in situ can be distinguished from adenomatous and microglandular hyperplasia of the endocervix immunohistochemically: in most cases adenocarcinoma in situ reacts positively with anti-CEA (Figs. 134, 135), whereas adenomatous and microglandular hyperplasias react negatively (compare also Hurlimann and Gloor 1984). Distinction from invasive adenocarcinoma is not possible from a small biopsy, but rather requires examination of larger areas of the endocervical mucosa. In contrast to invasive carcinoma, adenocarcinoma in situ is limited to the glands; a stromal response is lacking, and normal glands are constantly admixed with neoplastic glands (Östör et al. 1984).

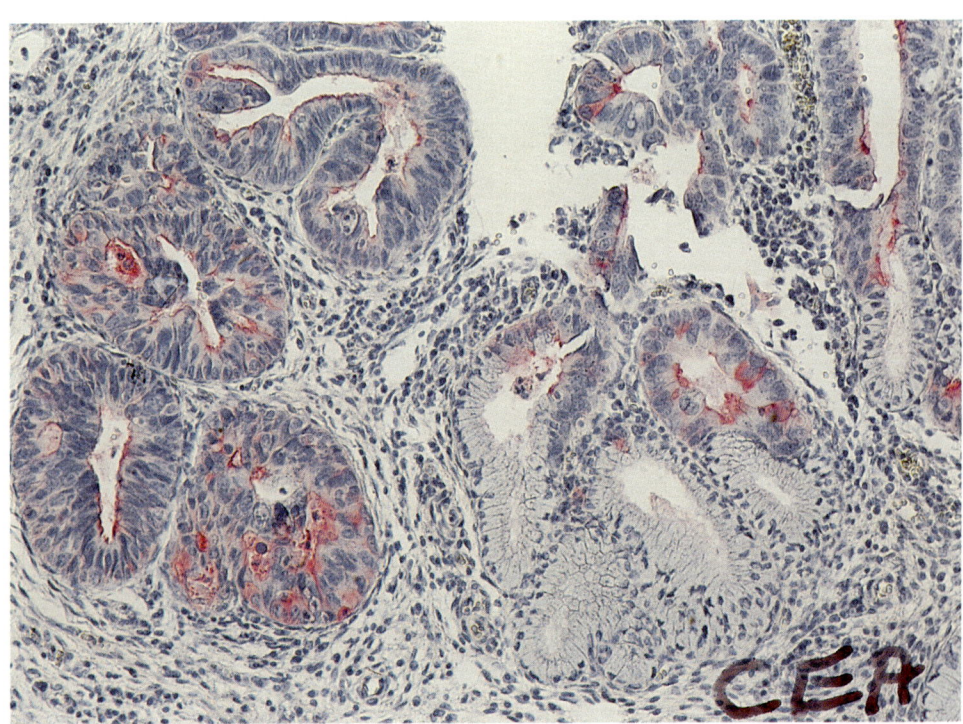

Fig. 134. Adenocarcinoma in situ, positive reaction with anti-CEA (normal glands react negatively)

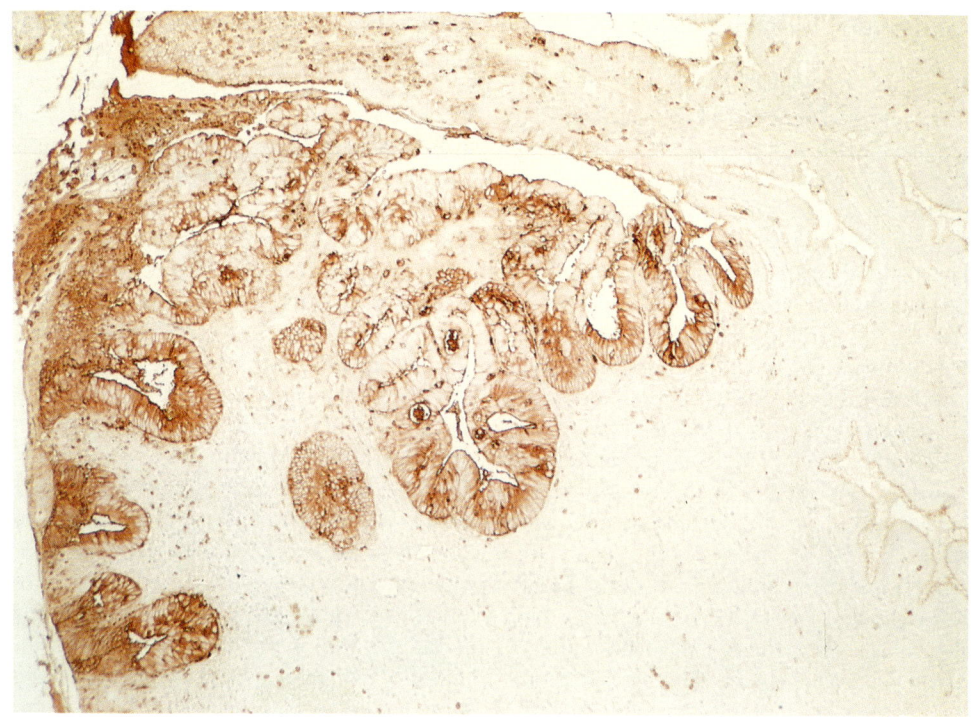

Fig. 135. Adenocarcinoma in situ, positive reaction with anti-CEA

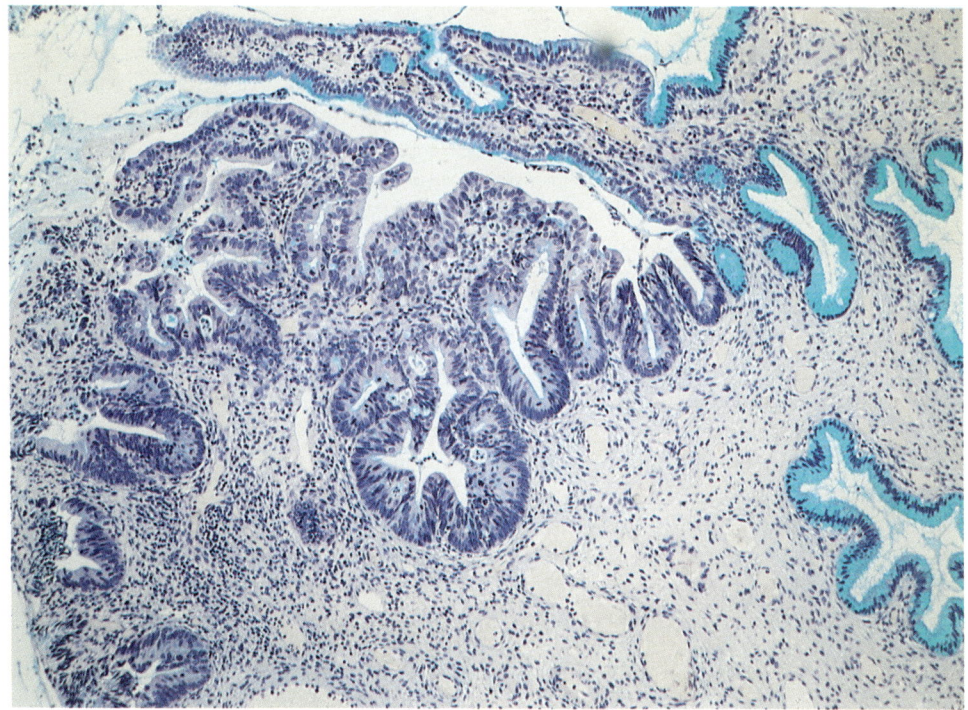

Fig. 136. Adenocarcinoma in situ, negative reaction with alcian blue (normal glands react positively)

Biological Behavior

The biological behavior of dysplasia and carcinoma in situ has been studied for several decades. Previous follow-up studies and epidemiological investigations have indicated that early lesions, as mild dysplasia, gradually evolved through increasing degrees of dysplasia to carcinoma in situ. Follow-up studies by cytology and colpomicroscopy have shown that patients with mild dysplasia developed severe dysplasia/carcinoma in situ in about 50% of cases after 9 years (Nasiell et al. 1983). The rate of progression, however, increased with the severity of the lesion, and the evolution time became shorter.

If left untreated, carcinoma in situ is known to progress to invasive carcinoma in a high percentage of patients (30%-70%) after a number of years. In an unpublished paper, based on a revision of Petersen's material (1955) of multiple biopsies, patients with carcinoma in situ of the cervix had a 34% risk of developing invasive carcinoma after 10 years and a 47% risk after 20 years (J. Clemmesen, H. W. Nielsen and H. Poulsen, in preparation). A few patients had unchanged carcinoma in situ for more than 25 years.

Further recent studies, however, indicate that the pathological behavior of cervical cancer in young women has dramatically changed, suggesting that the disease is becoming more severe (Elliot at al. 1989). Those differences in behavior may be in part explained by geographic variations. In this context, it must be emphasized how important it is to separate the rapidly progressing type of severe dysplasia and carcinoma in situ (HPV 16 or 18) from the more benign (p. 78). In a study by Syrjänen (1979), all of the precancerous cervical lesions in young girls below the age of 21, and 86.8% of those in women under the age of 41 were of the koilocytic (HPV-induced) type. These findings support the conclusion that the carcinogenic progression is more rapid in subtype 16 and 18 HPV-infected lesions than in those of other causes.

In addition, in their studies of cervical neoplasia developing in women in the United States and Brazil, Kurman et al. (1988) showed that, when they analyzed HPV types 16 and 18 separately, they found a highly significant correlation between the type of papilloma virus and the histologic grade of neoplasia. Since HPV 18 was rarely detected in preinvasive tumors (3%) but often in invasive carcinomas (22%) - as compared with HPV 16 found in 37% of preinvasive and in 41% of invasive carcinomas - they suggested that the HPV type 18 might initiate a rapidly progressive carcinoma of the cervix, the evolution of which would escape detection by the usual routine of cytological screening. Accordingly, the mean age of patients with invasive carcinoma associated with HPV 16 was 49 years, as contrasted with 37 years for patients with invasive carcinoma associated with HPV 18. Similar observations were made by Walker at al. (1989), who observed rapid recurrences in 45% of patients with carcinomas containing HPV 18 compared with 16% of patients with HPV 16 associated tumors. Even after treatment with conization or hysterectomy, patients with carcinoma in situ of the cervix have an increased risk of developing invasive carcinoma. In their large patient collective followed from 5 to 25 years, Mc Indoe et al. (1984) found that 22% with recurrent abnormal cytology developed carcinoma of the cervix or vaginal vault, and even among patients with normal cytology during the first 2 years after surgery, carcinoma arose later in 1.5%.

The behavior of dysplasia and carcinoma in situ can now be predicted with a high degree of accuracy for the individual patient. It is therefore of paramount importance to pursue appropriate precautions to prevent an invasive carcinoma from evolving once the diagnosis of a preinvasive lesion is made.

Malignant Tumors

Epithelial Tumors

Squamous and Reserve Cell Types
(Figs. 137–163)

Microinvasive Carcinoma (Figs. 137–144)
A microinvasive carcinoma (MIC; FIGO stage I a) was originally defined as an early invasive carcinoma that could not be detected grossly, only histologically (Mestwerdt 1947). Attempts to define its maximal size in millimeters in order to distinguish it from frank invasive carcinoma resulted in controversial opinions (Ferenczy and Winkler 1987). Since microinvasion often develops from precancerous epithelium located on the surface, as well as from that located in the glands, measurements cannot be made from the mucosal surface, but instead must be made from the intact basal membrane of the dysplastic epithelium bordering the carcinoma. According to the 1985 modification of FIGO staging, a MIC was defined as a carcinomatous invasion not exceeding 5 mm in depth and 7 mm in horizontal spread. Despite these strictures, the clinical outcome of patients with MIC was found to vary considerably, depending upon the variations in depth of stromal invasion, and upon the presence or absence of vascular invasion. To date it is widely accepted that a microinvasive squamous carcinoma is a lesion that invades no greater than 3 mm (as measured from the basement membrane of its point of origin) and does not show vascular invasion (Tsukamoto et al. 1989). According to several large clinical studies (cited by Ferenczy and Winkler 1987), when these criteria for MIC are applied, the rate of recurrence or of pelvic node metastases is less than 1%.

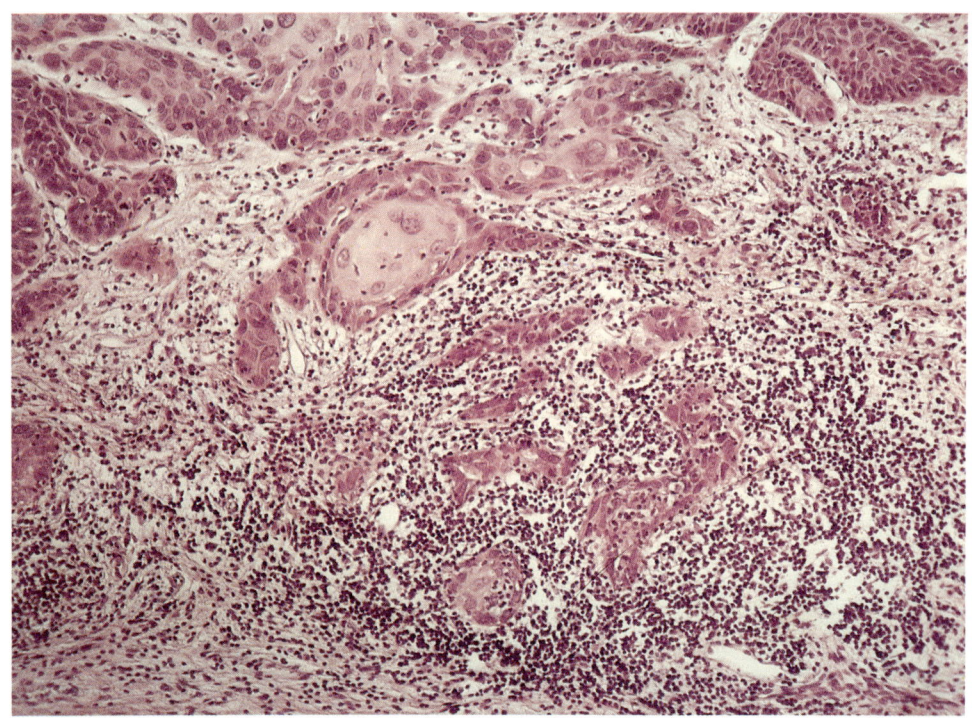

Fig. 137. Microinvasive carcinoma, netlike infiltration. H & E

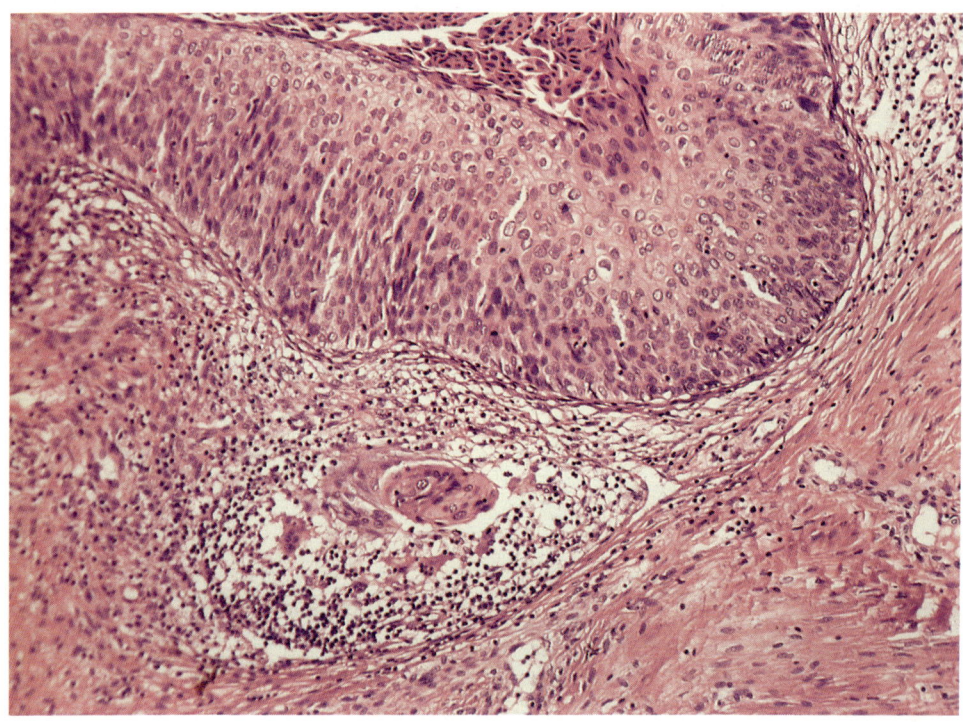

Fig. 138. Microinvasive carcinoma, netlike spread of individual cells. H & E

The type of stromal invasion of the carcinoma depends upon the type of cell from which it arises: MIC developing from dysplasias and carcinoma in situ of squamous cell type generally show an early branching invasion, whereby tumor cells separate, ramify, and form slender cords that penetrate between the stroma cells (Figs. 137–139).

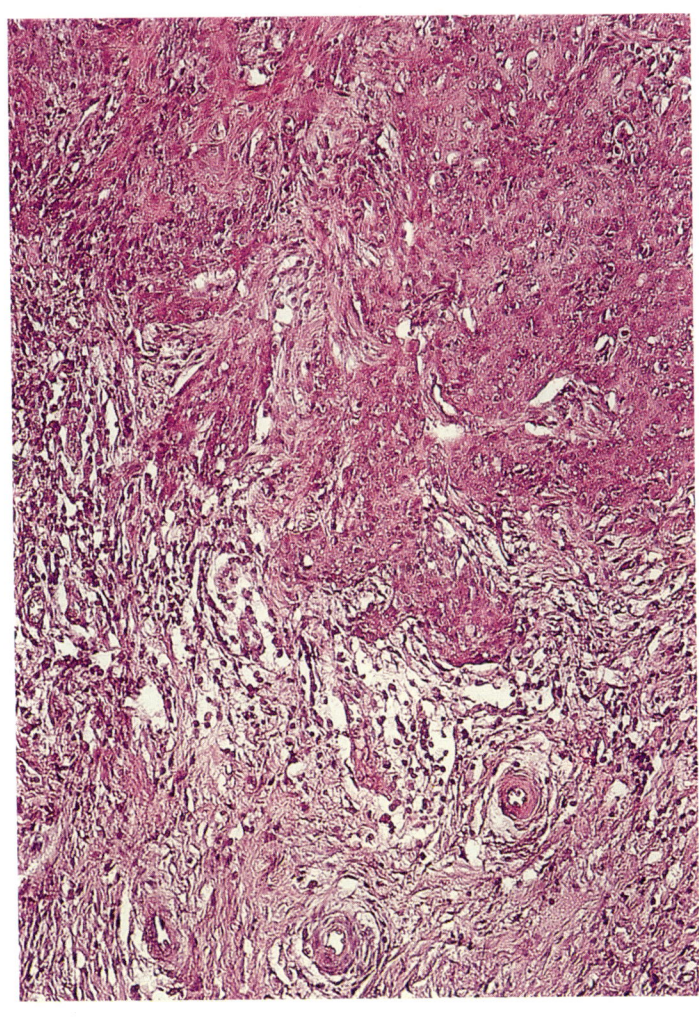

Fig. 139. Microinvasive carcinoma, netlike spread. H & E

In contrast, MIC developing from a carcinoma in situ of the reserve cell type grows as a plump bulky coherent infiltration, which bulges out from the confines of the endocervical glands, breaking through the basal membrane and pushing the surrounding stroma aside (Figs. 140–144). Both types of invasion show similar characteristic cellular changes at the site of early invasion: The nuclei become larger with prominent nucleoli, and the abundant eosinophilic cytoplasm may even start to keratinize. As a result, the invading carcinoma cells appear to be more differentiated than those of their noninvasive counter parts. In addition, the sites of microinvasion are often surrounded by dense lymphoplasmocytic infiltrates. Detection of lymphatic or vascular invasion is important for recognizing a more advanced stage of carcinoma (I b) and for differentiating it from a microinvasion. As one might expect from these differences in type of invasion, the reserve cell type carcinoma may extend over large areas of the cervix within an expanded field of endocervical glands, yet still be microinvasive (Fig. 143), whereas a carcinomatous invasion of the squamous cell type penetrating more than 3 mm in depth or invading vascular channels has to be classified as invasive carcinoma stage I b. In our expe-

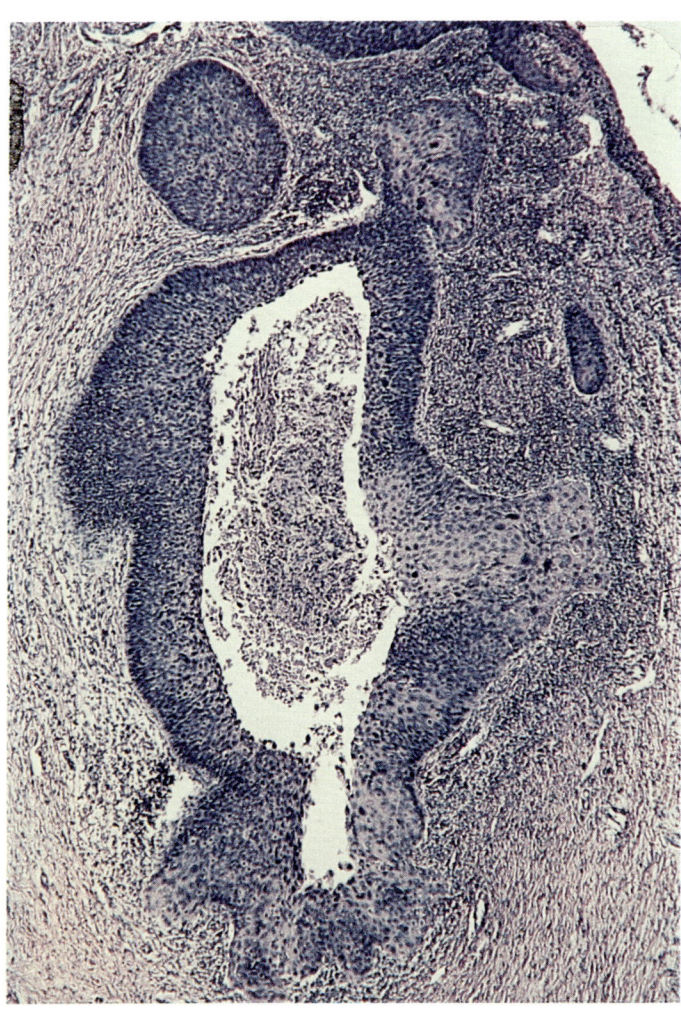

Fig. 140. Microinvasive carcinoma, plump infiltration. H & E

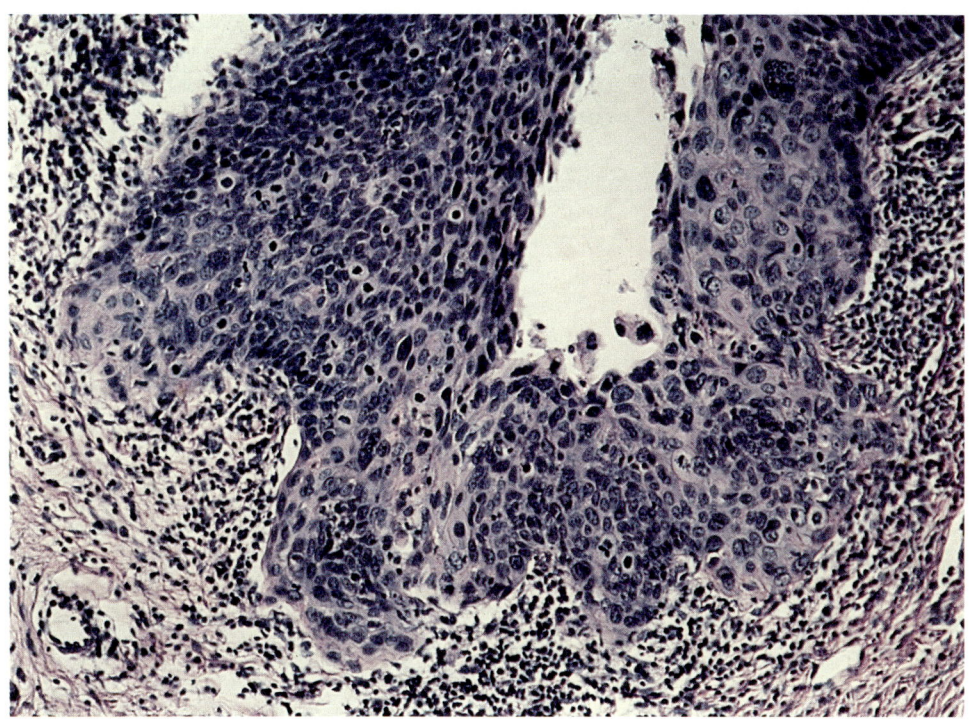

Fig. 141. Microinvasive carcinoma, plump infiltration. H & E

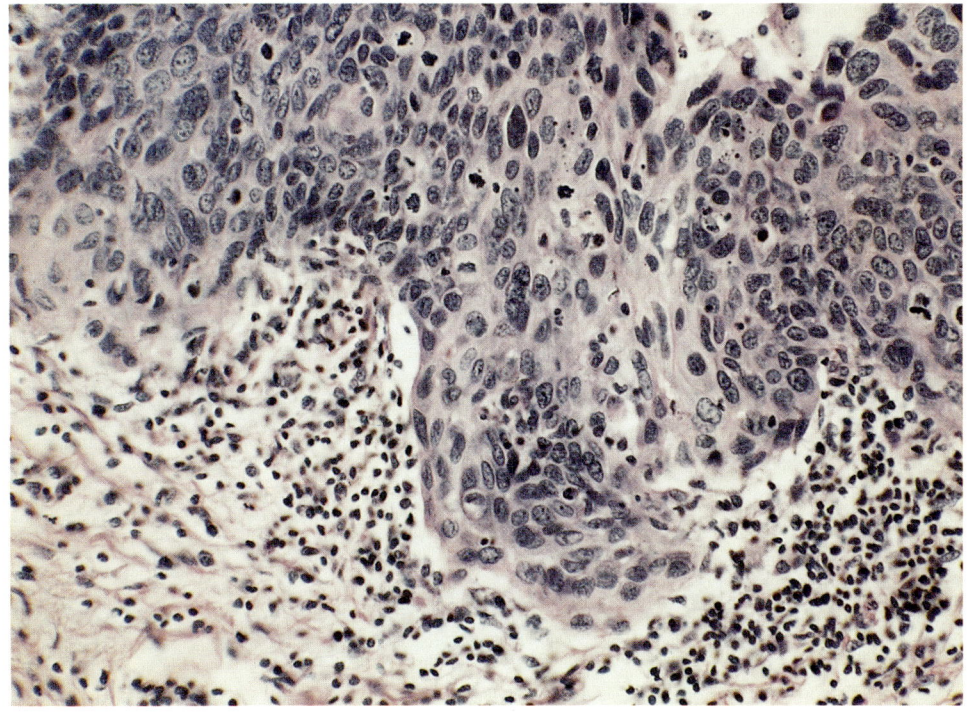

Fig. 142. Microinvasive carcinoma, plump infiltration. H & E, higher magnification

rience, this staging seems justified, since the netlike invasion of the squamous cell type often involves the lymphatic vessels early, whereas the bulky infiltration of reserve cell type spreads widely, but usually invades lymphatic vessels late. As our studies show, approximately 80% or even more of all invasive carcinomas are of the reserve cell type. This corresponds to the observation that up to 90% of all squamous cell carcinomas of the cervix start in the glandular area of the endocervix (Clement and Scully 1982).

Differential Diagnosis. It is of clinical importance to distinguish between the squamous and the reserve cell types because that distinction is important in deciding appropriate surgical therapy. If an MIC of the squamous cell type is found at the margins of a cervical cone, a Wertheim radical hysterectomy is recommended, since there is no guarantee that the carcinoma has not already invaded lymphatic channels or extended beyond the confines of the cone. On the other hand, a simple hysterectomy will almost always be sufficient for an MIC of the reserve cell type.

The two types of microinvasion can be distinguished histologically or immunohistochemically. As in the dysplasias preceding the carcinoma, the squamous cell type is positive with anticytokeratin 13 only; in contrast, the reserve cell type shows a coexpression of cytokeratin 13, 8, 18, and CEA.

Microinvasive carcinoma must be distinguished from invasive carcinoma stage I b by measuring the depth of invasion and by searching for vascular involvment, if the invasion is less than 3 mm. Differentiation from benign or preinvasive lesions is possible by noting whether the basal membrane is intact or not, as well as by noting an absence of stromal reaction or cellular maturation at the base of the atypical epithelium.

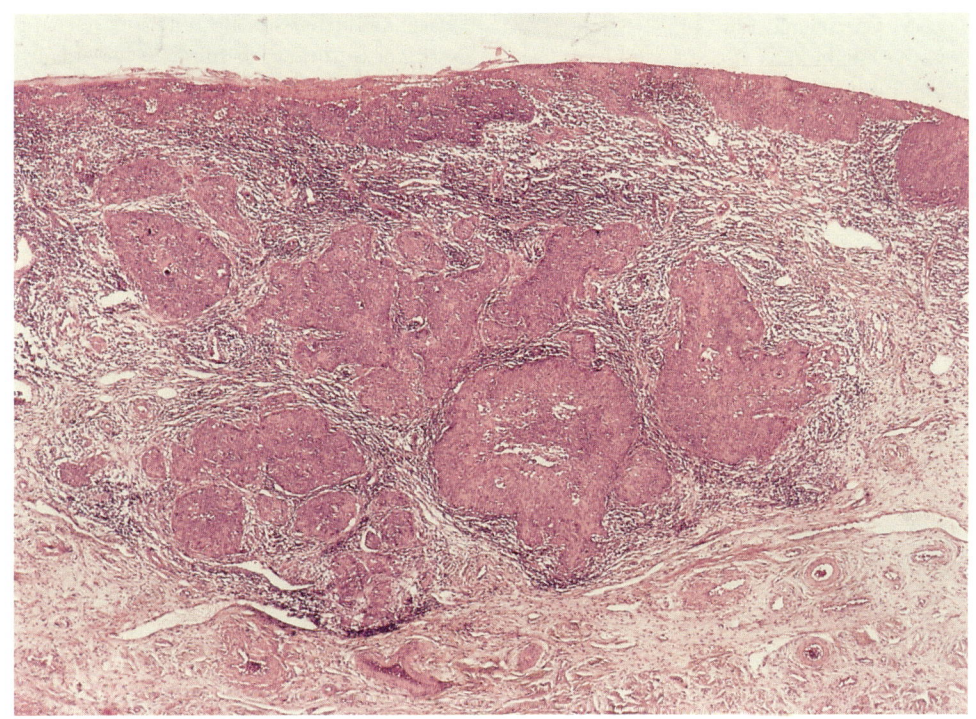

Fig. 143. Microinvasive carcinoma, extensive plump infiltration. H & E

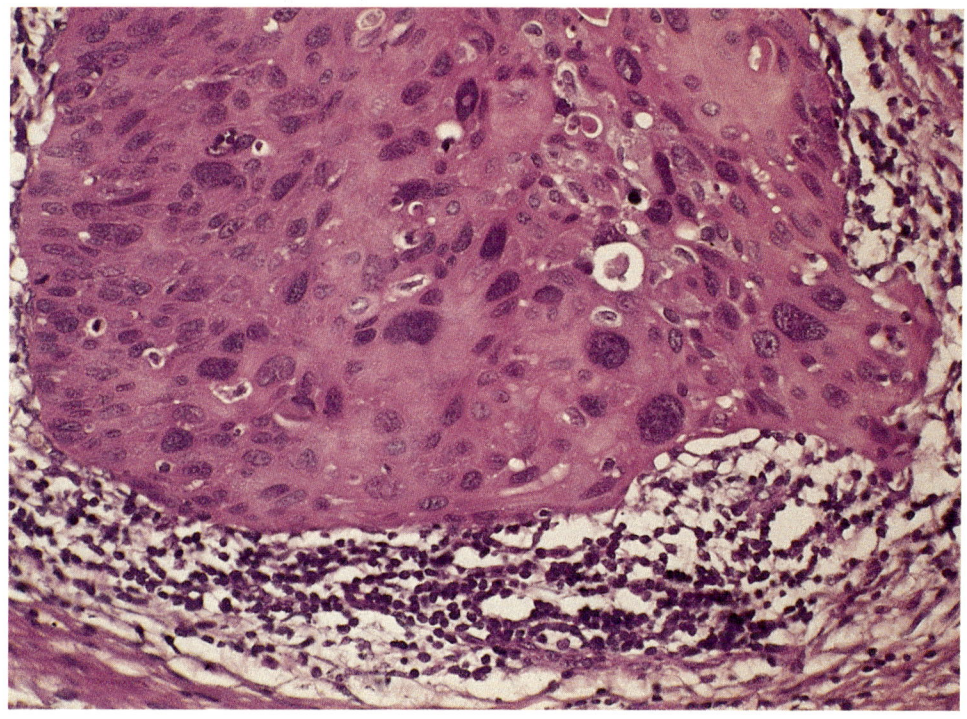

Fig. 144. Microinvasive carcinoma, plump infiltration. H & E, higher magnification

Invasive Carcinoma (Figs. 145–163)

Invasive carcinomas also show a broad spectrum, from microinvasion (up to 3 mm in depth) to clinically occult invasive carcinoma (measuring from 3 mm to more than 1 cm in depth (Boyes et al. 1970), and to grossly visible invasive carcinoma with endophytic or exophytic growth and spread throughout the cervical wall. As in the preinvasive stages, HPV DNA has also been detected in 89% of cervical squamous cell carcinomas (Gissmann 1984; Lorincz et al. 1987).

On histological examination three major types can be distinguished: small cell carcinoma, large cell nonkeratinizing carcinoma, and large cell keratinizing carcinoma. The *small cell carcinoma* (representing approximately 5%), as the least differentiated type, consists of diffusely infiltrating small or larger strands and nests of tumor cells with hyperchromatic oval nuclei in a sparse cytoplasm (Figs. 145–148). An intense stromal inflammatory reaction is characteristic (Fig. 146), and there is usually extensive lymphatic invasion (Fig. 148).

The *large cell nonkeratinizing carcinoma* (representing about 70%) is composed of broader cords of moderately differentiated tumor cells with large, often irregular nuclei. The cytoplasm varies in amount and differentiation (Figs. 149–154). Some of these carcinomas grow in rather uniform strands, whose spindle-shaped cells are vertically oriented towards the basal membrane resembling the preceding carcinoma in situ of reserve cell type (Fig. 153).

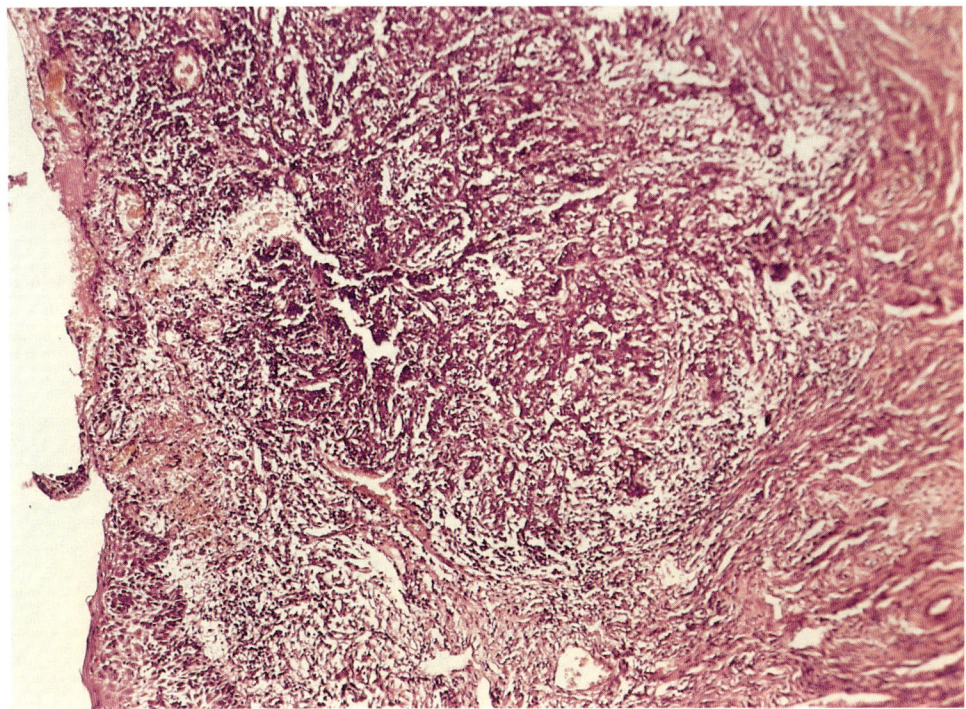

Fig. 145. Small cell carcinoma. H & E

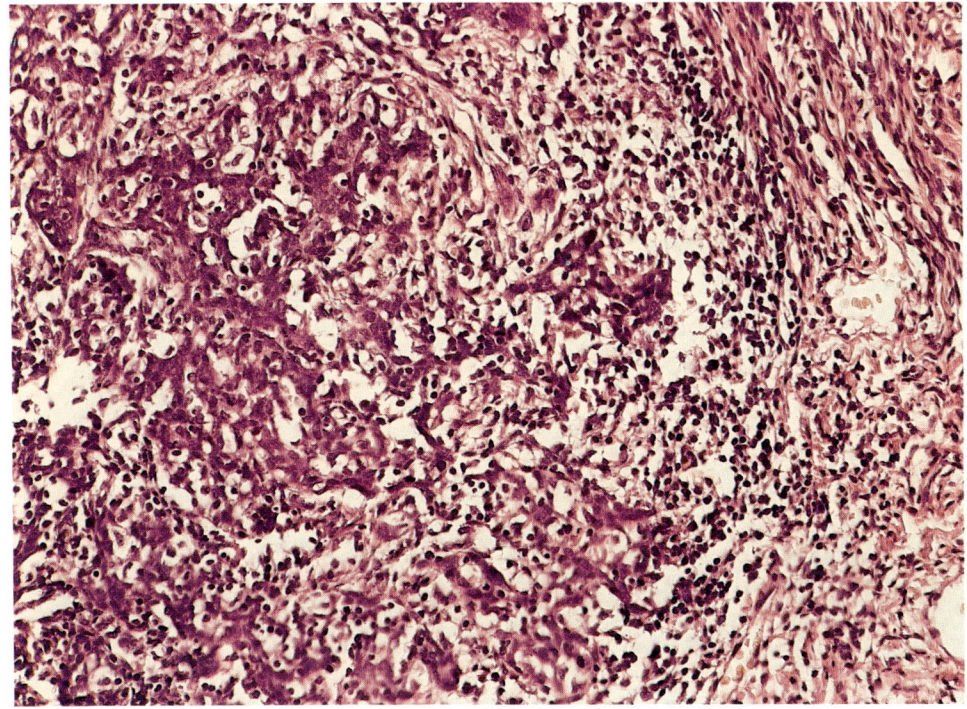

Fig. 146. Small cell carcinoma. H & E, higher magnification

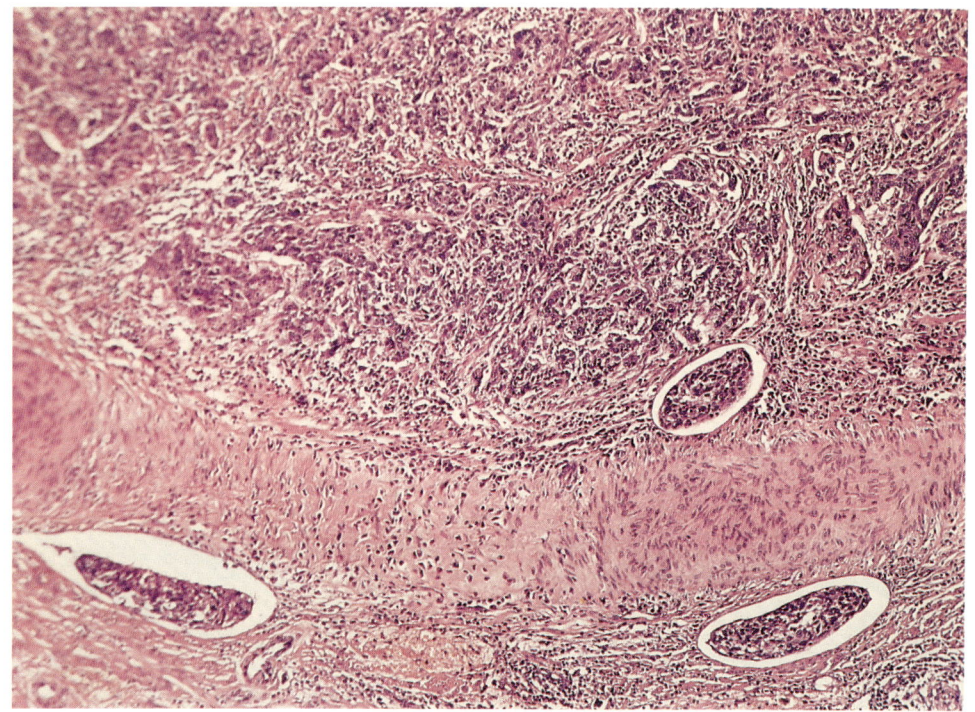

Fig. 147. Small cell carcinoma, extensive lymphatic invasion. H & E

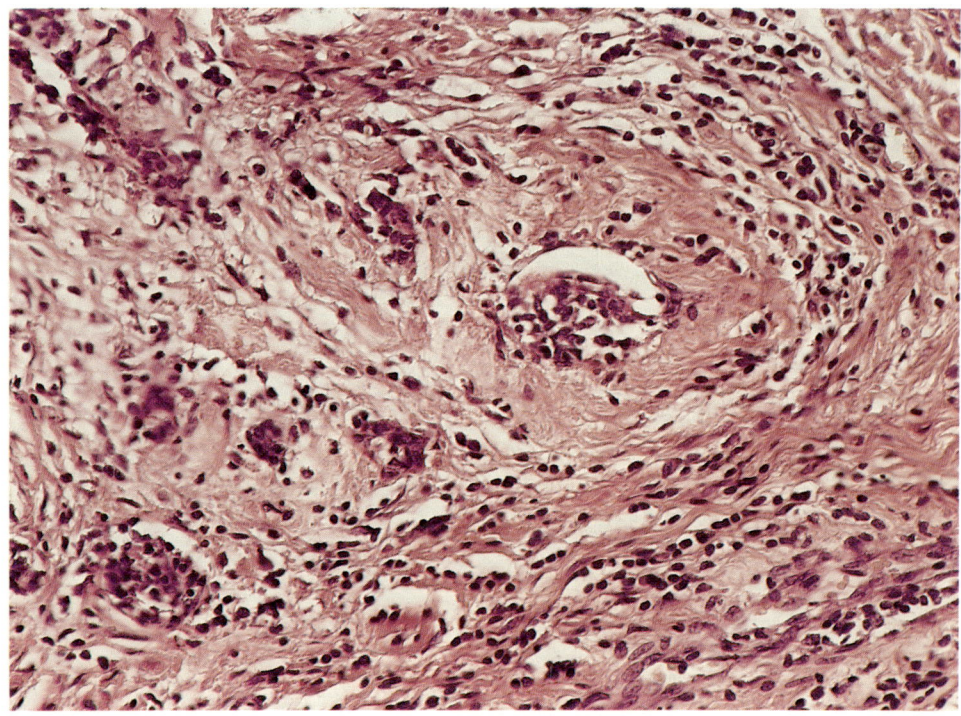

Fig. 148. Small cell carcinoma, extensive lymphatic invasion. H & E

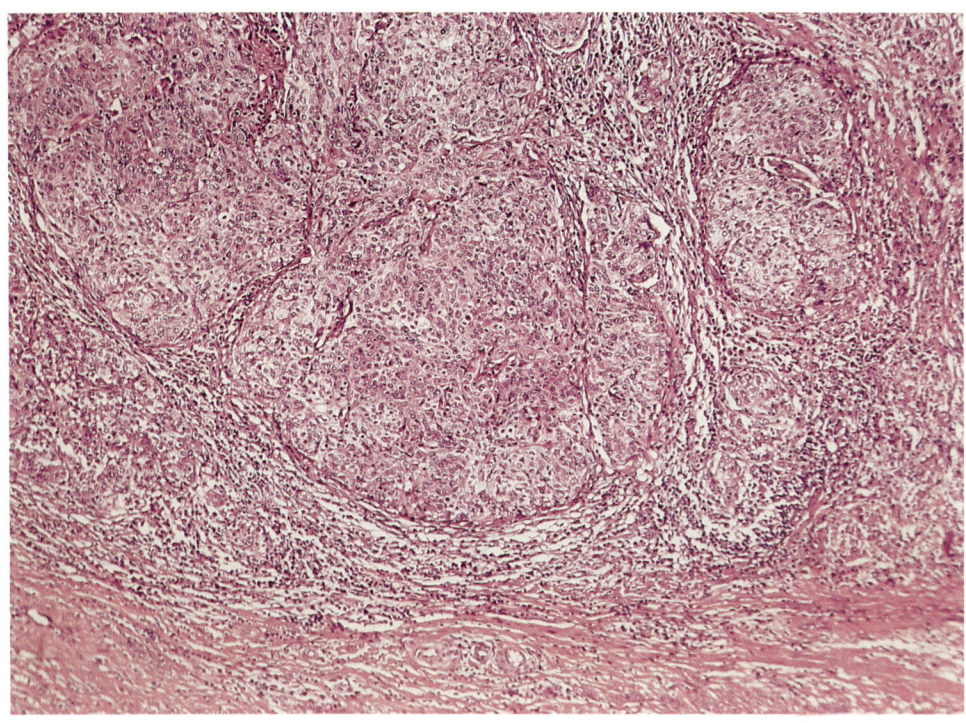

Fig. 149. Large cell nonkeratinizing carcinoma. H & E

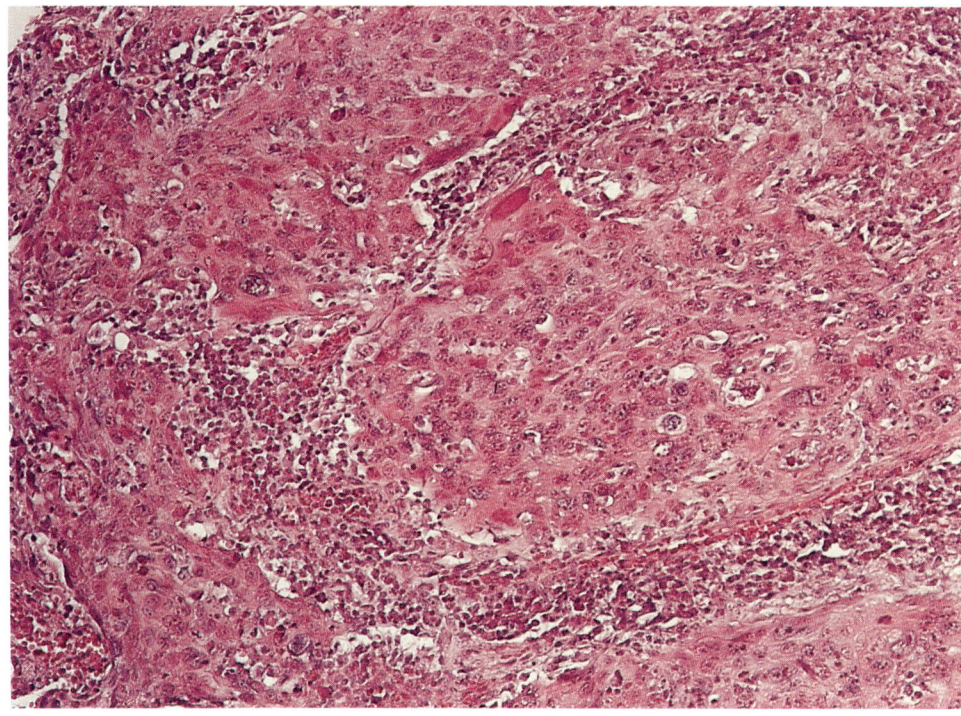

Fig. 150. Large cell nonkeratinizing carcinoma with slight nuclear polymorphism. H & E

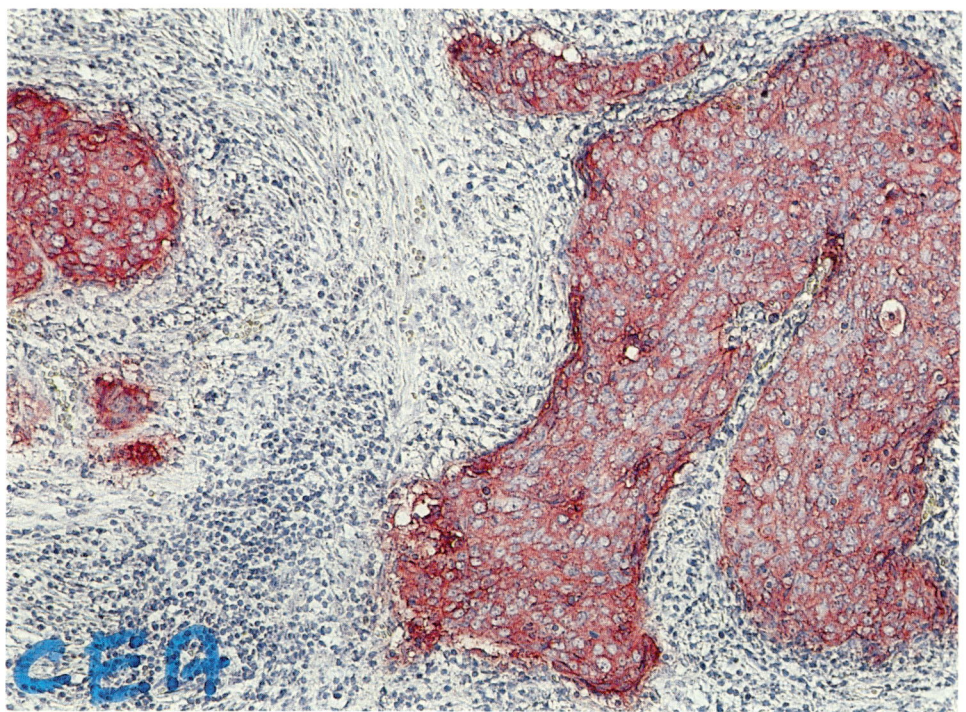

Fig. 151. Large cell carcinoma of reserve cell type. Immunohistochemical reaction with anti-CEA

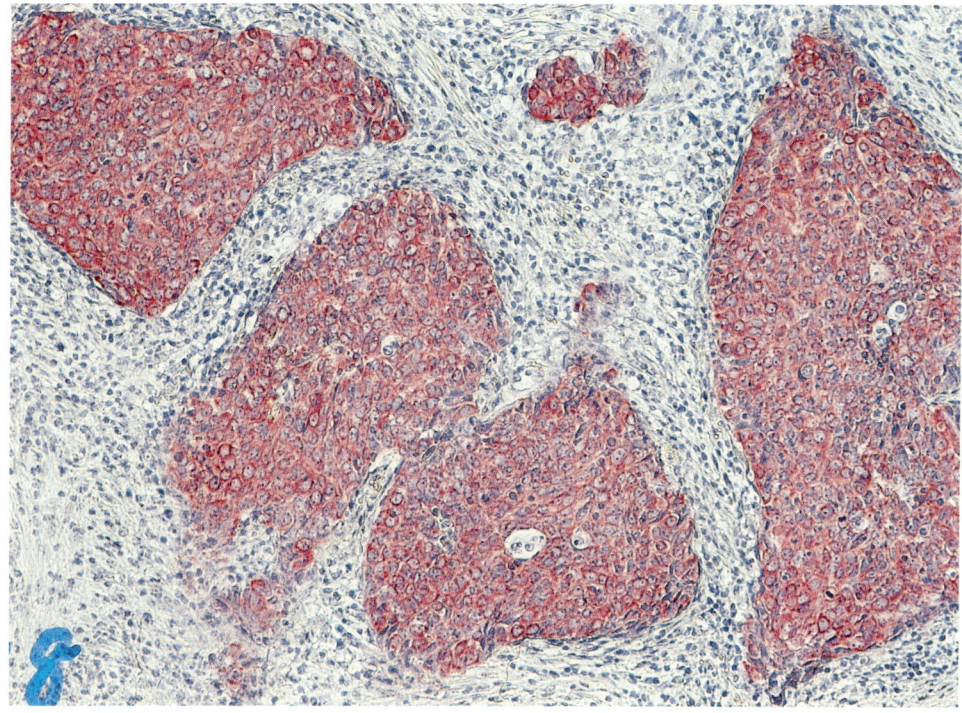

Fig. 152. Same as in Fig. 151. Immunohistochemical reaction with anticytokeratin 8

The *large cell keratinizing carcinoma* (representing about 25%) consists of small or large nests of mature epithelial tumor cells that adhere to one another by intercellular bridges. The nuclei are large, round or irregular, often hyperchromatic. The cytoplasm is abundant, eosinophilic or pale. Besides the keratin pearls in the center of epithelial nests (Fig. 157), a scattered monocellular keratinization is frequently seen (Figs. 155, 156).

As to be expected, these three types do not always occur alone. Combinations or mixtures may be seen, indicating again that we are dealing with a spectrum of biological changes. An intermediate form between small cell and large cell carcinoma is shown in Figs. 159–161; a special form consisting of nonkeratinizing and keratinizing carcinoma may result in a pleomorphic type of carcinoma (Fig. 162).

With invasive carcinoma, it is difficult to trace the cell of origin and to differentiate on routine histological examination between the squamous cell and reserve cell types. With immunohistochemistry, such a distinction is possible in the majority of carcinomas (Moll et al. 1983). As in the preinvasive stages, the *invasive carcinoma of the reserve cell type* shows a coexpression of cytokeratin 13, 8, 18, and CEA (Figs. 151, 152, 158, 160 and 161), whereas the *invasive carcinoma of the squamous cell type* reacts positively only with the squamous epithelial cytokeratins and negatively with anticytokeratin 8 and 18 and with anti-CEA (Dallenbach-Hellweg and Lang 1990).

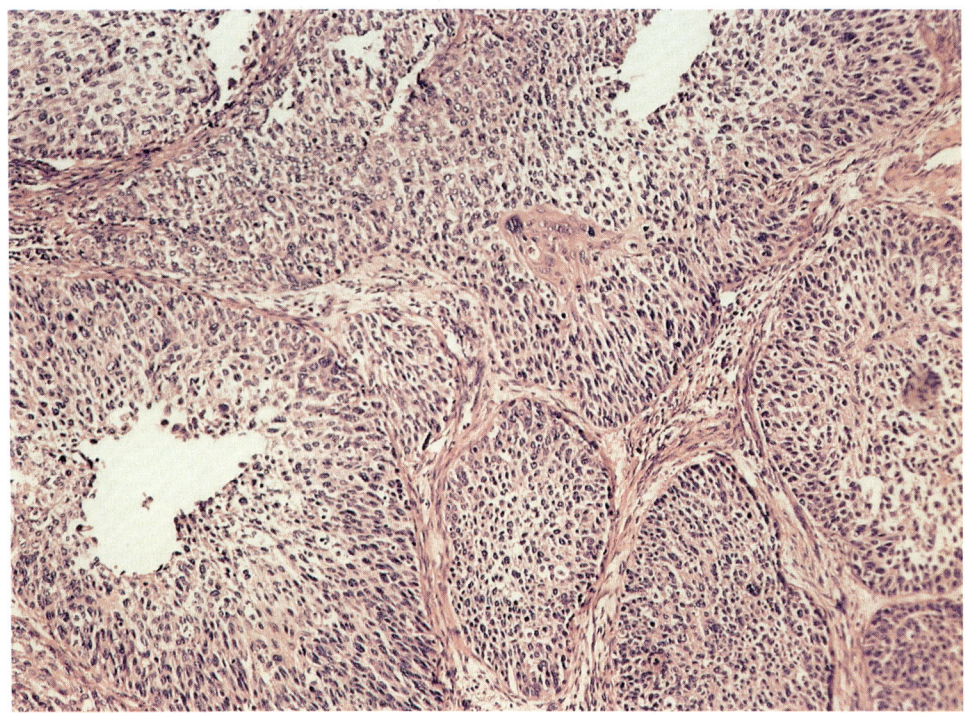

Fig. 153. Large cell nonkeratinizing carcinoma, poorly differentiated, with spindle-shaped cellular appearence. H & E

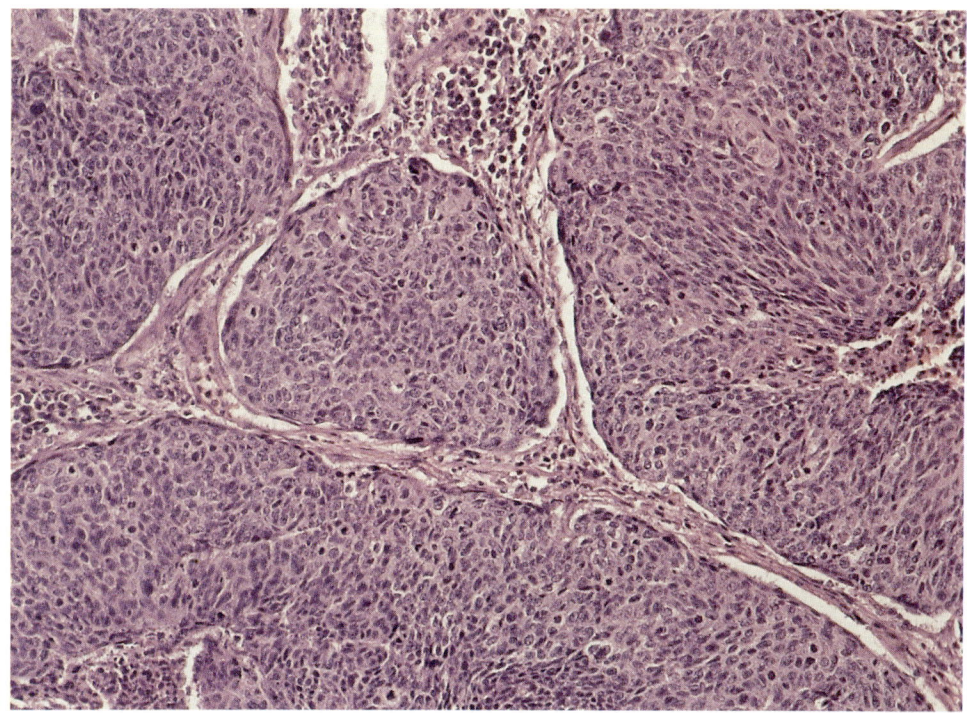

Fig. 154a. Large cell nonkeratinizing carcinoma, moderately differentiated. H & E

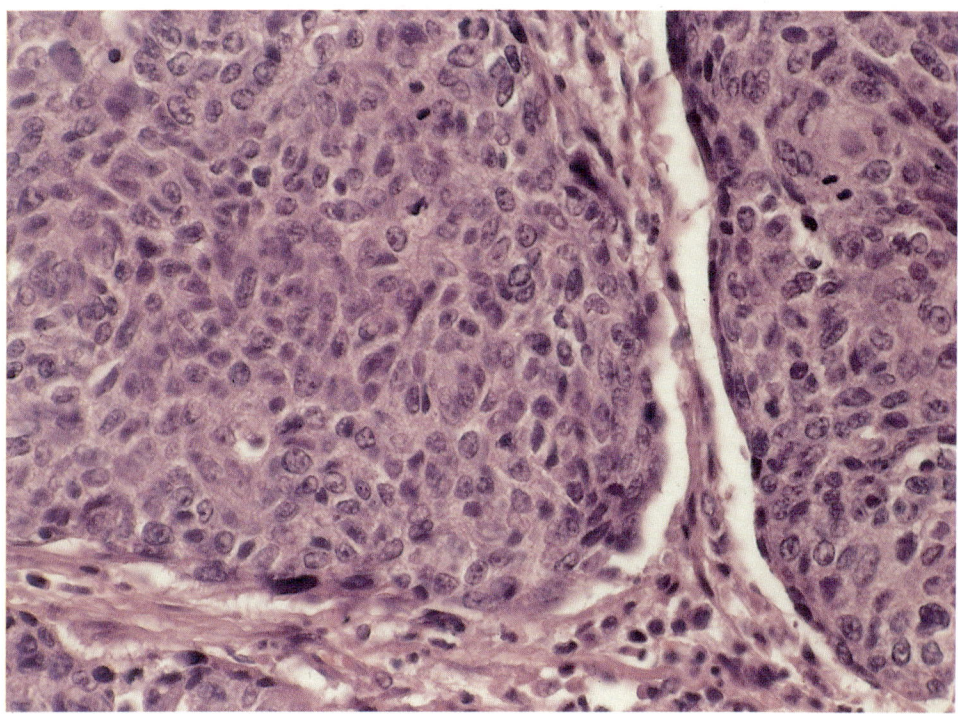

Fig. 154b. Same as Fig. 154a. H & E, higher magnification

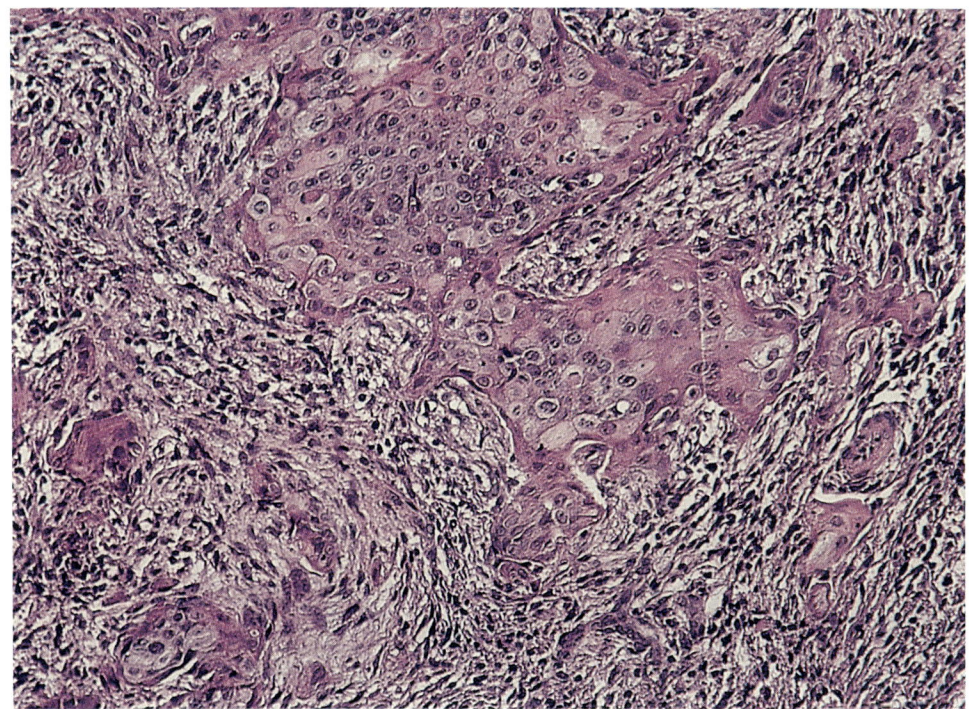
Fig. 155. Large cell keratinizing carcinoma. H & E

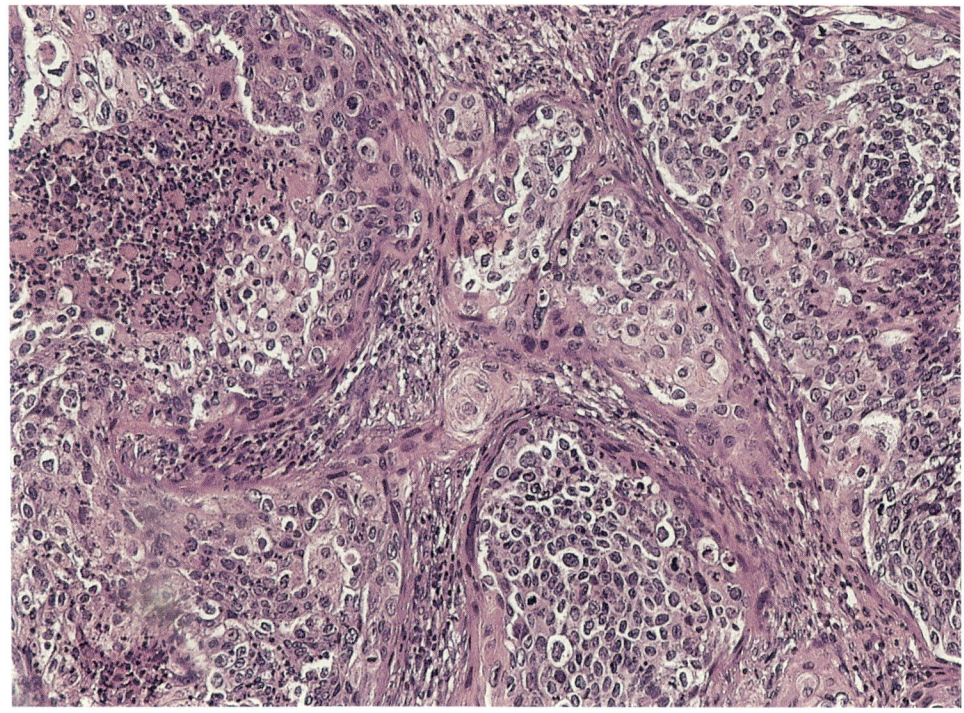
Fig. 156. Large cell keratinizing carcinoma. H & E

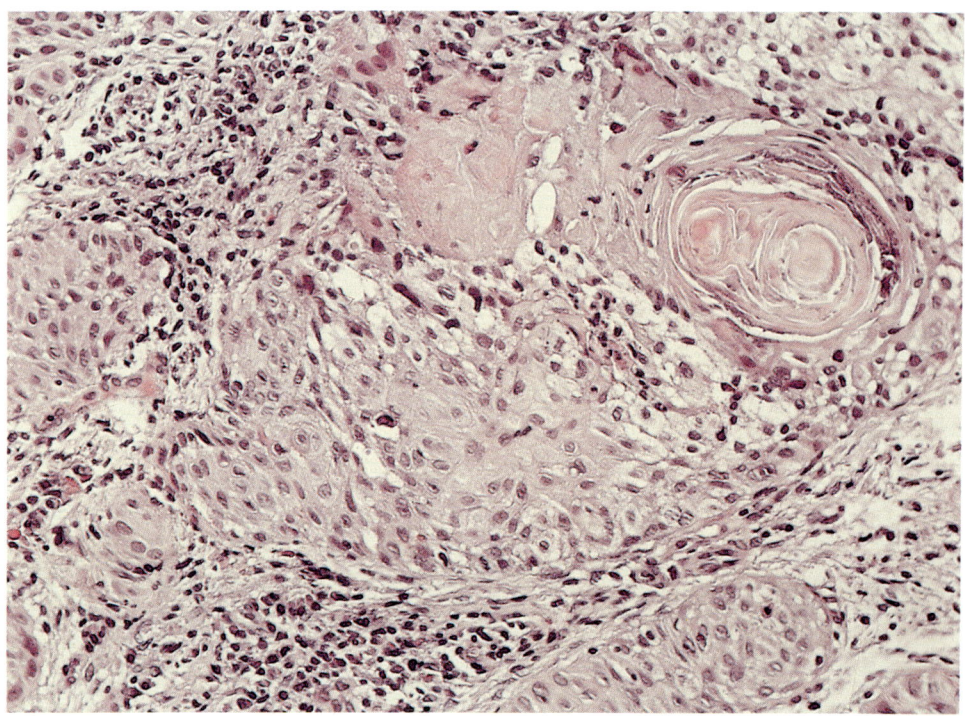

Fig. 157. Large cell keratinizing carcinoma. H & E

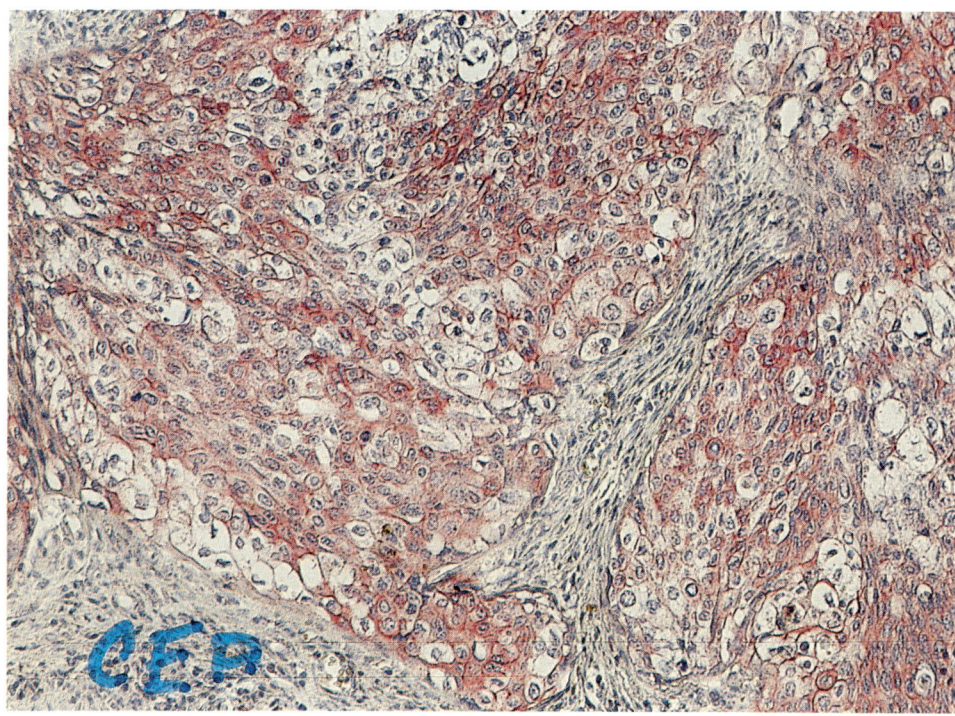

Fig. 158. Large cell keratinizing carcinoma of reserve cell type. Immunohistochemical reaction with anti-CEA

With these techniques, of which the CEA-reaction is the most important, it becomes obvious that both histogenetic types of invasive carcinoma, the squamous and the reserve cell type, may occasionally consist of small or large cells and may or may not keratinize. Despite their structural alteration, they retain the cytokeratin pattern shown by their cells of origin. In addition, the reserve cell carcinomas acquire a coexpression for CEA just as the adenocarcinomas, which may also arise from reserve cells. The expression for CEA indicates malignant change. In applying these stains it becomes apparent that most invasive cervical carcinomas arise from reserve cells, which are the most susceptible cells for HPV infections of type 16 and 18. To determine the rate of growth (cell proliferation index) in each type of carcinoma, KI 67 is the most reliable marker for measuring not only cells in mitosis, but in all stages of cell division not detectable in routine stains (Fig. 163).

Both the small cell and the large cell types of carcinoma vary in their mode and speed of invasion and spread: as in the microinvasive stages, the squamous type carcinoma shows early root- or netlike stromal infiltration with rapid lymphatic invasion and spread beyond the uterus. In the reserve cell type, the bulky infiltration usually remains confined to the uterine cervix until it has largely replaced the cervical wall. Since apparently none of the conventional histological parameters, such as degree of keratinization, nuclear pleomorphism, number of mitoses, cell size, or stromal reaction, can reliably predict patient survival (Beecham et al. 1978; Crissman et al. 1987), the differentiation of these two types of carcinoma by identifying their histogenetic origins is much more important than distinguishing between small or large cell types with or without keratinization.

Differential Diagnosis. The small cell carcinomas must be distinguished from the small cell neuroendocrine (carcinoid) type of carcinoma (see p. 155). This is possible with neu-

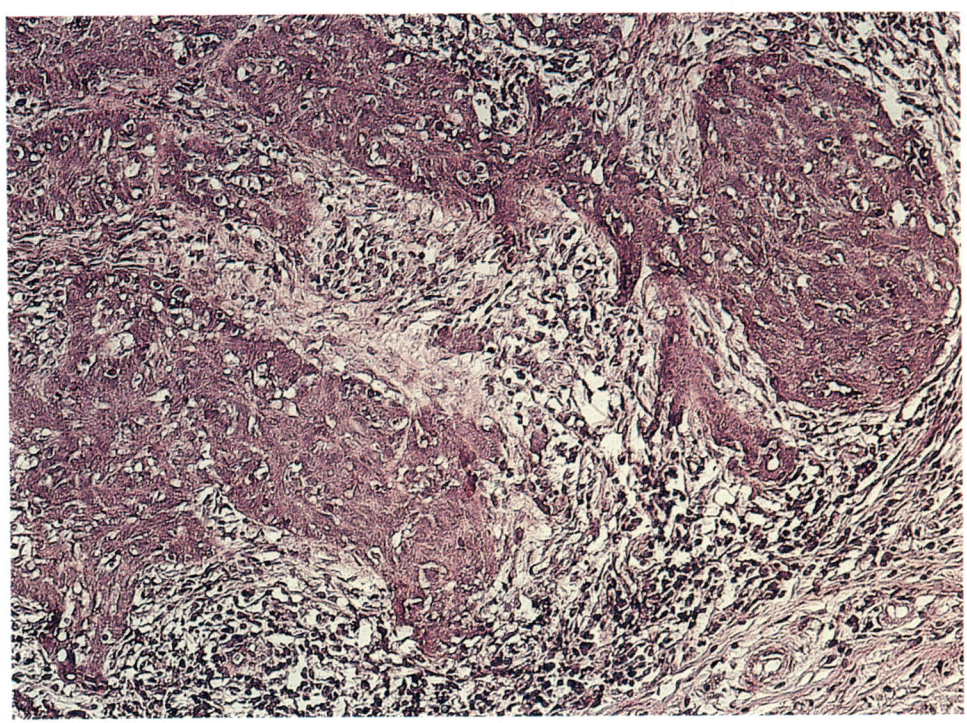

Fig. 159. Intermediate form between small and large cell carcinoma. H & E

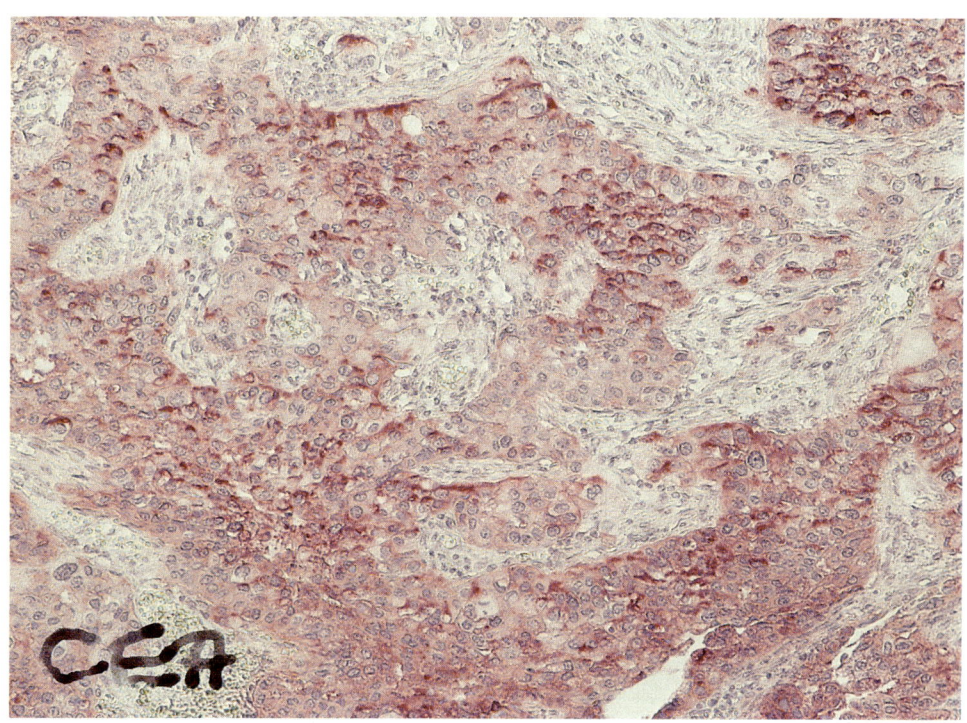

Fig. 160. Same as Fig. 159. Immunohistochemical reaction with anti-CEA

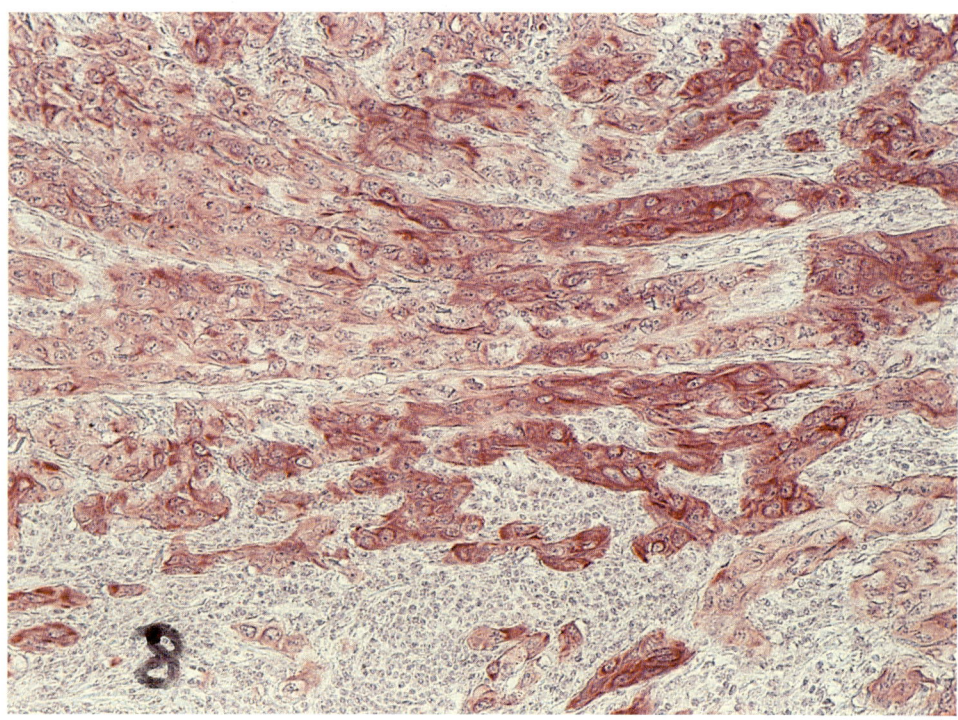

Fig. 161. Same as Fig. 159. Immunohistochemical reaction with anticytokeratin 8

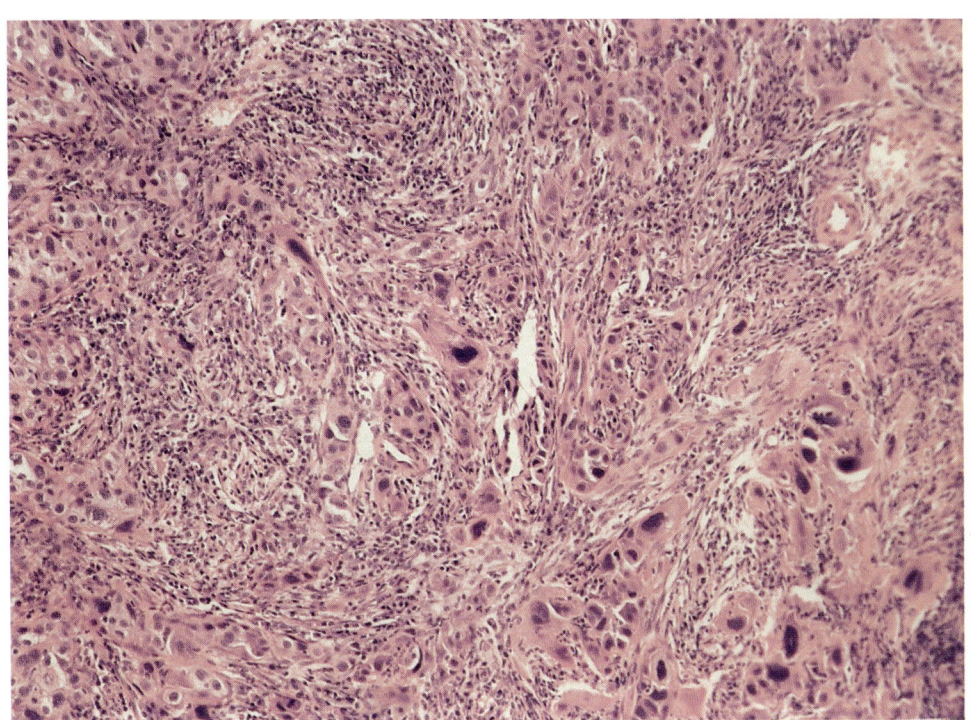

Fig. 162. Large cell pleomorphic carcinoma. H & E

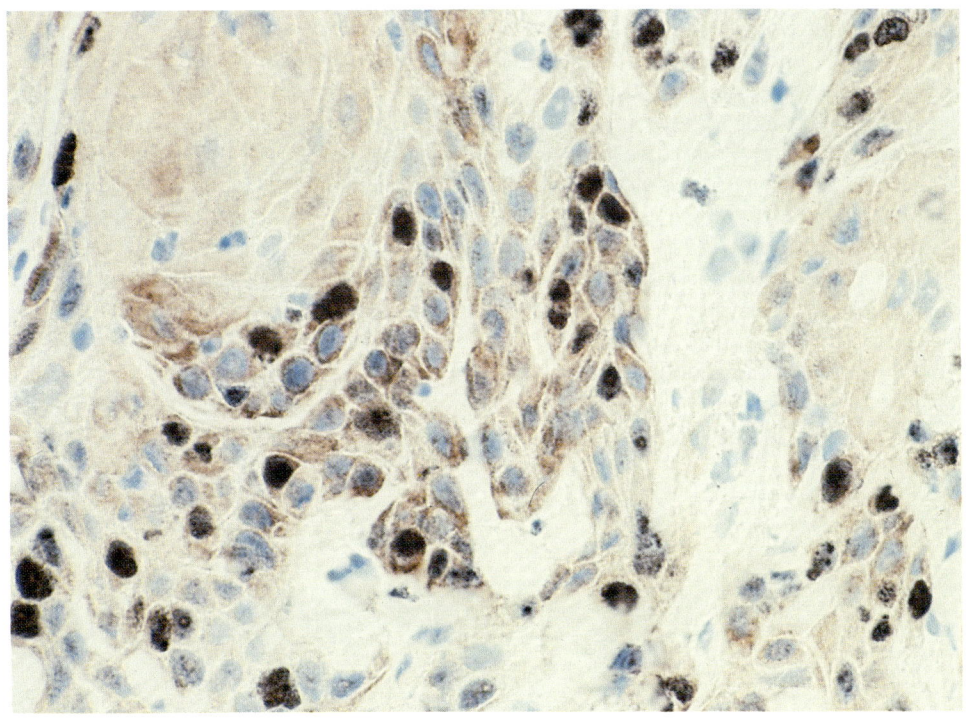

Fig. 163. Large cell keratinizing carcinoma. Immunohistochemical reaction with KI 67

roendocrine markers or with a Grimelius stain, which is positive in neuroendocrine tumors but negative in the small cell carcinoma of reserve cell origin. Primitive neurogenic tumors closely resembling small cell carcinomas are negative with all markers for cytokeratin and for CEA, but show a distinctly positive reaction for NSE (see p. 157). – Occasionally a chronic granulomatous inflammation may be confused with a small cell carcinoma. A careful cytological evaluation should help to reveal the nature of such granulomas, which will give negative reactions for cytokeratins.

Verrucous carcinoma is a rare variant of cervical squamous cell carcinoma composed of very well-differentiated keratinizing squamous cells growing in frondlike papillae. Stromal invasion is always bulky; lymphatic involvement or distant spread is rare. This tumor is more common in the vulva and has been found to be associated with HPV infection of type 6 (Okagaki et al. 1984).

Distinction from large papillomas, on one hand, and from the large cell keratinizing type of invasive carcinoma, on the other hand, may be difficult unless the entire tumor is studied (Rorat et al. 1978). The presence of small groups of anaplastic cells in the underlying stroma excludes verrucous carcinoma. Verrucous carcinoma has a tendency to recur locally, and the therapy of choice is wide local excision.

Papillary squamous cell carcinoma is another rare variant of cervical carcinoma, presenting the gross and histological appearance of a benign papilloma undergoing dysplastic cellular change (compare Figs. 113 and 114). Beneath the papillary dysplasia, strands of invasive carcinoma can be detected (Randall et al. 1986). Diagnosis of invasion, therefore, depends upon examining the entire papillary lesion.

Glandular Type (Figs. 164–190)

All types of adenocarcinomas of the endocervix have become more common over the past two decades (Schwartz and Weiss 1986). Their proportion among all cervical cancers has increased from 4.6% to over 30%. As already mentioned, the great majority of endocervical adenocarcinomas contain HPV 18. This virus infects both the reserve cells and the glandular epithelial cells when these are hyperplastic, that is, excessively stimulated with synthetic gestagens taken as the major component of oral contraceptives (Gallup and Abell 1977; Dallenbach-Hellweg 1984). This concept is in agreement with recent epidemiological studies (Brinton et al. 1986; Peters et al. 1986). Both infected and hyperstimulated cell types: reserve cells and glandular cells, may under such conditions develop into in situ and invasive adenocarcinoma.

The prognosis of all types of endocervical adenocarcinomas is generally less favorable than that of squamous carcinomas (Eide 1987). It depends more on the degree of nuclear ploidy, the stage of the disease, and the lymph node status than on the histological appearance (Fu et al. 1982; Hopkins et al. 1988).

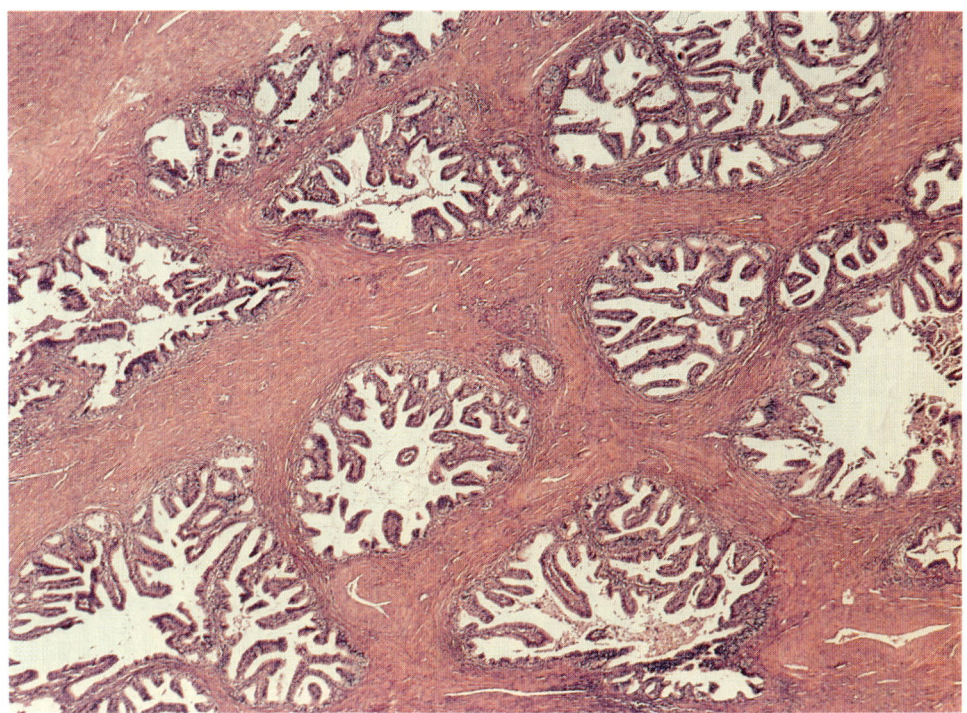
Fig. 164. Minimal deviation adenocarcinoma. H & E

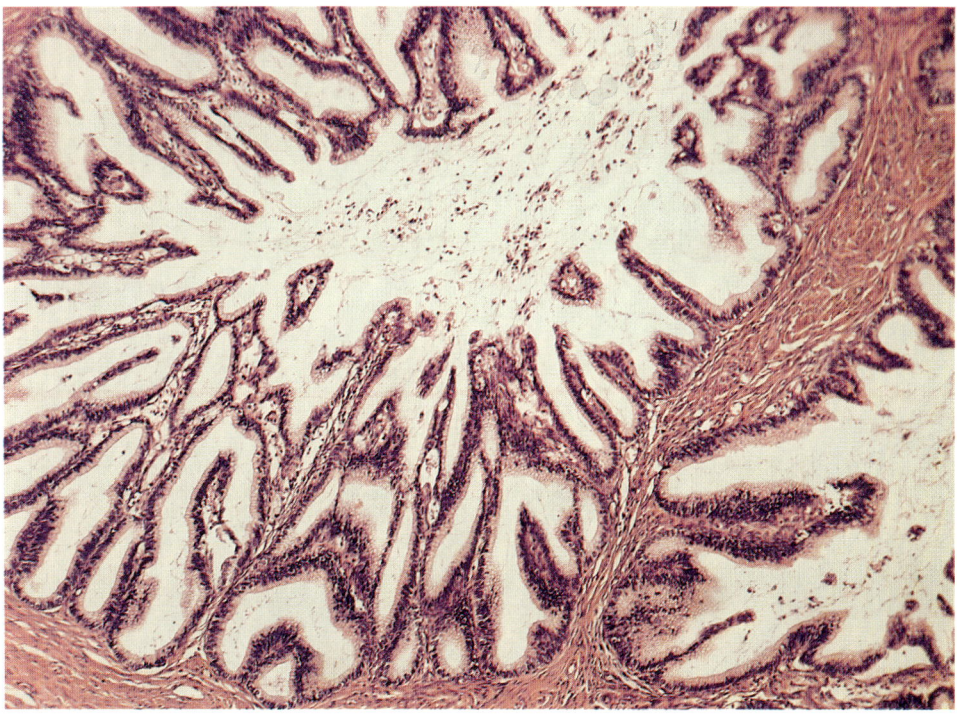
Fig. 165. Minimal deviation adenocarcinoma. H & E, higher magnification

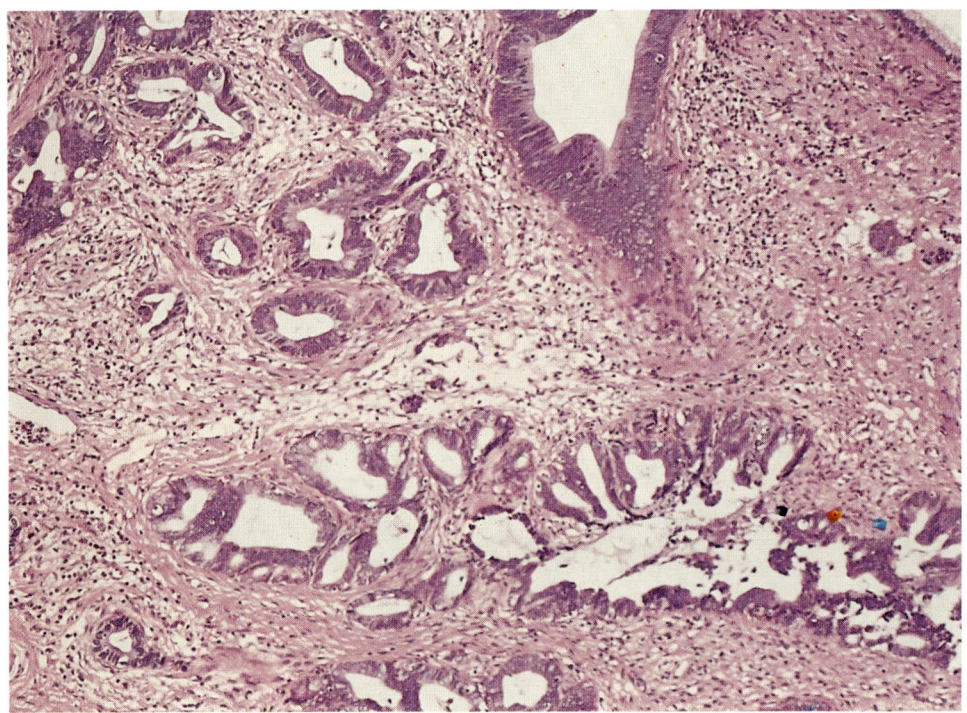

Fig. 166. Mucinous adenocarcinoma, grade 1. H & E

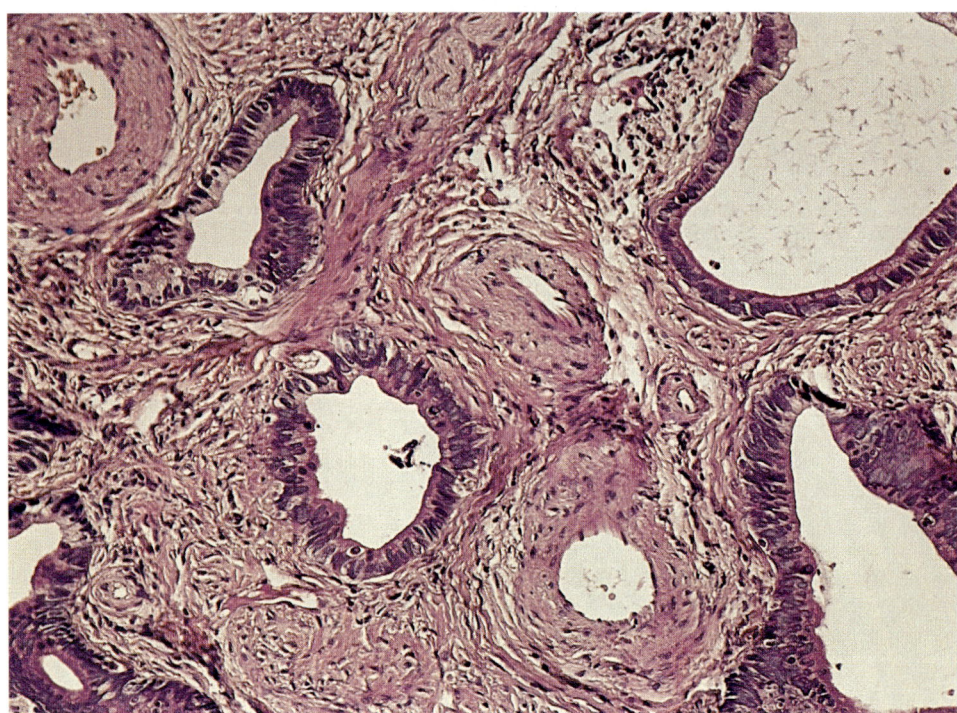

Fig. 167. Mucinous adenocarcinoma, grade 1. H & E, higher magnification

Mucinous Adenocarcinoma

The mucinous (endocervical) type of adenocarcinoma (Figs. 164–177) is most frequently encountered. All degrees of differentiation can be found. The amount of mucin roughly follows the degree of differentiation. Most of the mucinous adenocarcinomas are well or *moderately differentiated*. (Figs. 166–171) Their interbranching glands may show microglandular changes (Fig. 171) and contain variable amounts of intracytoplasmic mucin (Fig. 174). In the poorly differentiated type, (Figs. 172, 173) solid strands of tumor cells predominate with pseudorosette formation or palisading of nuclei. There is very little intracytoplasmic mucin, but monocellular or microcystic accumulation of mucin may be found scattered within cellular strands. All types of mucinous carcinomas, regardless of their degree of differentiation, almost always stain positively for CEA (Figs. 175, 176).

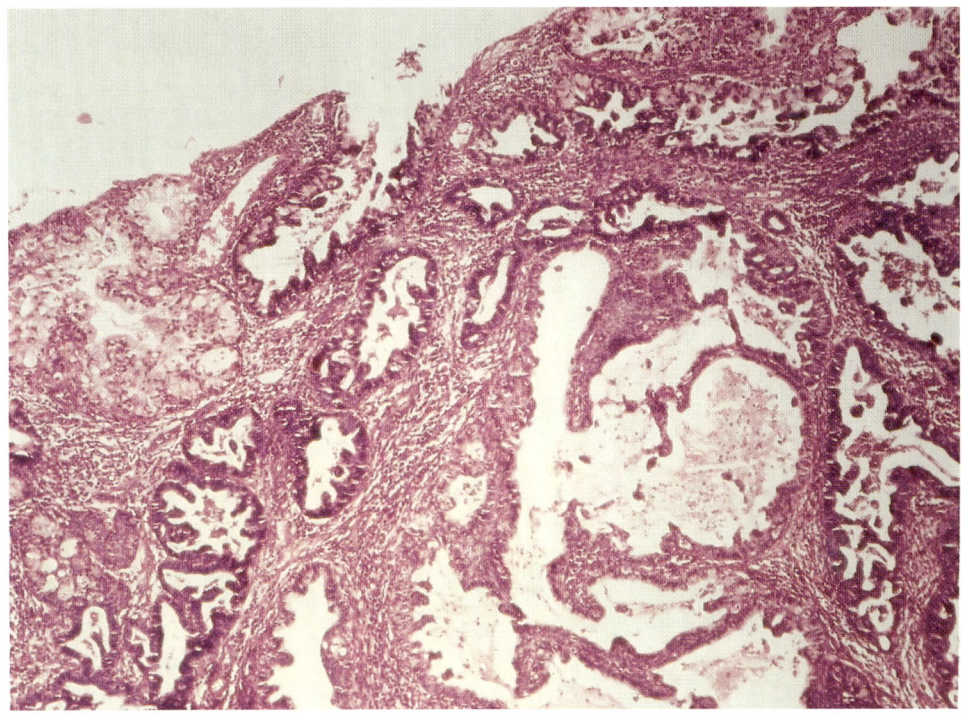

Fig. 168. Mucinous adenocarcinoma, grade 1, glandular-papillary. H & E

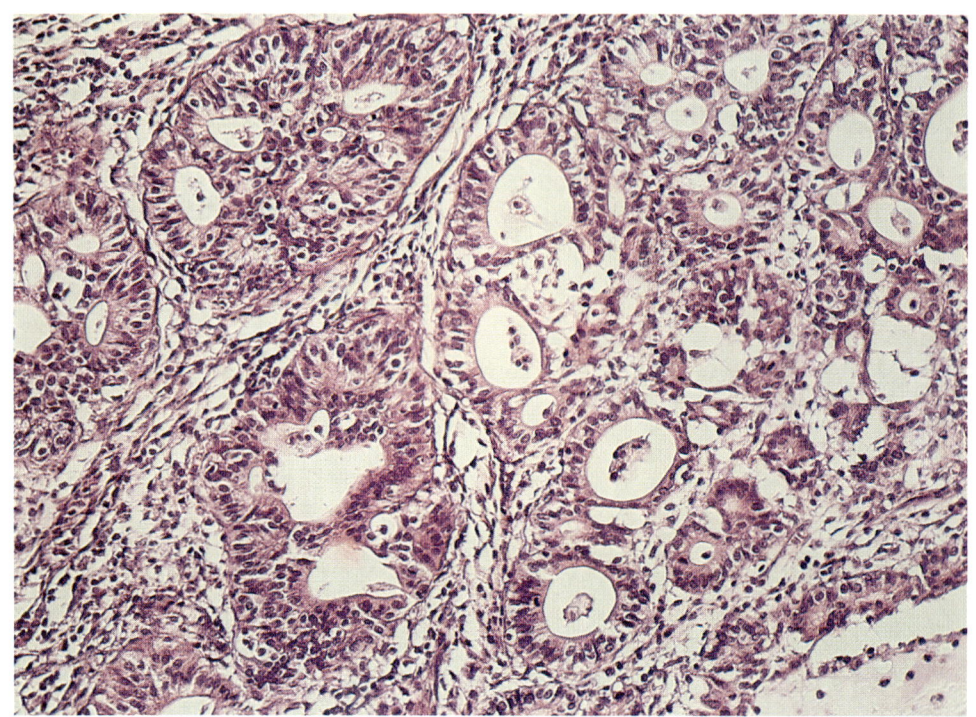

Fig. 169. Mucinous adenocarcinoma, grade 2. H & E

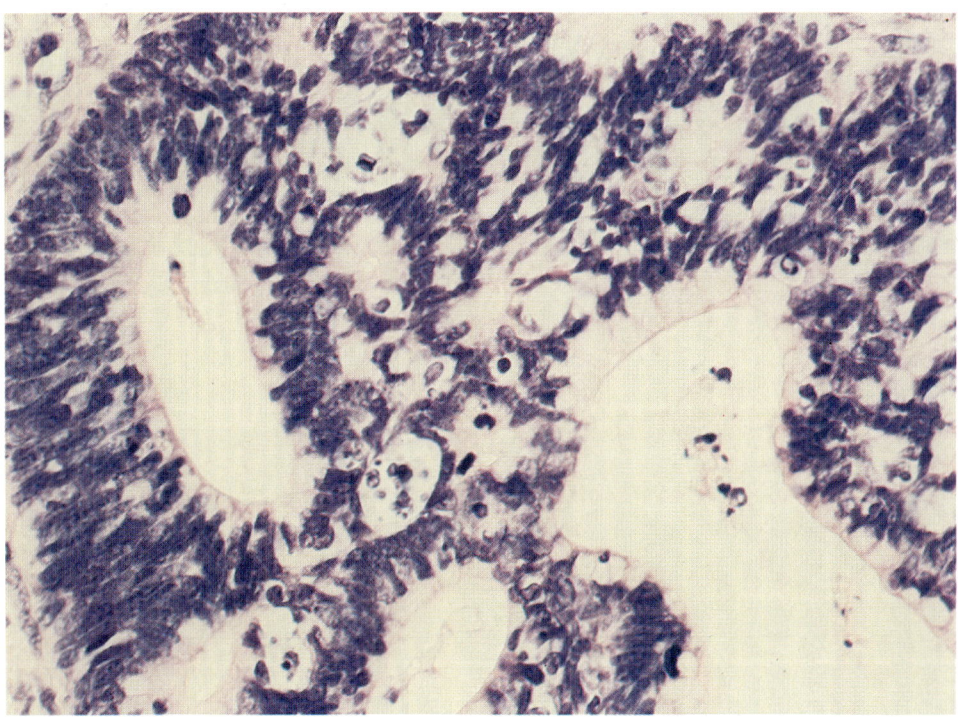

Fig. 170. Mucinous adenocarcinoma, grade 2. H & E, higher magnification

Minimal Deviation Adenocarcinoma (adenoma malignum, Figs. 164, 165) is extremely well differentiated, but nonetheless has a poor prognosis, often despite radical therapy (Silverberg and Hurt 1975; Kaku and Enjoji 1983; Kaminski and Norris 1983; Michael et al. 1984). This particular type of endocervical adenocarcinoma may be associated with a Peutz-Jegher's Syndrome and with a second primary ovarian mucinous adenocarcinoma (Young and Scully 1988; Gilks et al. 1989). Cytological abnormalities are absent or subtle, consisting of slight nuclear enlargement, chromatin clumping, loss of nuclear polarity, and increased mitotic activity. The carcinomatous glands are lined by a single layer of columnar mucinous epithelium generally similar to that seen in normal glands. There may be a weak desmoplastic or edematous reaction around some glands. Necrosis is absent. Architectural abnormalities are the main distinguishing features: the endocervical glands, excessively convoluted with papillary projections into their lumina, are randomly distributed in the cervical wall, which they invade beyond the area in which glands are normally found. In most cases, vascular and perineural invasion is already evident.

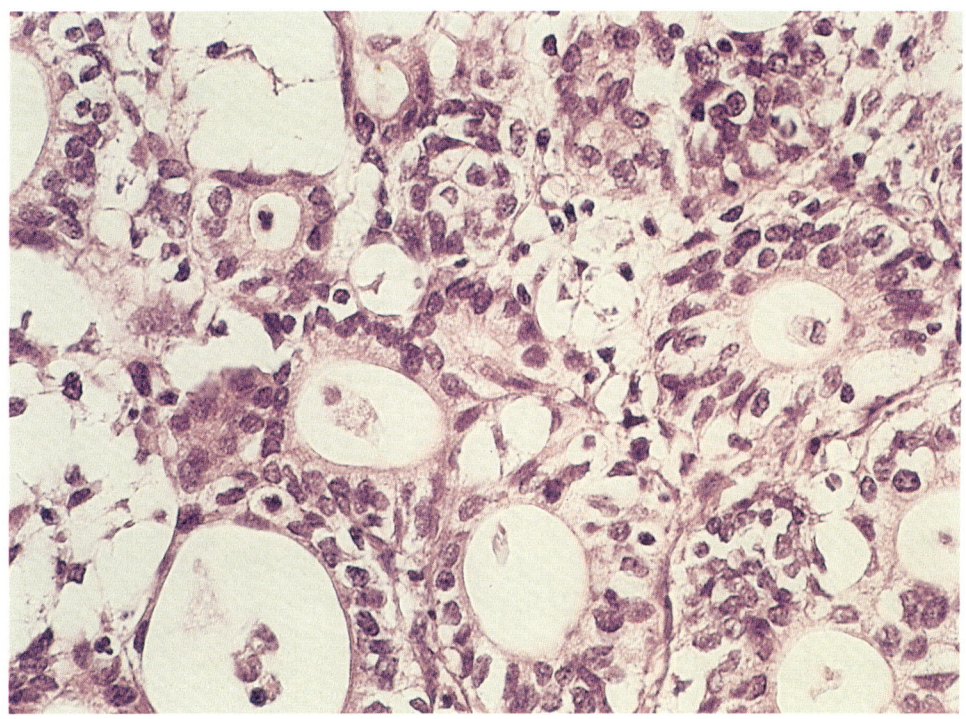

Fig. 171. Mucinous adenocarcinoma, grade 2-3. H & E

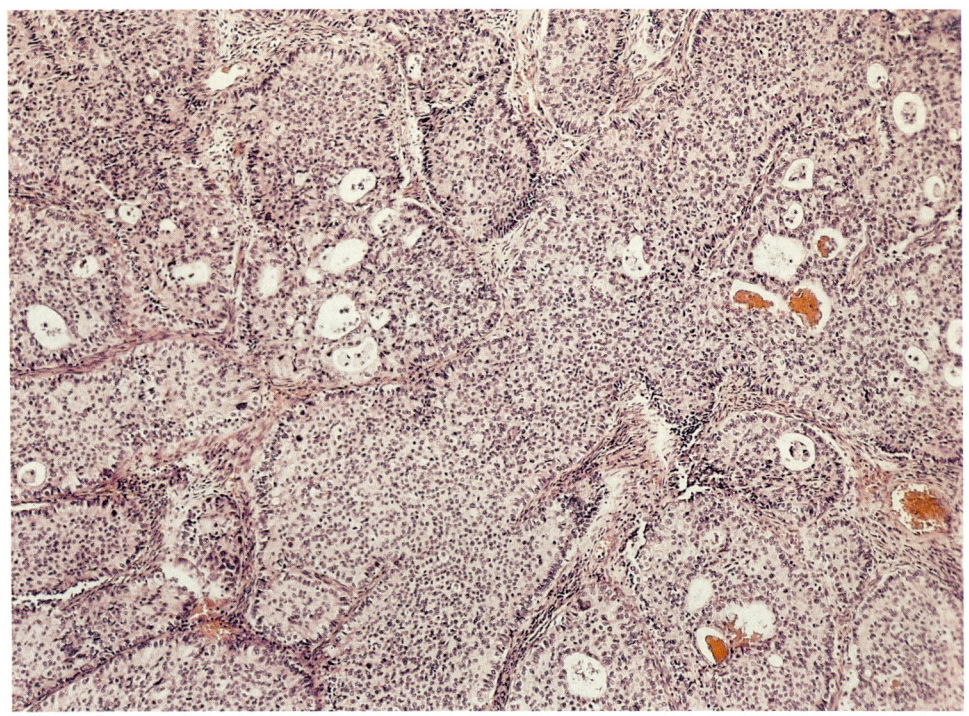

Fig. 172. Mucinous adenocarcinoma, grade 3. H & E

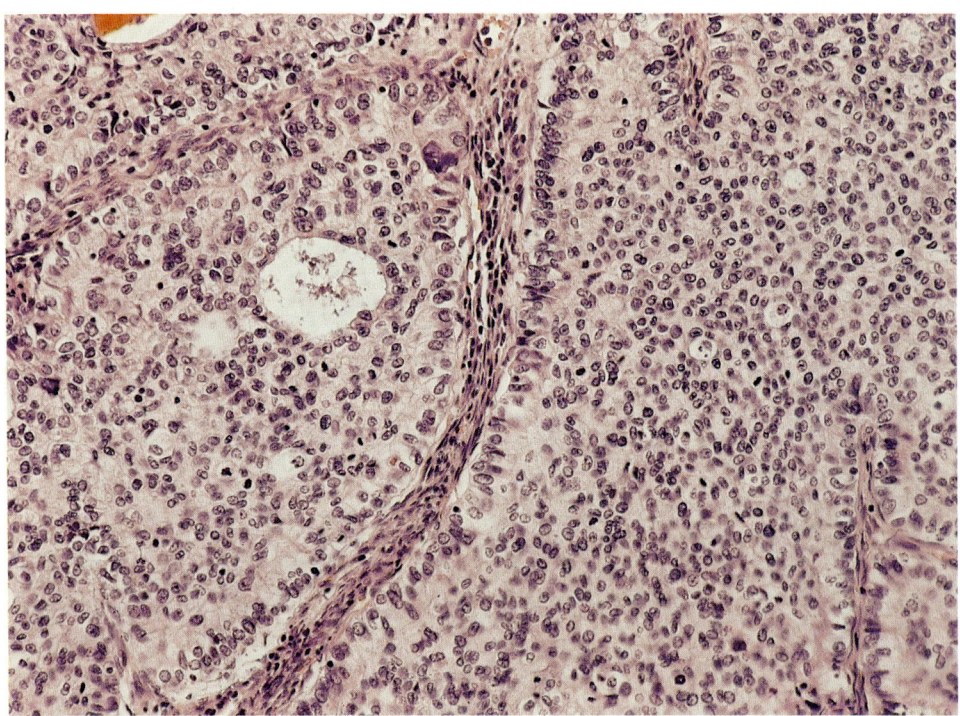

Fig. 173. Mucinous adenocarcinoma, grade 3. H & E, higher magnification

Differential Diagnosis. It may be very difficult to distinguish affected glands from normal or hyperplastic endocervical glands and even impossible if only a small biopsy is available. In such cases, immunohistochemical stains with anti-CEA may be very helpful: all or part of the carcinomatous glands are positive for CEA in most instances, whereas normal and hyperplastic endocervical glands stain negatively (Speers et al. 1983; Steeper and Wick 1986; Nanbu et al. 1988; Gilks et al. 1989).

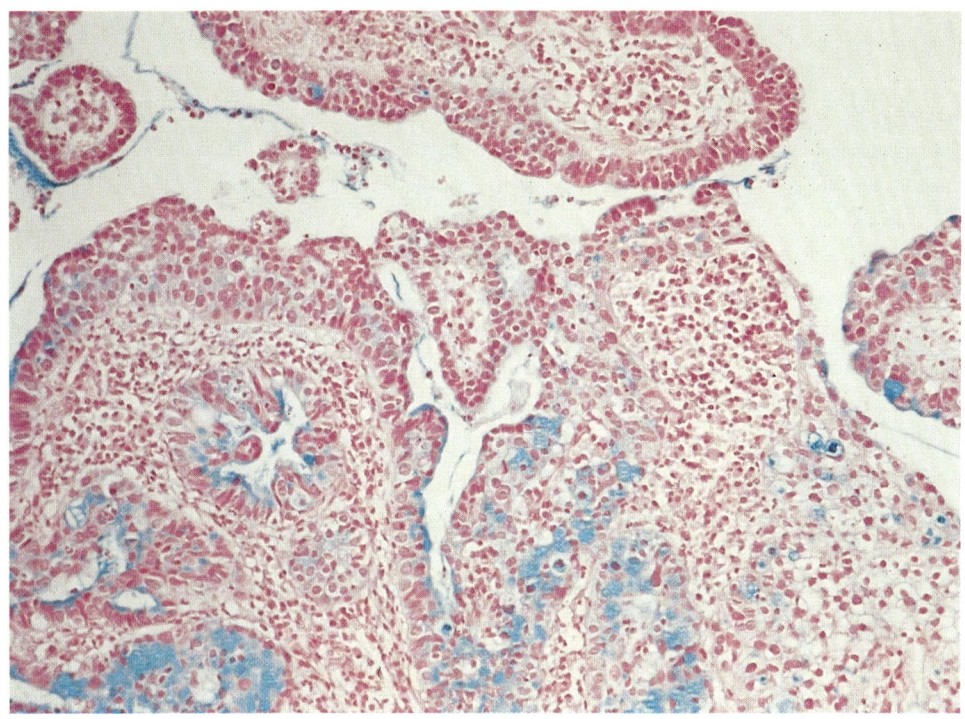

Fig. 174. Mucinous adenocarcinoma, grade 2. Alcian blue reaction

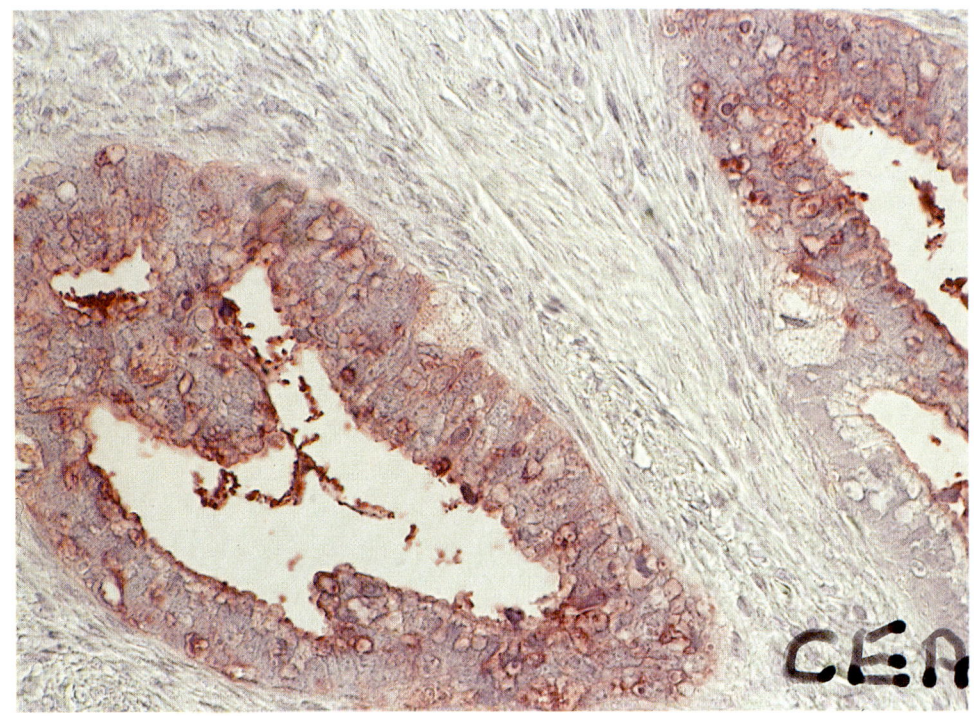

Fig. 175. Mucinous adenocarcinoma, grade 1. Immunohistochemical reaction with anti-CEA

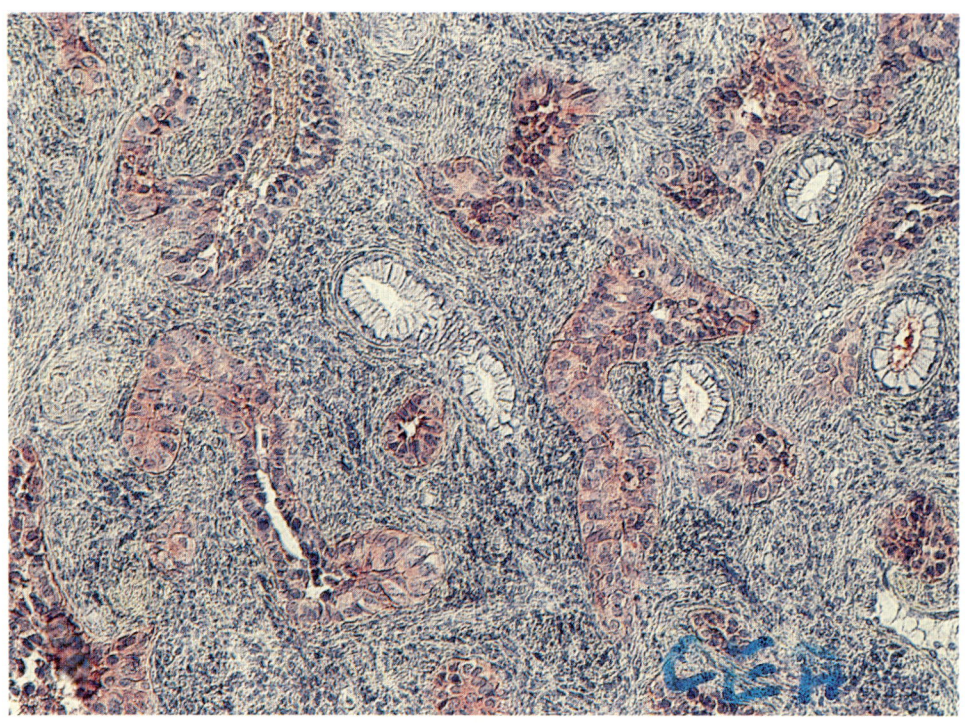

Fig. 176. Mucinous adenocarcinoma, grade 3. Immunohistochemical reaction with anti-CEA (normal glands react negatively)

Intestinal Mucinous Adenocarcinoma. The intestinal type of mucinous adenocarcinoma (Fig. 177) contains goblet cells resembling those of adenocarcinoma of the colon, and occasionally argentaffin and Paneth's cells. Such an intestinal-type change may be found diffusely or only focally within a mucinous carcinoma, which has developed from an intestinal metaplasia of the endocervical mucosa.

Various other types of müllerian metaplasia may give rise to special forms of endocervical adenocarcinomas (Lauchlan 1984). A villoglandular papillary type of well-differentiated adenocarcinoma has a more favorable prognosis (Young and Scully 1989). A combination of mucinous adenocarcinoma and epidermoid carcinoma may be seen and should be distinguished from adenosquamous carcinoma.

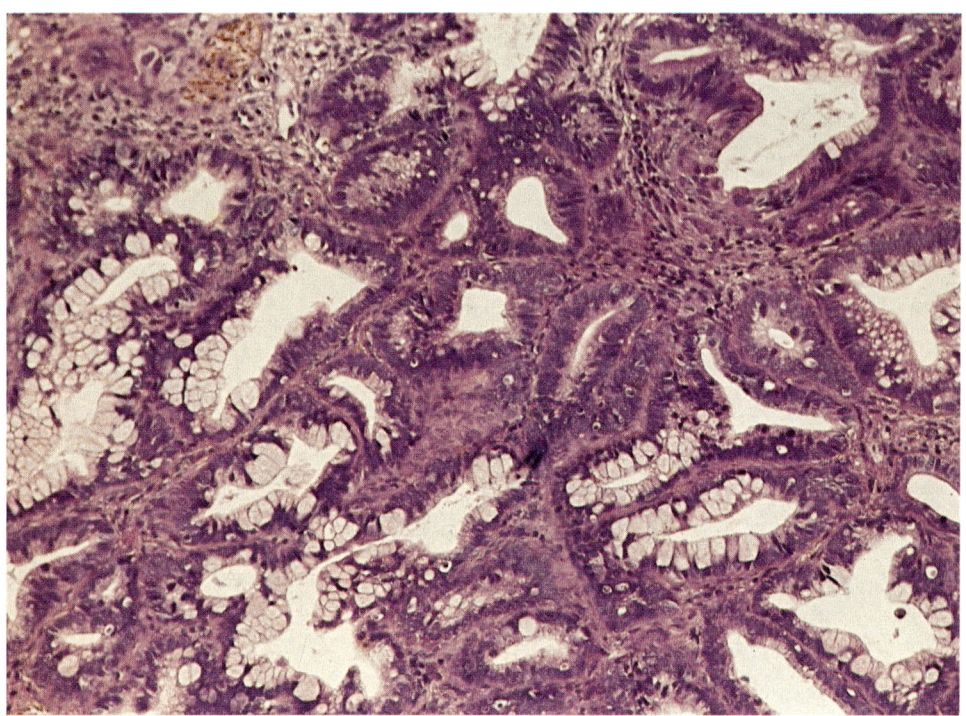

Fig. 177. Mucinous adenocarcinoma, intestinal type. H & E

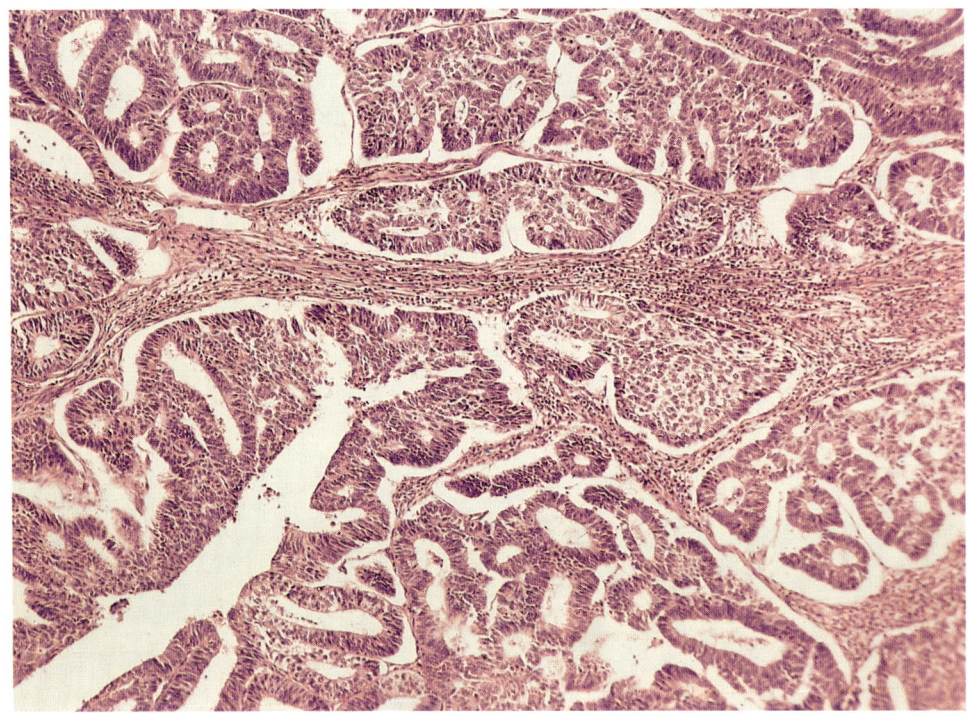
Fig. 178. Adenocarcinoma of endocervix, endometrioid type. H & E

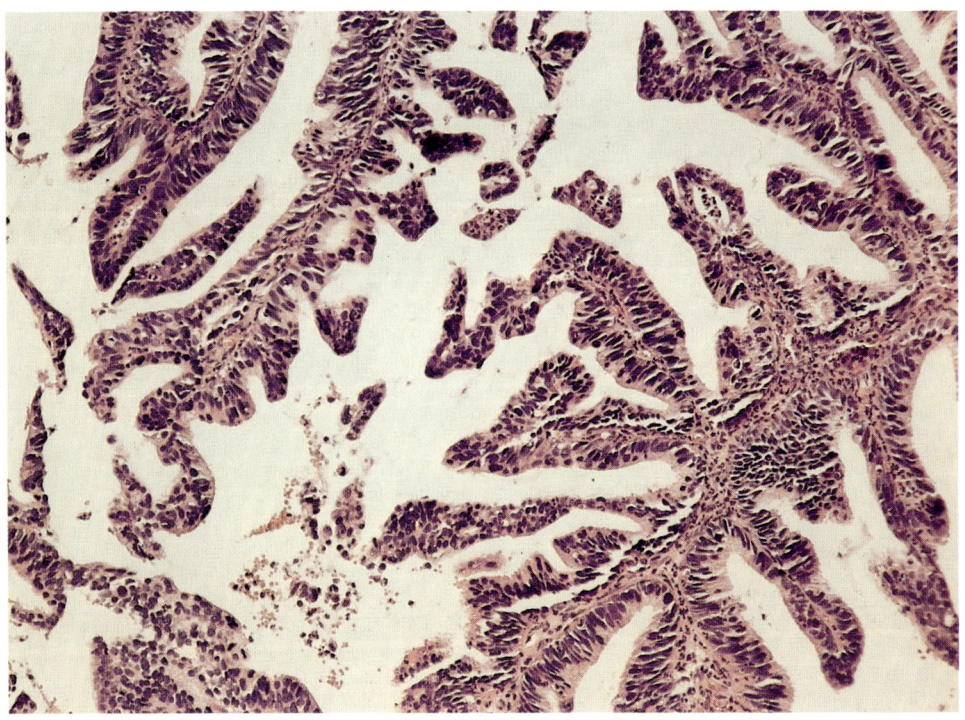
Fig. 179. Adenocarcinoma of endocervix, endometrioid type, glandular-papillary. H & E

Endometrioid Adenocarcinoma

The endometrioid type of adenocarcinoma (Figs. 178–180) may arise from metaplasia or from ectopic endometrial glands, representing embryological remnants displaced in the deeper portions of the cervical wall (Noda et al. 1983; Teshima et al. 1985). Its histological structure is like that of the endometrial-type adenocarcinoma arising from the corpus mucosa. PAS positive and diastase resistant secretions may be found in the glandular lumina, but not in the cytoplasm. There may be foci of squamous metaplasia, as in adenoacanthoma of endometrial origin (Dallenbach-Hellweg and Poulsen 1985).

Differential Diagnosis. Distinguishing an endometrioid type of adenocarcinoma from a primary endometrial adenocarcinoma that has extended or metastasized to the cervix may be impossible in routine histological examination of curettings or biopsies, even when mucin stains are used. Immunohistochemical stains, however, may help considerably: endometrioid type adenocarcinomas of endocervical origin, in contrast to primary endometrial carcinomas, are negative with antivimentin (Fig. 180) and positive with anti-CEA in most instances (Dabbs et al. 1986; Cohen et al. 1982; Dallenbach-Hellweg and Lang 1990).

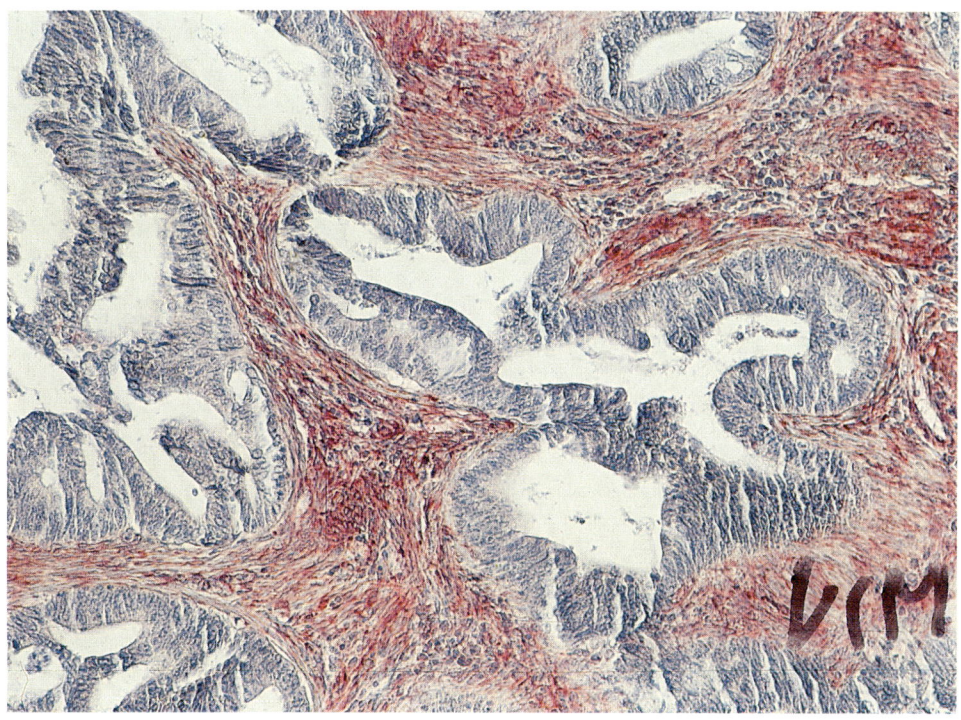

Fig. 180. Adenocarcinoma of endocervix, endometrioid type. Immunohistochemical reaction with antivimentin

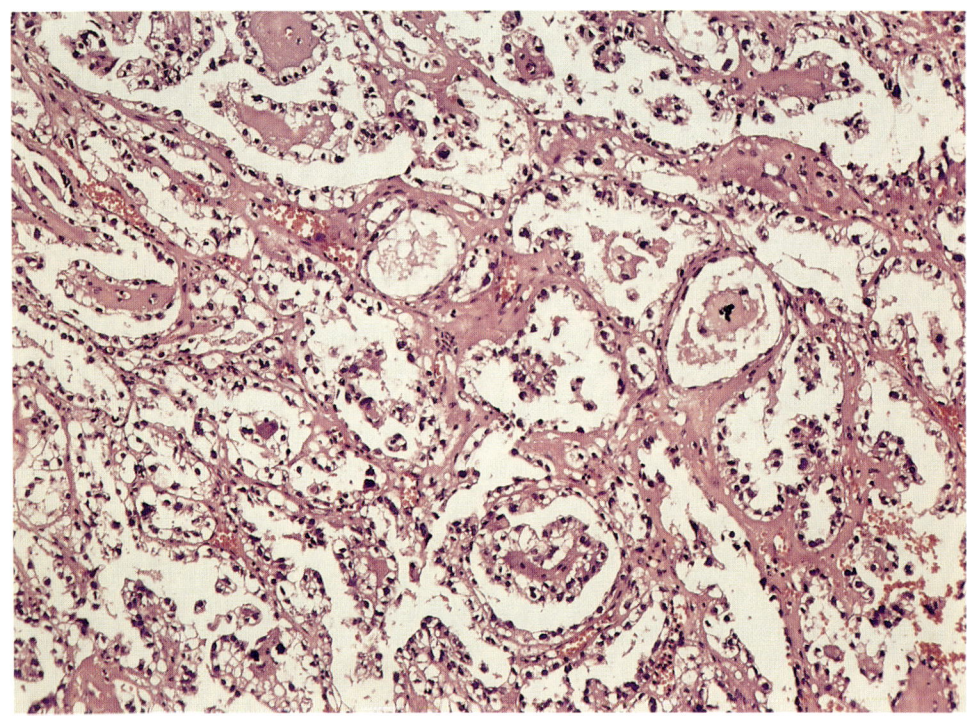

Fig. 181. Clear cell adenocarcinoma, glandular type. H & E

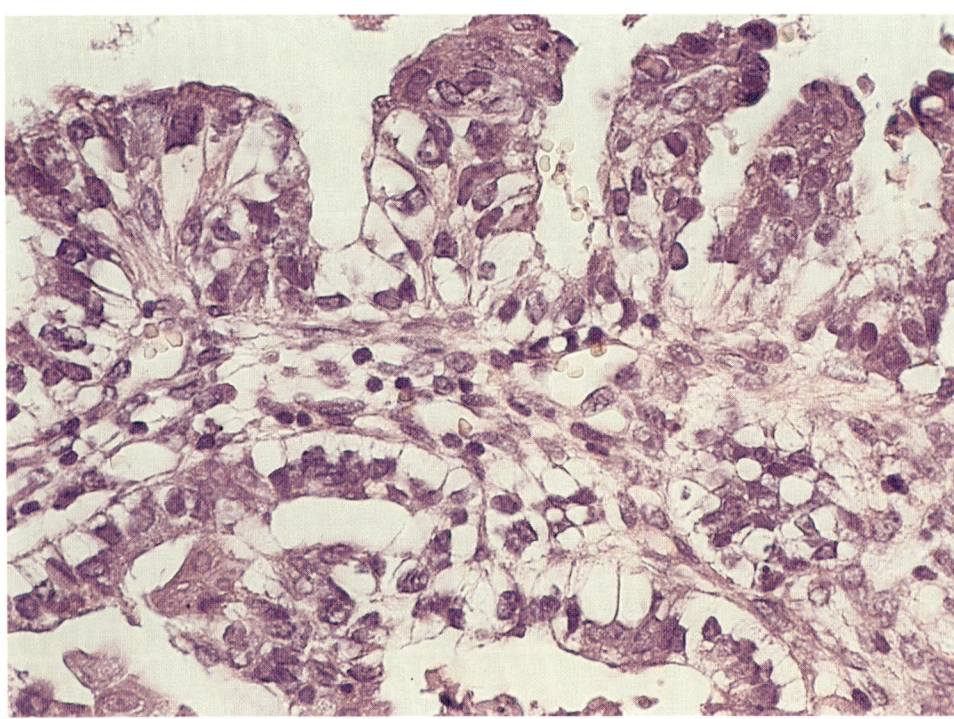

Fig. 182. Clear cell adenocarcinoma, glandular-papillary type. H & E

Clear Cell Adenocarcinoma

The clear cell adenocarcinoma (Figs. 181–183) may be mainly solid (Fig. 183) or glandular (Fig. 180) with papillary protrusions (Fig. 182), hobnail cells, and a glycogen-rich cytoplasm (Fig. 181). It resembles closely the clear cell carcinomas of ovarian, endometrial, or vaginal origin. The endocervical clear cell adenocarcinomas most likely arise from reserve cells, which presumably through faulty differentiation remain at an intermediary stage of development between incomplete keratinization and the secretion of mucins (Dallenbach-Hellweg and Lang 1990).

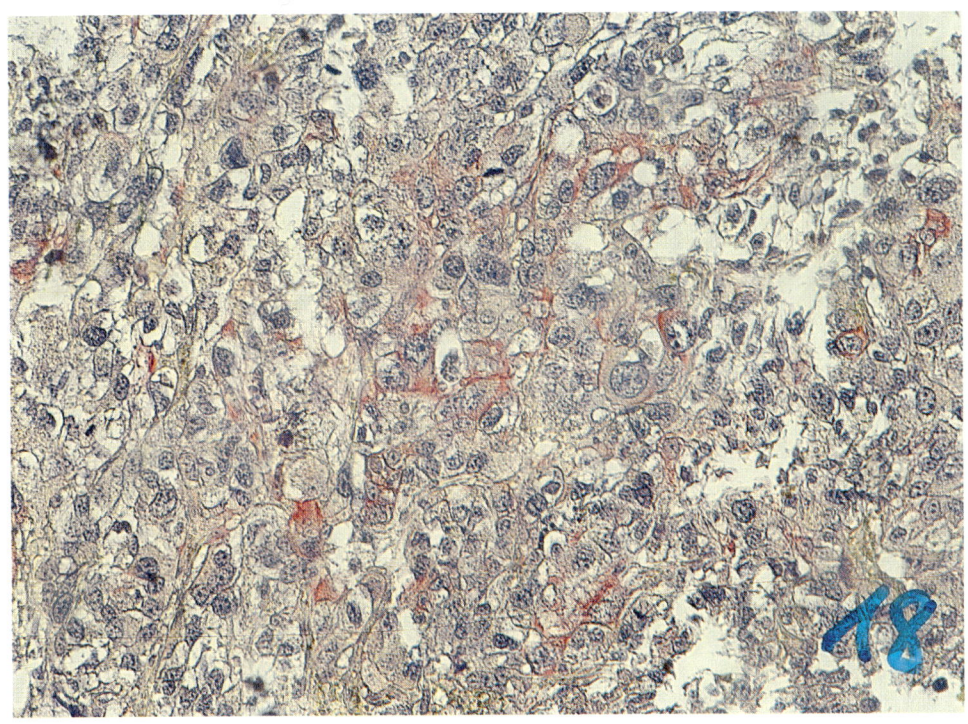

Fig. 183. Clear cell adenocarcinoma, solid type. Immunohistochemical reaction with anticytokeratin 18

Serous Papillary Carcinoma

The serous papillary carcinoma (Figs. 184, 185), too, closely resembles those originating in the ovaries and endometrium (Dallenbach-Hellweg and Poulsen 1985). It may also contain psammoma bodies.

Differential Diagnosis. Clear cell and serous papillary carcinomas can be distinguished from atypical microglandular endocervical hyperplasia in most cases by showing their positive reaction with anti-CEA; microglandular hyperplasia reacts negatively. Distinction from an Arias-Stella reaction should not be difficult, since that reaction is noninvasive and limited to the endocervical mucosa, and mitoses are rare or absent.

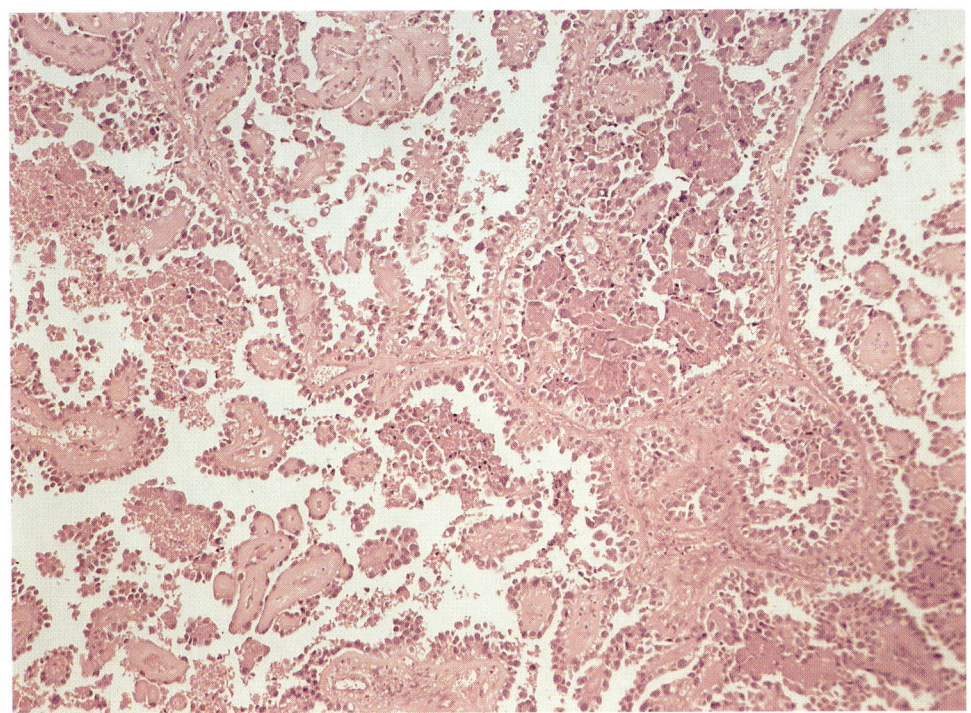

Fig. 184. Serous papillary carcinoma. H & E

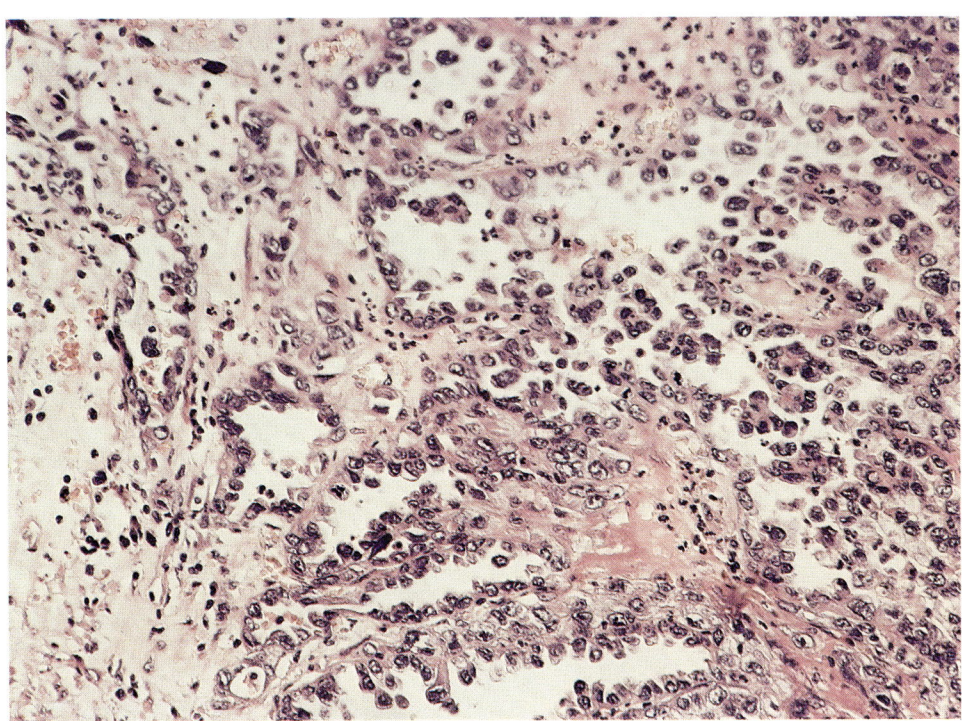

Fig. 185. Serous papillary carcinoma. H & E, higher magnification

Mesonephric Adenocarcinoma

The mesonephric adenocarcinoma (Figs. 186-190) is a rare cervical tumor (Mc Gee et al. 1962; Buntine 1979), representing approximately 3% of the adenocarcinomas of this location (Hart et al. 1972). Whereas the adenocarcinomas described above are of müllerian origin, this type is not. Reports in the literature about incidence are conflicting, since this tumor has been confused with other types, mainly with clear cell carcinomas. The true mesonephric adenocarcinoma is a well-defined tumor, which originates from remnants of the mesonephric duct in the lateral wall of the cervix. Hence it is localized deeper in the cervical wall than the other types of adenocarcinoma. It consists of very characteristic small, round glandular lumina lined by a low cuboid epithelium usually devoid of cytological atypia (Figs. 186-188).

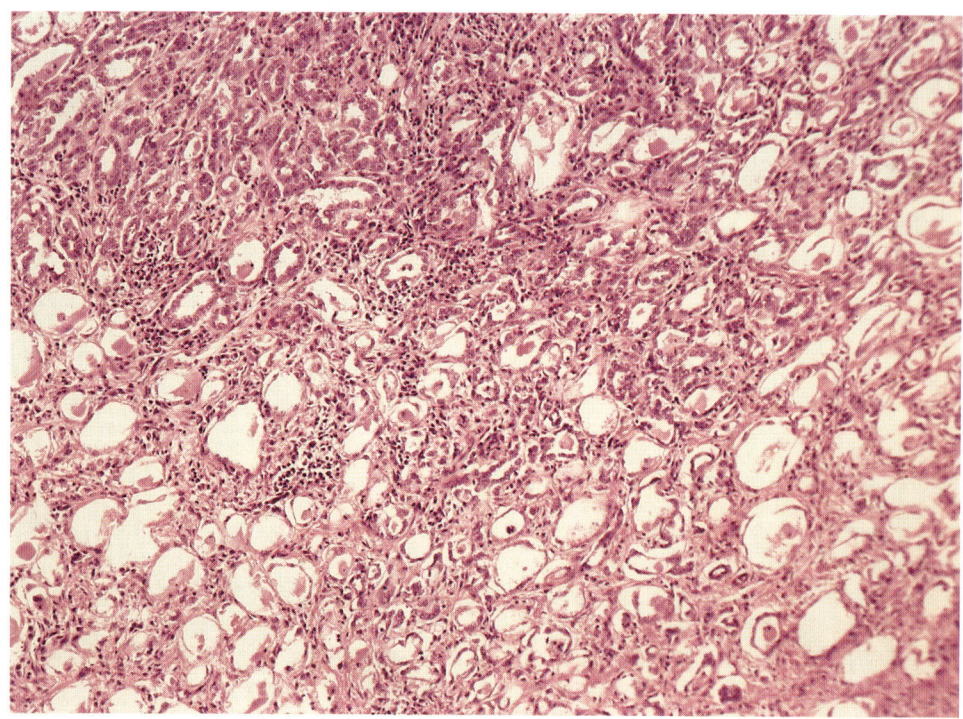

Fig. 186. Mesonephric adenocarcinoma. H & E

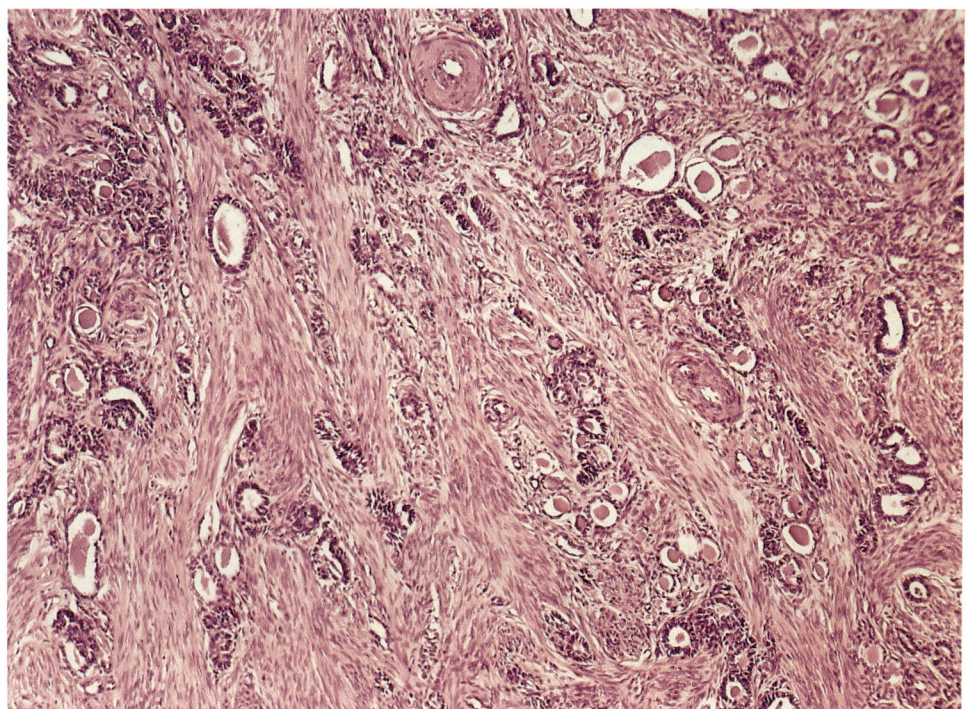

Fig. 187. Mesonephric adenocarcinoma. H & E

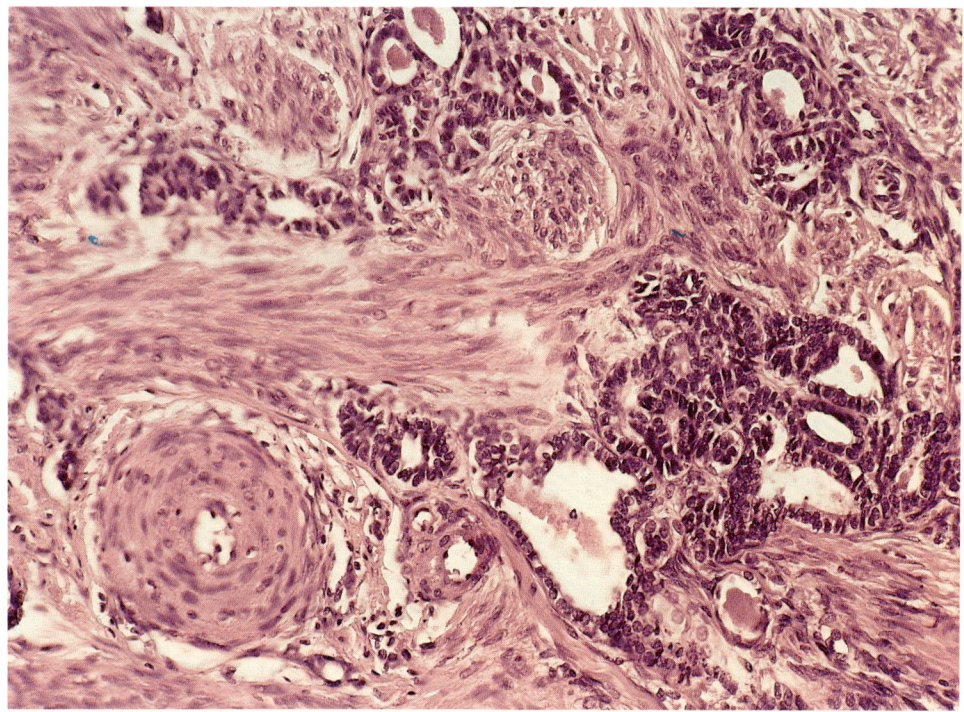

Fig. 188. Mesonephric adenocarcinoma. H & E, higher magnification

Mucin is absent in the sparse cytoplasm, but a small amount of PAS-positive material may be detected in the glandular lumina (Fig. 189). Solid strands of tumor cells may occasionally be seen between the small glands. Despite their bland appearance, the carcinomatous glands spread early and diffusely, invading all parts of the uterus. Both mesonephric hyperplasia and carcinoma have been observed more frequently during the past few years. They are often associated with microglandular hyperplasia of the endocervix or with in situ or invasive endocervical-type adenocarcinomas as well. Since the mesonephric ducts require testosterone for further development during ontogenesis, it has been suggested that an association exists between nortestosterone derivatives as components of oral contraceptives and an enhanced proliferation of mesonephric remnants in the cervix (Lang and Dallenbach-Hellweg 1990).

Differential Diagnosis. It is usually possible to distinguish mesonephric adenocarcinomas from endocervical and heterotopic müllerian type adenocarcinomas by the characteristic histological appearances of their carcinomatous glands alone. Important and distinct differences in their immunohistochemical reactions, however, assist in the differentiation: the mesonephric adenocarcinoma reacts consistently negatively with anti-CEA (Ayroud et al. 1985), but shows a weak expression of vimentin (Fig. 190) and a coexpression of cytokeratin 13, 8 and 18. Distinguishing it from florid mesonephric hyperplasia may be difficult, if not impossible, unless the whole uterus is available for examination.

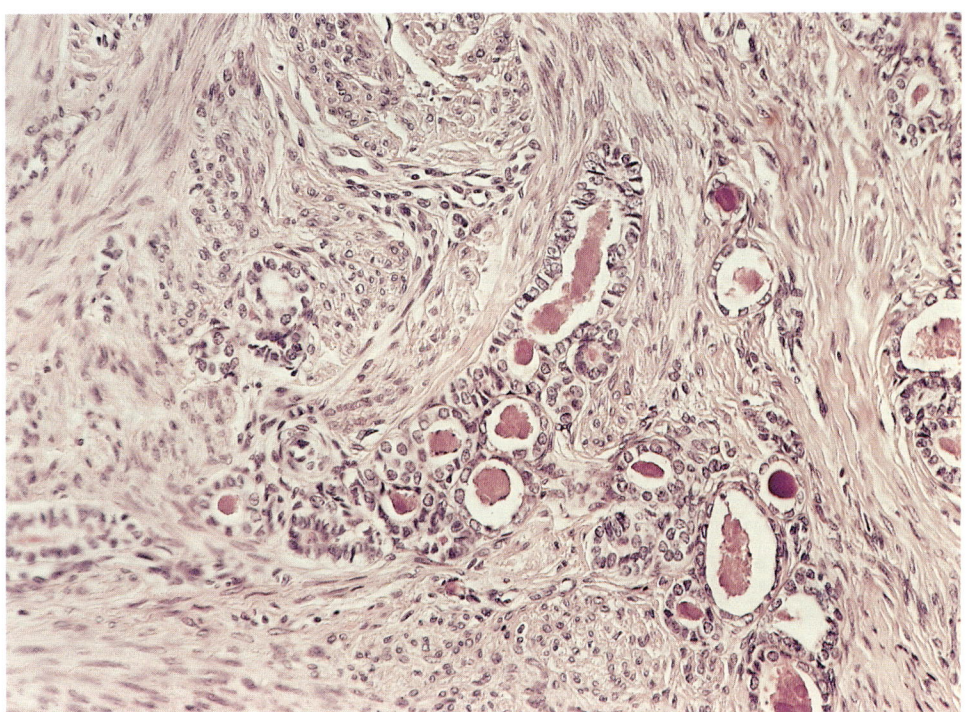

Fig. 189. Mesonephric adenocarcinoma. PAS reaction

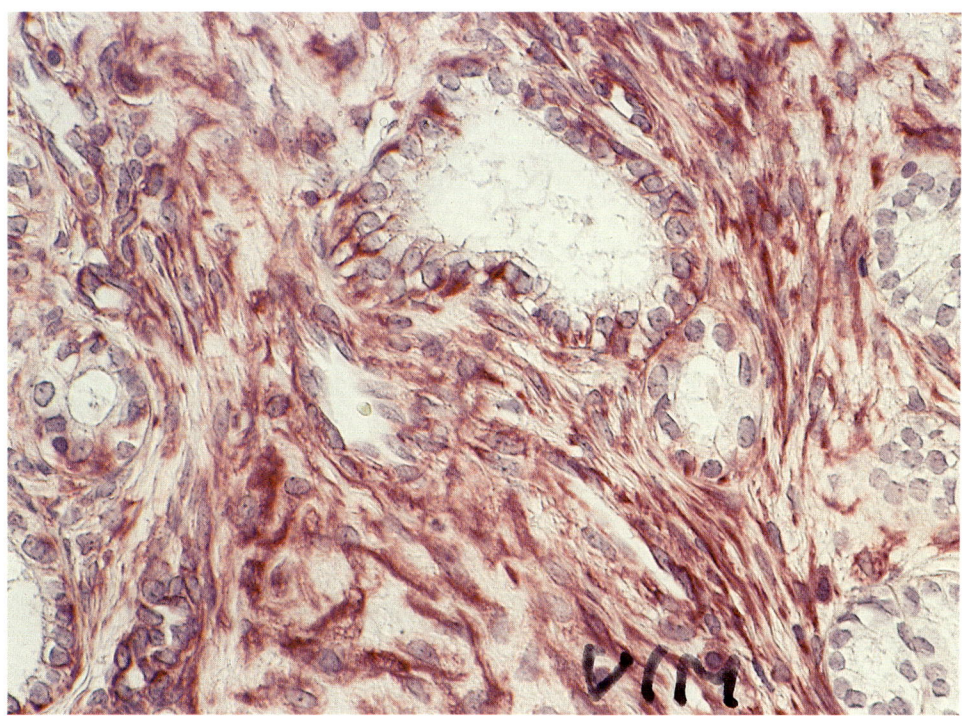

Fig. 190. Mesonephric adenocarcinoma. Immunohistochemical reaction with antivimentin

Mixed Type (Figs. 191-196)

Adenosquamous Carcinoma

The incidence of *adenosquamous carcinoma* (Figs. 191, 192) has significantly increased during the past few years, particularly in younger women (Adcock et al. 1982). Since it originates from the bipotential reserve cells, and since it is most frequently associated with HPV infection type 18 (Smotkin et al. 1986) or the equally frequent type 16 (Tase et al. 1988), this increase is explainable by hormonal overstimulation and the resulting increased susceptibility of the reserve cells already mentioned. Besides, the endogenous hormonal overstimulation during pregnancy may explain why 50% of all invasive cervical carcinomas in pregnant women are of the adenosquamous type (Glücksmann 1957). Furthermore, refined histological, immunohistochemical, and ultrastructural methods have helped to recognize mixed epithelial patterns more readily. For instance, using these new methods glassy cell carcinomas of the endocervix, characterized by large cells with abundant finely granular, ground-glass-type cytoplasm, prominent nuclei and lack of intercellular bridges and resembling clear cell carcinomas, have been recognized as poorly differentiated adenosquamous carcinomas with a very unfavorable prognosis (Richard et al. 1981; Ulbright and Gersell 1983; Tanaka et al. 1984; Wells and Brown 1986). Even in the moderately differentiated types of adenosquamous carcinomas, both glandular and squamous elements are intimately mixed (Fig. 192). Either keratinization (Fig. 191) or mucin formation (Fig. 192) may predominate.

Differential Diagnosis. Distinguishing an endocervical carcinoma from a primary adenosquamous carcinoma or adenoacanthoma of the endometrium is possible immunohistochemically. The endocervical carcinomas are nearly always positive for CEA and always negative for vimentin.

Mucoepidermoid Carcinoma

The mucoepidermoid carcinoma (Figs. 193-196) differs from the adenosquamous carcinoma by its mono- or multicellular production of mucin within solid strands of squamoid cells. Mono- or multicellular keratinization is often evident in cells neighboring mucin-secreting cells (Figs. 195, 196). Histogenetically, these carcinomas also originate from bipotential reserve cells that are intermixed (Figs. 193, 194). In poorly differentiated forms of mucoepidermoid carcinoma, mucin production may be discrete and only detectable when a PAS reaction is used. With this stain, it readily becomes apparent that the percentage of mucin-secreting squamous carcinomas is surprisingly high (Hellweg 1957; Benda et al. 1985).

Differential Diagnosis. The distinction between mucoepidermoid (mixed) and squamous carcinomas is of clinical importance, since mixed carcinomas metastasize to pelvic lymph nodes in 30% of the patients compared with 7% in nonmucin-producing carcinomas (Benda et al. 1985). In comparison, the metastatic rate to pelvic lymph nodes for pure adenocarcinomas is said to be about 15%. In spite of this, the prognosis in patients with adenocarcinomas is even worse than in those with mixed mucin-producing tumors, apparently because of the early vascular invasion of the adenocarcinomas.

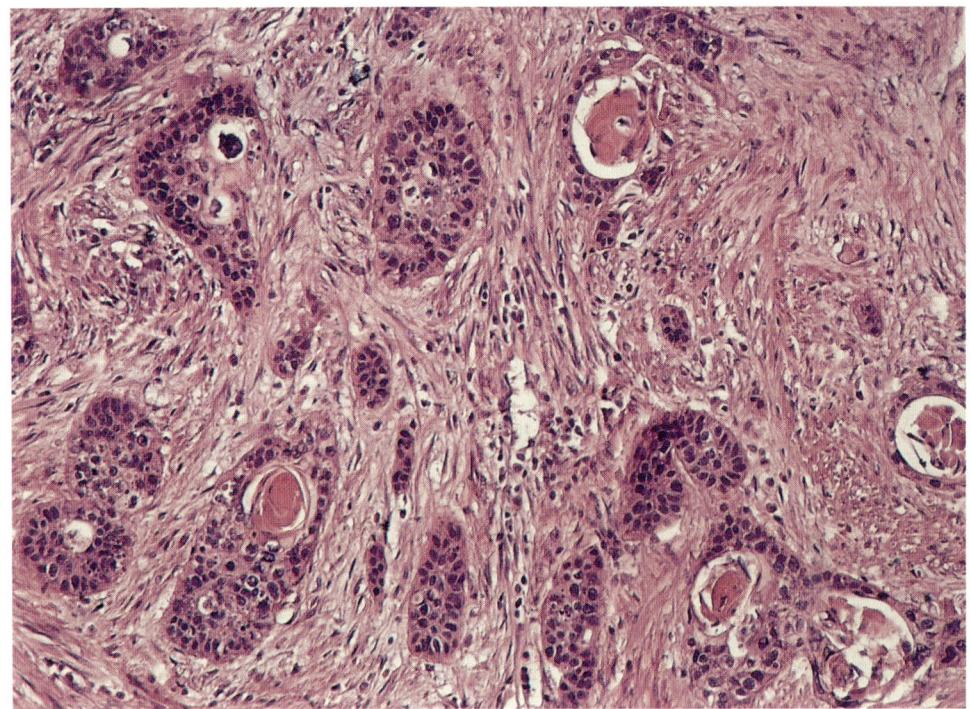

Fig. 191. Adenosquamous carcinoma, with formation of keratin pearls. H & E

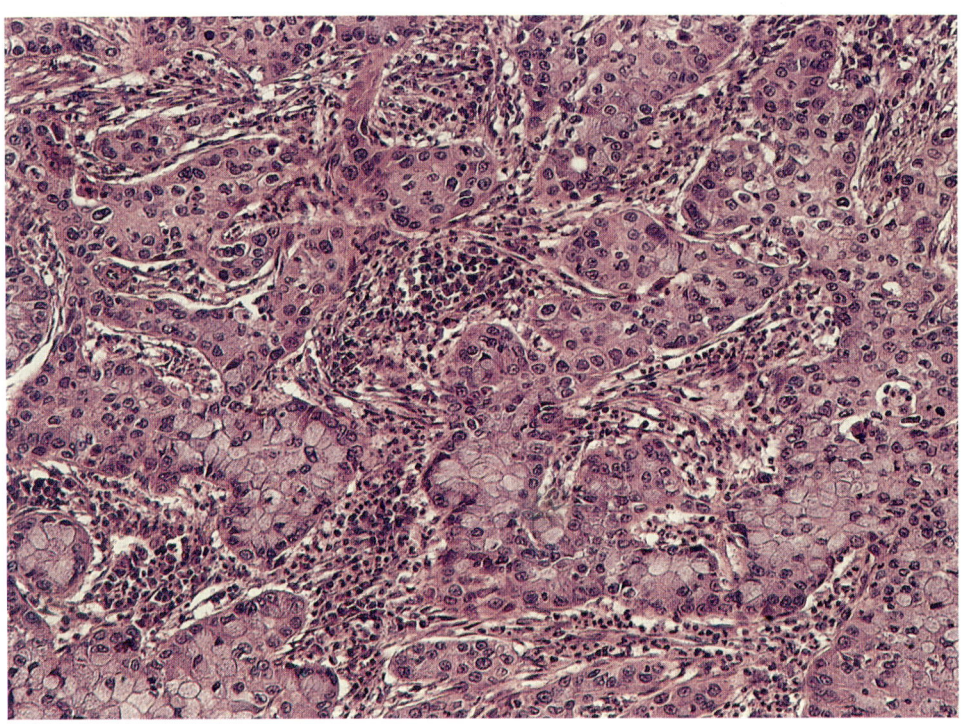

Fig. 192. Adenosquamous carcinoma, with predominant mucinous differentiation. H & E

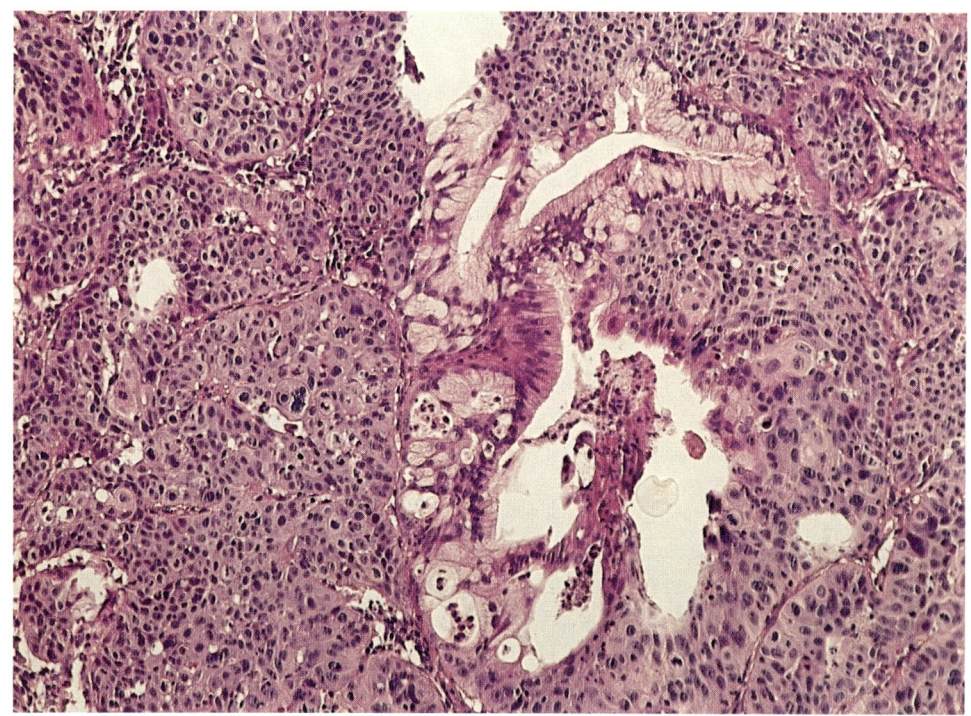

Fig. 193. Mucoepidermoid carcinoma. H & E

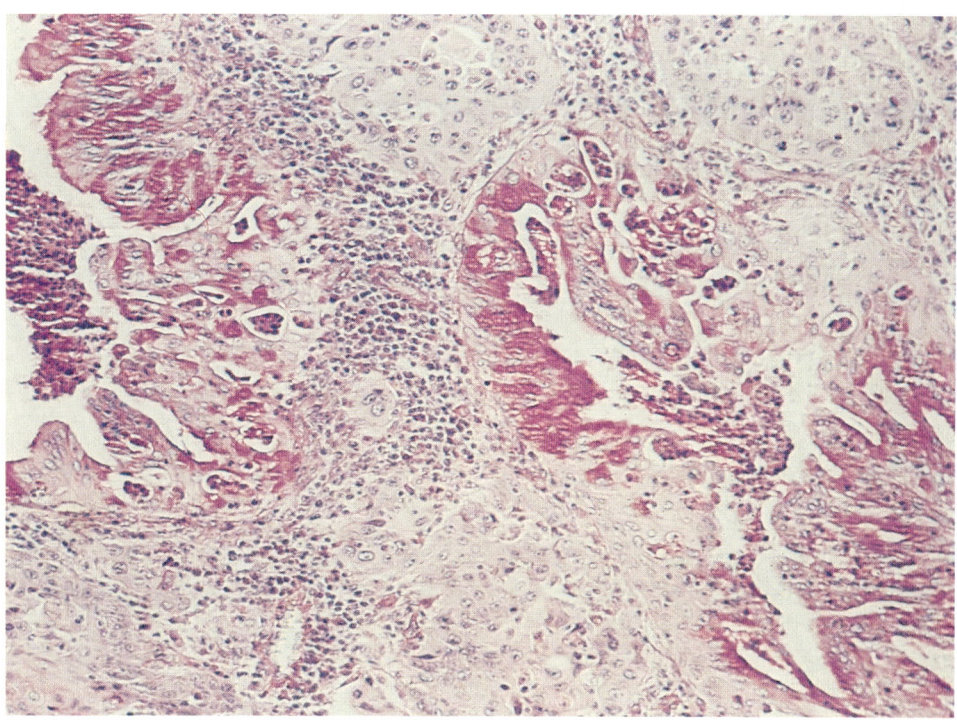

Fig. 194. Mucoepidermoid carcinoma. PAS reaction

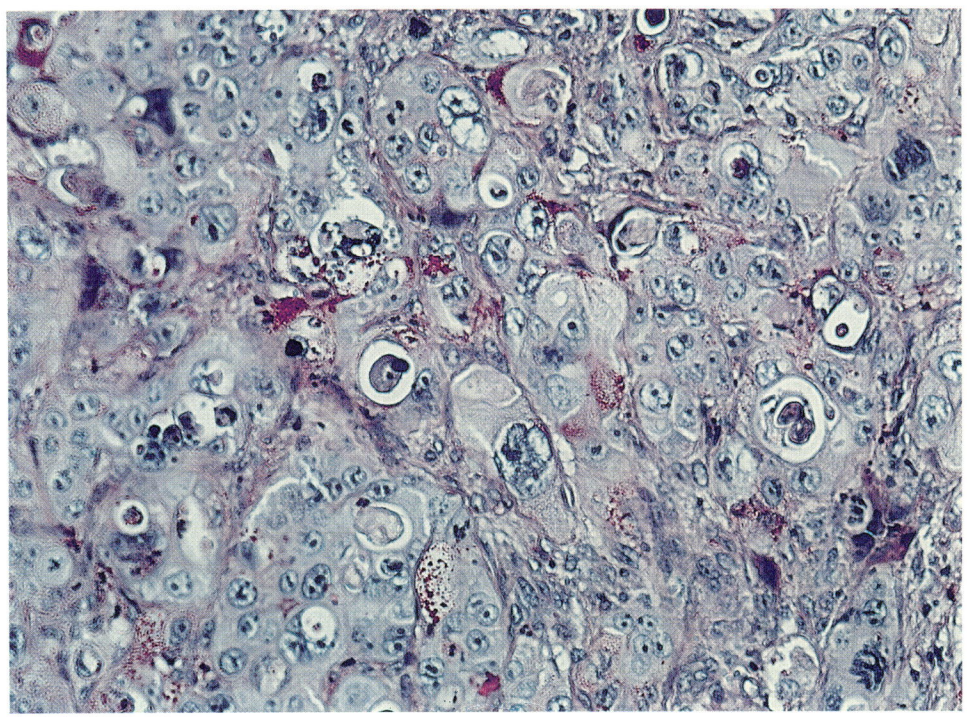

Fig. 195. Mucoepidermoid carcinoma, monocellular mucin formation. PAS reaction

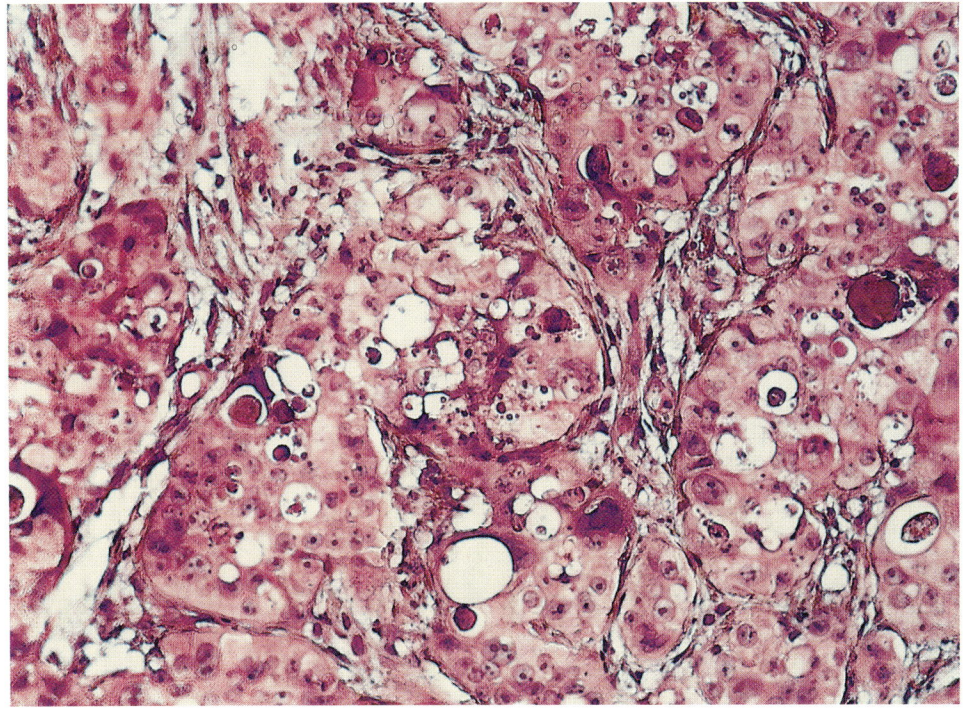

Fig. 196. Mucoepidermoid carcinoma, monocellular keratinization. Phloxine-tartrazine stain

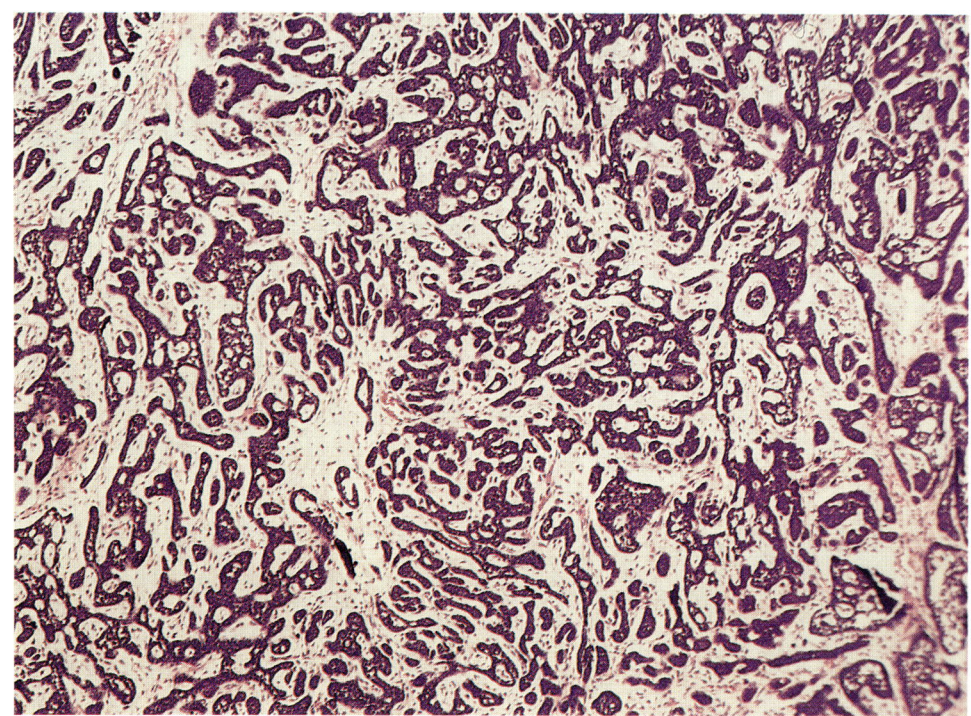

Fig. 197. Adenoid cystic carcinoma. H & E

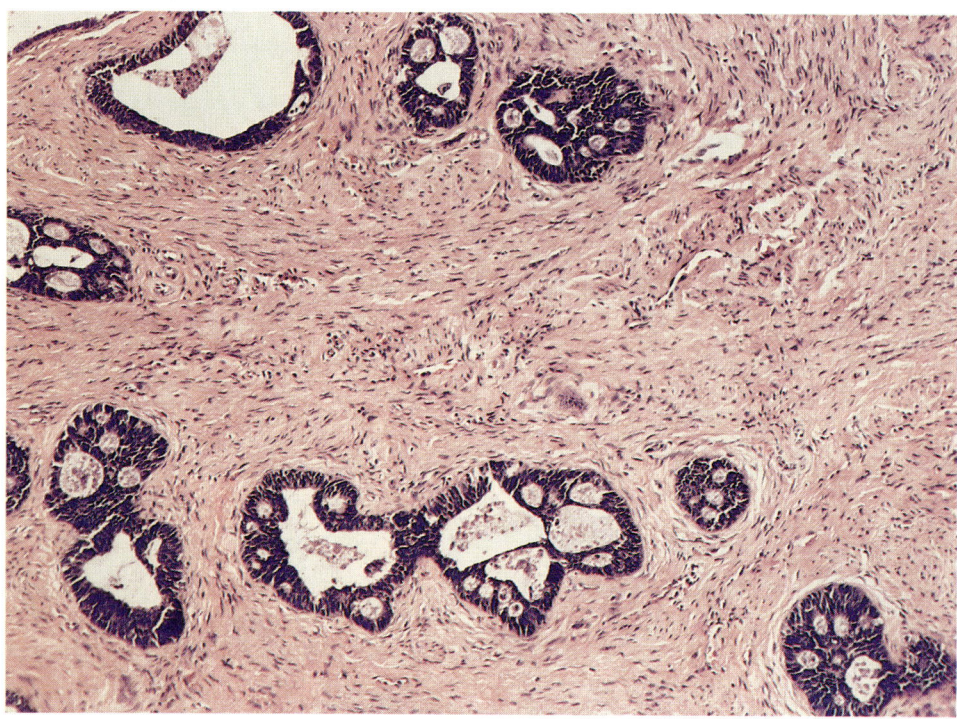

Fig. 198. Adenoid cystic carcinoma. H & E, higher magnification

Adenoid Type (Figs. 197-200)

Adenoid Cystic Carcinoma

The adenoid cystic carcinoma (Figs. 197-199) is characterized by a cribriform or cylindromatous pattern. It is composed of fairly uniform, small basaloid cells with scanty cytoplasm and rounded or angulated hyperchromatic nuclei. These cells form small branching (Fig. 197) or larger strands (Fig. 199), surround small or larger cysts (Fig. 198), or form small acini filled with a hyaline or basement membrane-like material rich in acid mucopolysacharides. This tumor is often associated with foci of squamous cell or adenocarcinoma. Adenoid cystic carcinomas show early lymphatic invasion and are more aggressive than most cervical adenocarcinomas (Hoskins et al. 1979).

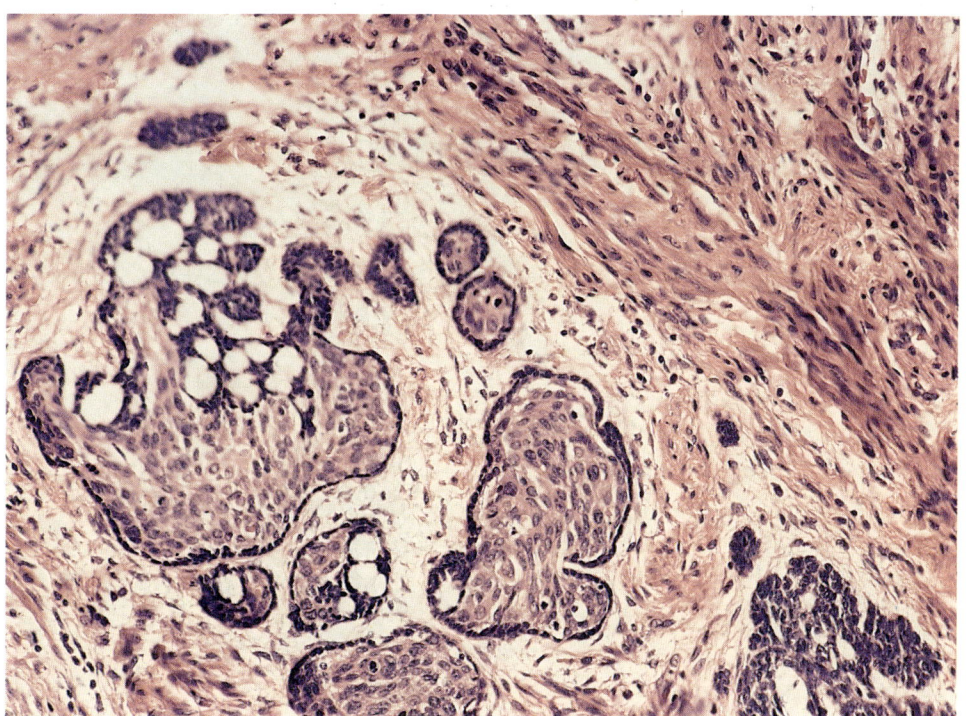

Fig. 199. Adenoid cystic carcinoma, with foci of squamoid differentiation. H & E, higher magnification

Adenoid Basal Carcinoma

The adenoid basal carcinoma (Fig. 200) must be differentiated from the adenoid cystic carcinoma. It consists of small, round to oval branching nests of cells, resembling those of basal cell carcinoma of the skin, with palisading of the peripheral cell layers. There are no or only rare cystic pseudoglands. The tumor cells are small and uniform, with rounded hyperchromatic nuclei in scanty cytoplasm. Mitoses are infrequent.

Adenoid cystic and adenoid basal carcinoma have a similar cytoskeleton of intermediate filaments, which indicates they apparently arise from pluripotent reserve cells of the endocervix (Ferry and Scully 1988).

Differential Diagnosis. It is important to distinguish adenoid basal from adenoid cystic carcinoma because a patient with adenoid basal carcinoma has a much more favorable prognosis; only a simple hysterectomy is required (van Dinh and Woodruff 1985). Histological differentiation is possible by applying the different architectural and cytological features described above.

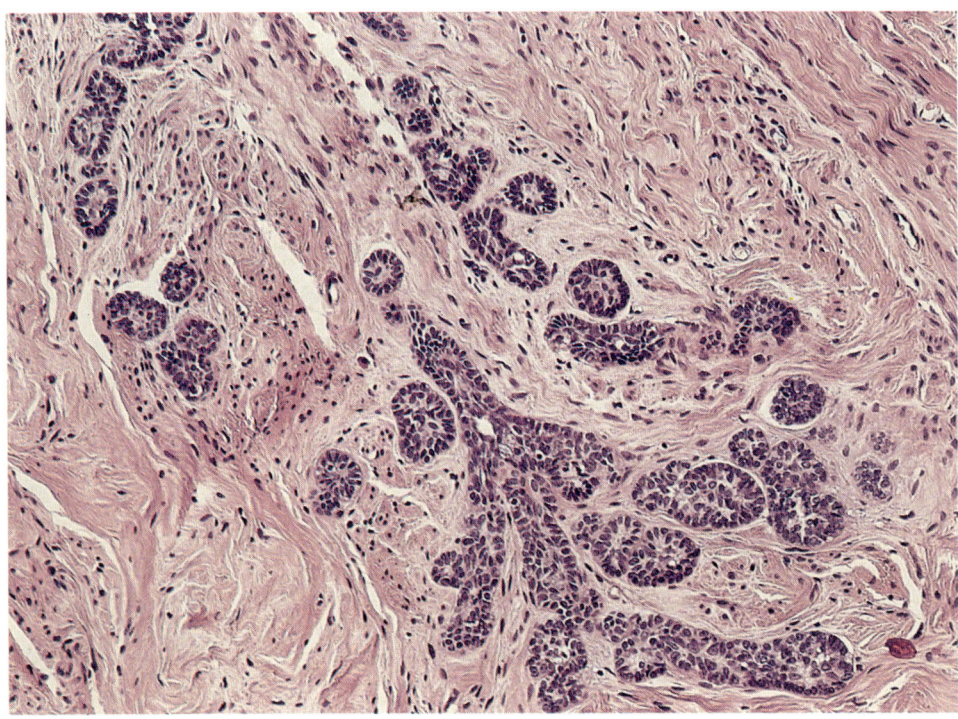

Fig. 200. Adenoid basal carcinoma. H & E

Heterotopic Type (Figs. 201-205)

Neuroendocrine Carcinomas

Neuroendocrine carcinomas most likely develop from neuroendocrine cells occurring in the normal endocervix (Scully et al. 1984; Fetissof et al. 1985), or from stimulated multipotential precursor cells of the endocervical epithelium undergoing neuroendocrine metaplasia and hyerplasia (Chan et al. 1989). They may be fairly well differentiated (carcinoids) or poorly differentiated (small cell carcinomas).

Carcinoid tumors of the cervix are thought to originate from endocervical argyrophil cells. The tumors consist of rather uniform, small, round or ovoid cells growing in solid sheets, small lobules, or trabeculae. Occasionally, flattened cells line glandlike, mucin-containing microcysts. The slightly elongated nuclei of the tumor cells have a coarse chromatin pattern. Mitoses are frequent. Vascular invasion is often obvious, giving evidence of the malignant behavior of these tumors.

Small cell carcinomas of neuroendocrine origin (Fig. 201) are considered to be the poorly differentiated variety of carcinoid tumors, resembling small cell carcinomas of the lung. The cells of these tumors are spindle shaped. Their scanty cytoplasm contains argyrophilic neurosecretory granules, demonstrable by the Grimelius stain (Yamasaki et al. 1984), S100, or by specific neuroendocrine markers such as neuron-specific enolase (NSE), chromogranin, and synaptophysin (Hachitanda et al. 1989). Mitoses are numerous.

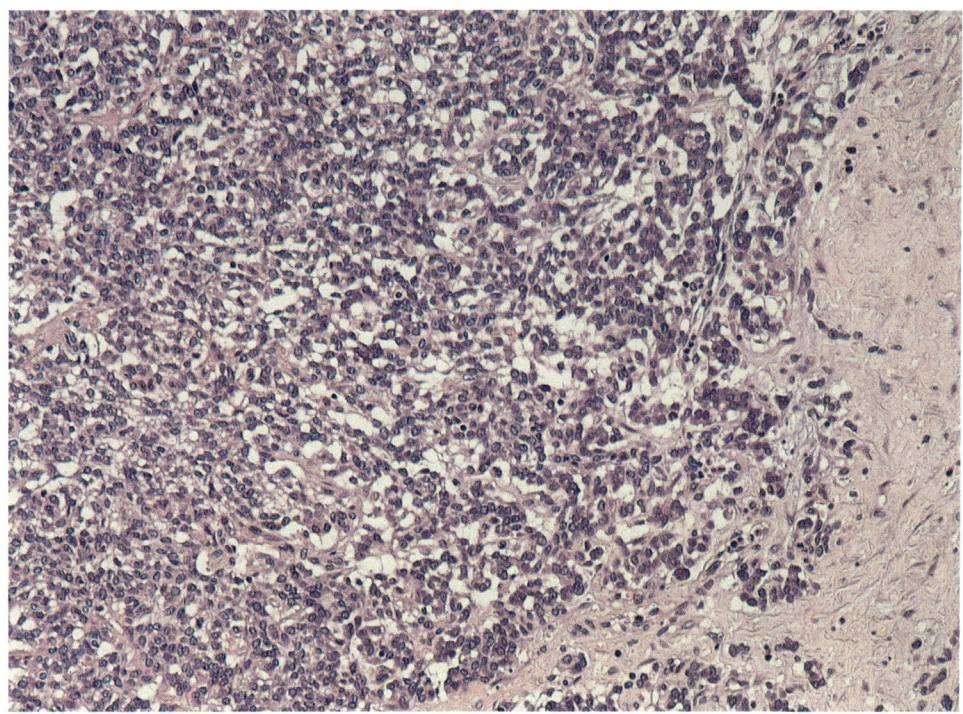

Fig. 201. Neuroendocrine (small cell) carcinoma. H & E

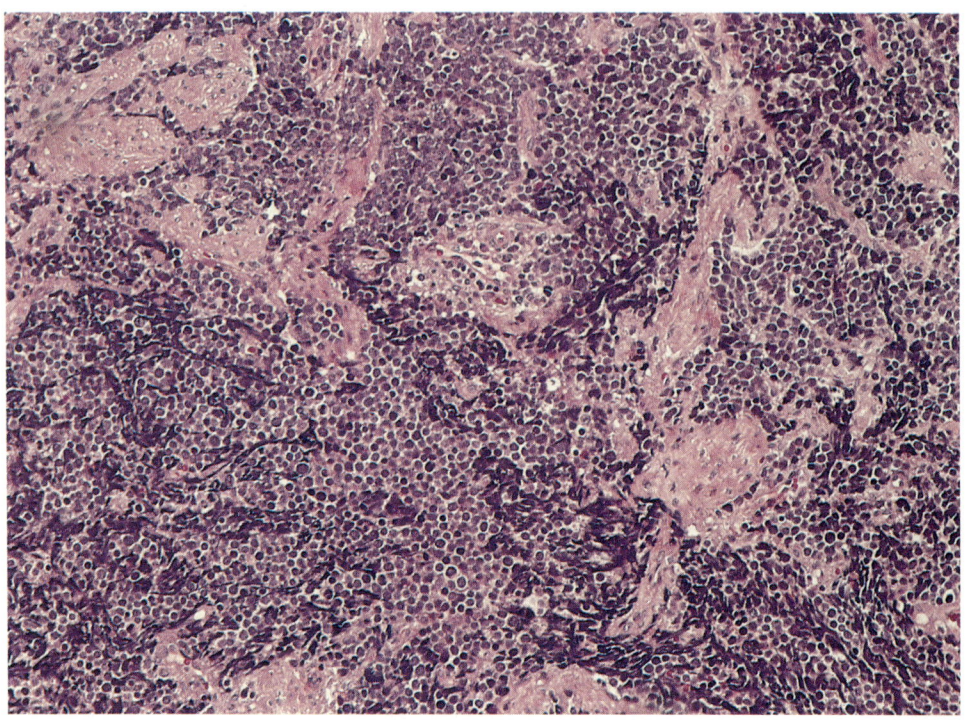

Fig. 202. Embryonal neuroblastoma (primitive neuroectodermal tumor). H & E

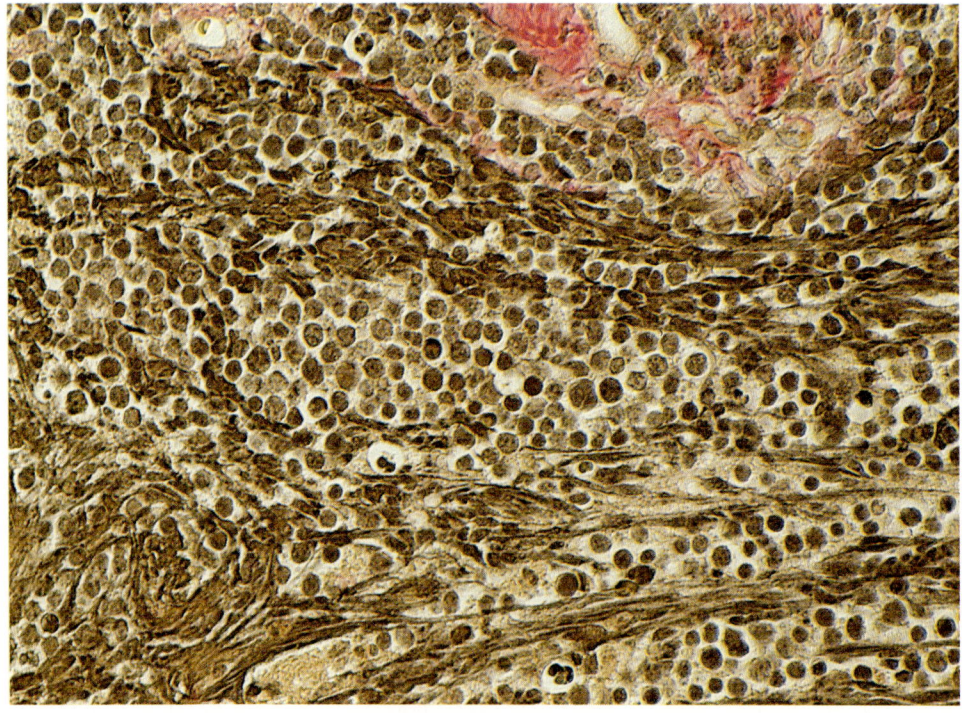

Fig. 203. Embryonal neuroblastoma (primitive neuroectodermal tumor). Van Gieson's stain

Neurogenic Tumors

Neuroblastomas (Figs. 202-204) of the cervix are very rare. We observed a very undifferentiated cervical tumor in a 29-year-old woman. The solid, round, and small-celled tumor was negative with most of the markers for intracytoplasmatic intermediate filaments, including cytokeratins, S100, and CEA, but showed a distinct immunohistochemical reaction for NSE and was classified as *embryonal neuroblastoma* (primitive neuroectodermal tumor).

Differential Diagnosis. Carcinoid tumors can be distinguished from adenosquamous carcinomas by detecting neuroendocrine granules in the carcinoid cells (Grimelius stain). Small cell neuroendocrine carcinomas must be differentiated from nonendocrine, poorly differentiated small cell carcinomas of the reserve cell type, with which they have often been confused (Groben et al. 1985), although the small cell carcinomas lack neuroendocrine differentiation (Fujii et al. 1986). With the aid of immunohistochemistry, it has become obvious that not all small cell carcinomas of the cervix are of neuroendocrine origin (Ulich et al. 1986; Ueda et al. 1989). Since most neuroendocrine carcinomas are also positive for CEA and cytokeratin (Gersell et al. 1988) a distinction from undifferentiated reserve cell carcinomas is only possible with markers for neurosecretory granules.

Neuroblastomas can be distinguished from small cell carcimomas and from neuroendocrine tumors by their negative reaction for cytokeratins, CEA, and S-100. Hence, one should not be satisfied in saying an undifferentiated tumor is unclassifiable before attempting to detect specific intermediate filaments with modern immunohistochemical methods.

In general, patients with neuroendocrine tumors of the cervix seem to have a poor prognosis, regardless of type (Walker et al. 1988). According to recent observations, however, patients with tumors of neural crest origin (neuroendocrine carcinomas), which reacted positively with S-100 had a much more fa-

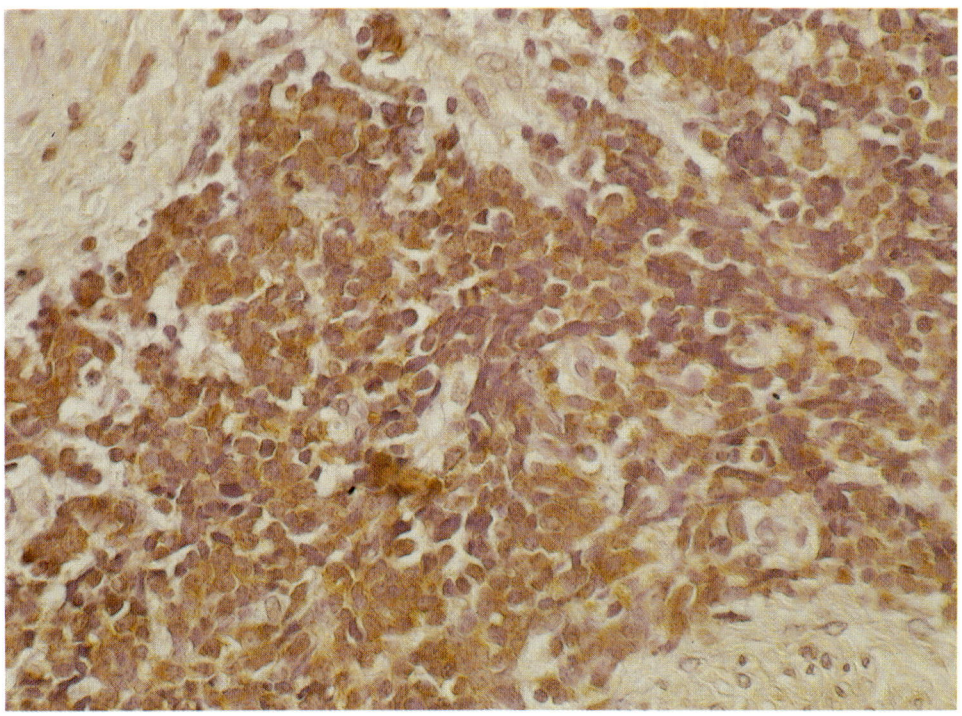

Fig. 204. Embryonal neuroblastoma (primitive neuroectodermal tumor). Immunohistochemical reaction with NSE

vorable prognosis than those with S-100 negative neuroblastic tumors (Aoyama et al. 1990). By collecting such observations differences in clinical behaviour between small cell carcinomas of neuroendocrine or reserve cell origin and neurogenic tumors may become obvious.

Malignant Melanoma

It is extremely rare for the cervix to be the primary tumor site for malignant melanoma (Fig. 205). Only a few cases have been reported in the literature (Hall et al. 1980) and recently summarized (Holmquist and Torres 1988). Histogenetically, the tumor apparently arises from neural elements. Occasional melanocytes can be found in the normal ectocervical epithelium (Stegner 1959). As in the skin, or elsewhere, the tumor is composed of pleomorphic round to spindle-shaped cells containing varying amounts of fine melanin pigment (Fig. 205). The tumor cells spread diffusely throughout the cervix, while the covering ectocervical epithelium usually remains intact. When melanin pigment is absent or very scanty, it is possible to distinguish the melanoma from undifferentiated carcinomas or sarcomas with the S-100 reaction, which is consistently positive in malignant melanoma.

Mesenchymal Tumors (Figs. 206–209)

Primary mesenchymal tumors of the cervix are rare compared with their counterparts in the uterine corpus with which they are structurally identical. *Leiomyosarcomas* (Fig. 206) consist of pleomorphic myoblasts with polyploid nuclei. *Rhabdomyosarcomas* and *chondrosarcomas* (Fig. 207) may occur in adults in the pure form or as part of a mesodermal mixed tumor (Fig. 213). The same holds true for *osteosarcoma* (Bloch et al. 1988) and *angiosarcoma*. The primary occurrence of an alveolar soft part sarcoma in the uterine cervix is extremely rare (Flint et al. 1985).

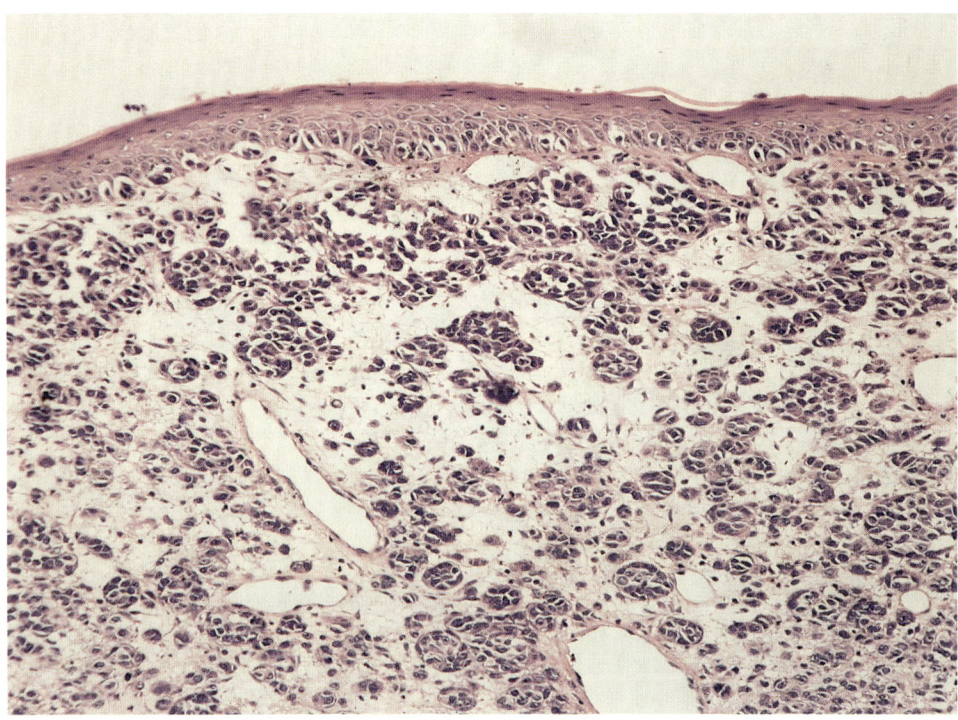

Fig. 205. Malignant melanoma. H & E

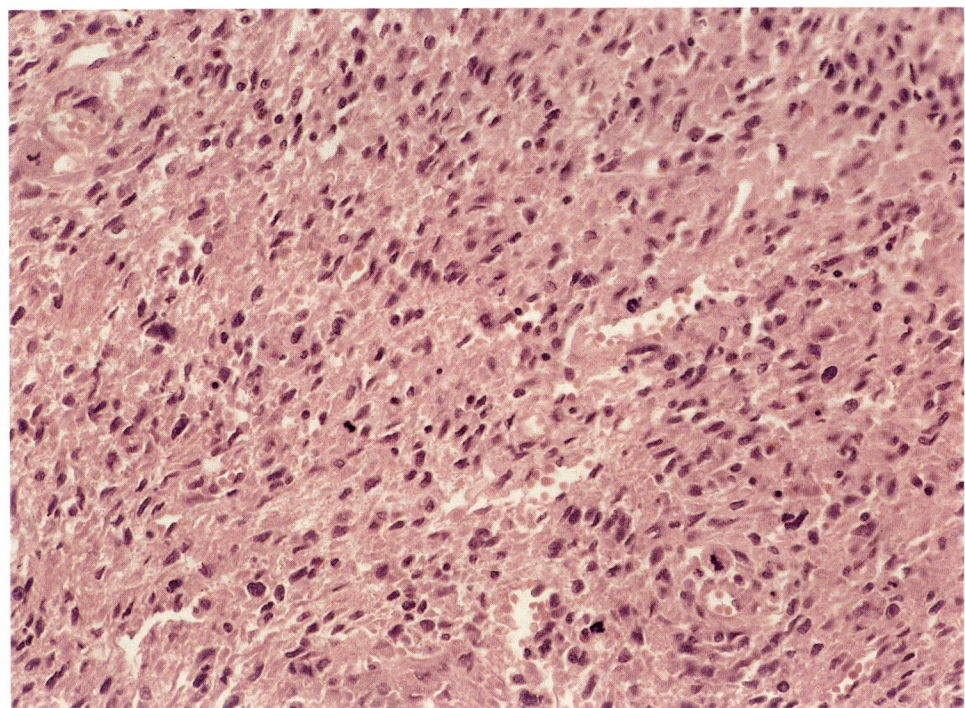

Fig. 206. Leiomyosarcoma. H & E

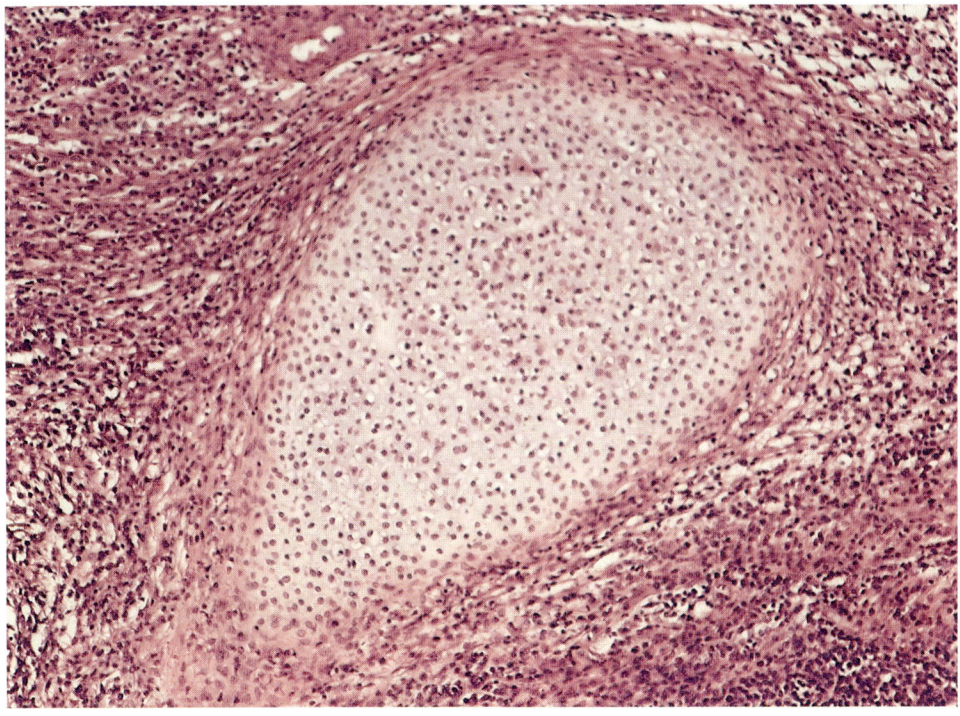

Fig. 207. Chondrosarcoma. H & E

Malignant lymphomas (Fig. 208) rarely occur in the cervix, either as nodular or diffuse lymphomas. Lesions with large cleaved cells are more often localized and have a better prognosis than large or small noncleaved and immunoblastic types (Harris and Scully 1984).

Differential Diagnosis. It is clinically important to distinguish lymphomas from undifferentiated small or large cell carcinomas, since malignant lymphomas may be treated successfully with irradiation (Komaki et al. 1984). Further subclassification of lymphomas permits ever more precise recommendations for therapy (Friederike Dallenbach, personal communication). This distinction is possible immunohistochemically with specific markers for lymphogenic cells, e.g., L 26 which is a B cell marker (Fig. 209). – Distinguishing malignant lymphoma from benign lymphoma-like lesions may be difficult (Young et al. 1985). Surface ulcerations and mixed infiltrates of acute inflammatory cells and plasma cells are rarely seen in lymphomas, whereas deep extension into the cervix and cellular monomorphism are usually absent in benign inflammatory conditions.

Granulocytic sarcoma of the cervix is an extremely rare local tumorous manifestation and precursor of myelogenous leukemia (Abeler et al. 1983; Banik et al. 1989). Its differentiation from malignant lymphoma or small cell carcinoma may be impossible in routine histological sections. Special stains, like the antilysozyme immunoperoxidase method, are useful.

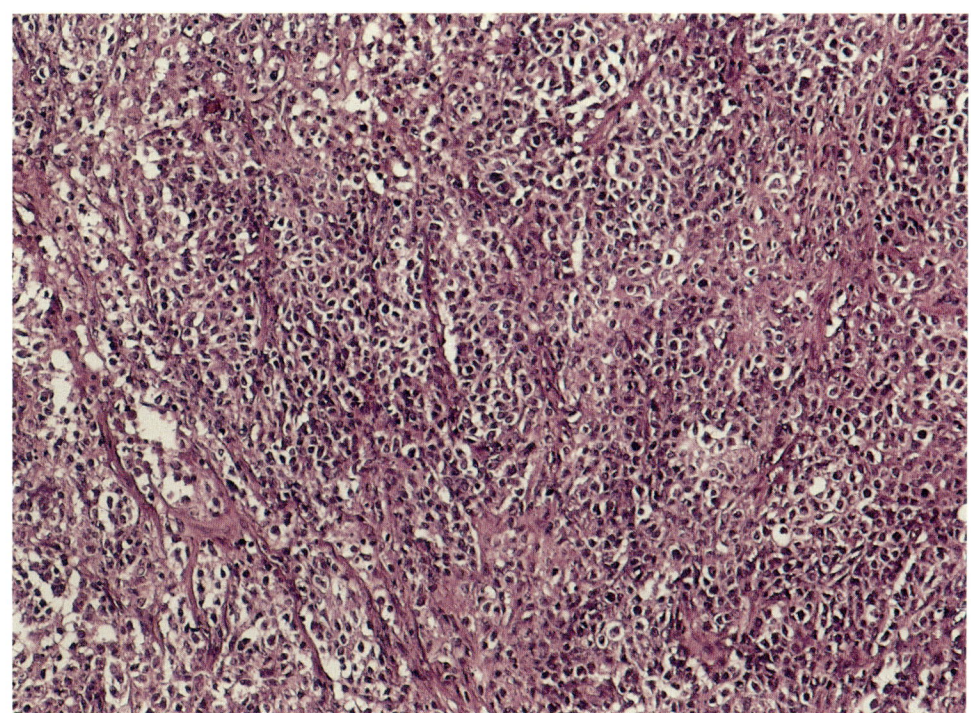

Fig. 208. Malignant B cell non-Hodgkin-lymphoma, multilobulated centroblastic type. H & E

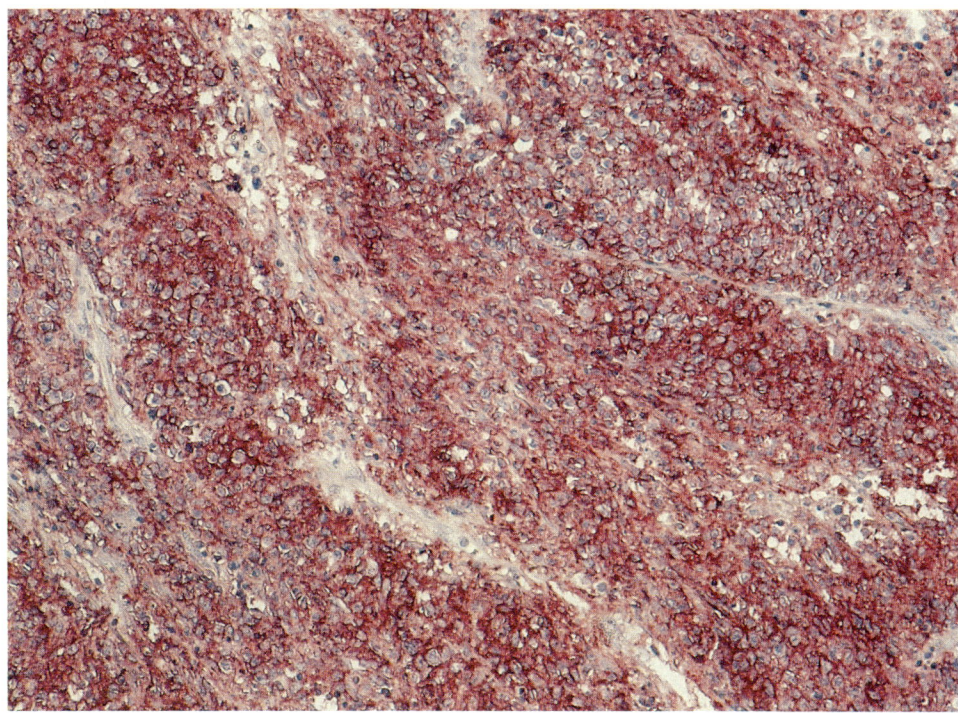

Fig. 209. Malignant non-Hodgkin-lymphoma, B cell type. Immunohistochemical reaction with L 26

Mesodermal Mixed Tumors
(Figs. 210–220)

Carcinosarcomas (Figs. 210, 211) and *malignant müllerian mixed tumors* (Figs. 212–214) are identical to and often part of the corresponding tumors of the uterine corpus. Carcinosarcomas consist of carcinomatous glands of endometrial, mucinous, or occasionally clear cell-type, and sarcomatous fibroblasts or stromal cells. The malignant müllerian mixed tumors, on the other hand, are composed of heterologous epithelial and mesenchymal elements, and may show a great variety of structures. The sarcomatous component, in particular, may be very pleomorphic, forming rhabdomyoblasts (Fig. 212), chondroblasts (Fig. 213), or osteoblasts (Fig. 214). When large enough sections are available for study, the recognition of a malignant müllerian mixed tumor is no problem.

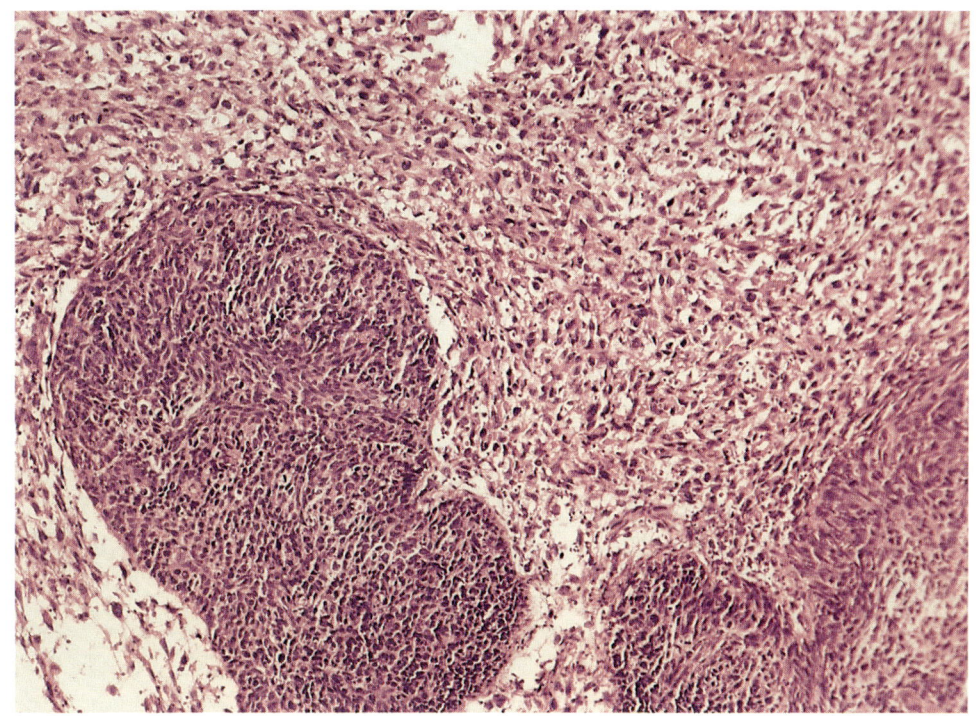

Fig. 210. Carcinosarcoma with solid epithelial nests. H & E

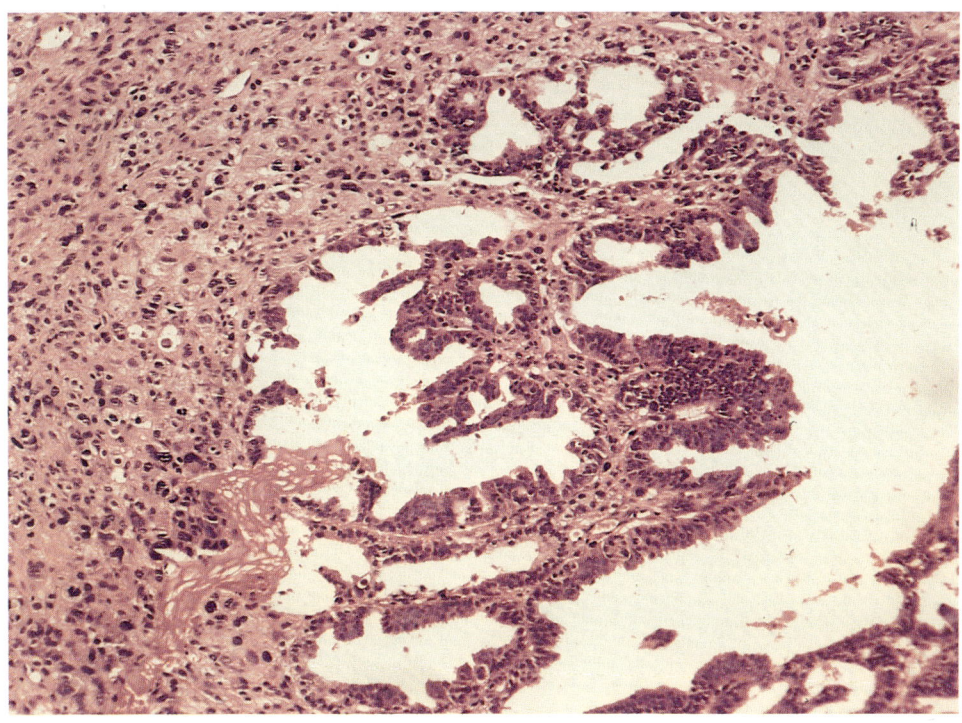

Fig. 211. Carcinosarcoma with gland formation. H & E

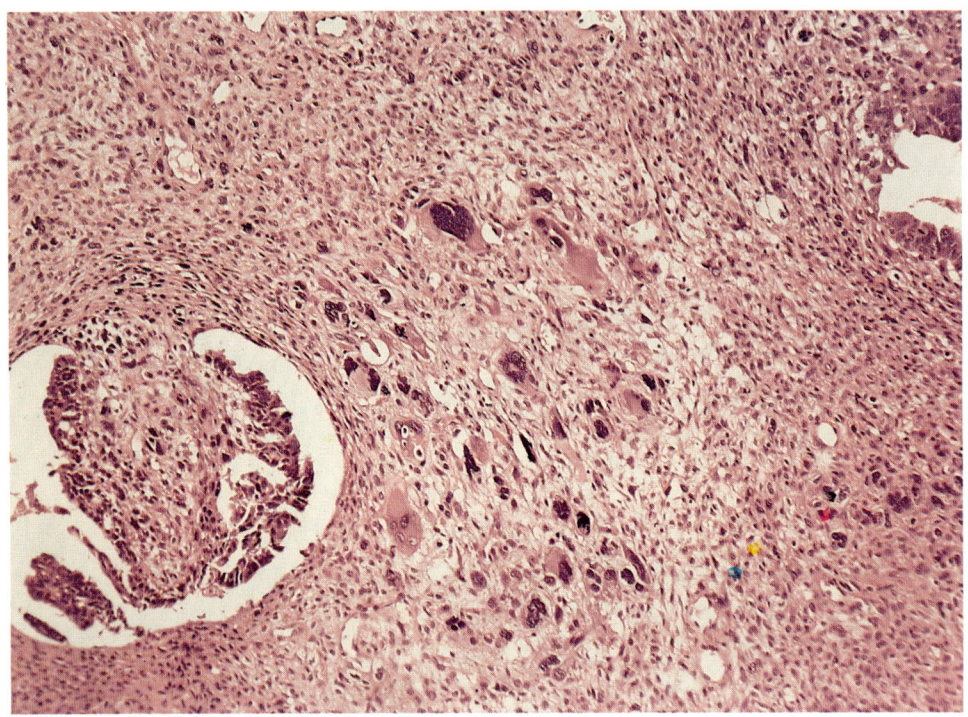

Fig. 212. Malignant müllerian mixed tumor, with rhabdomyoblasts. H & E

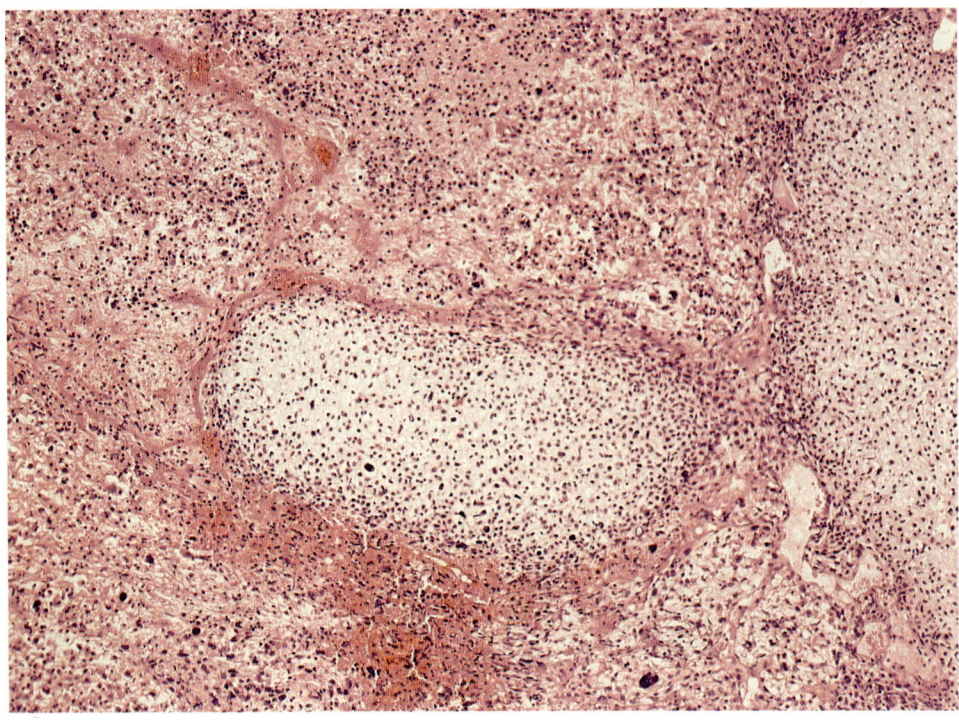

Fig. 213. Malignant müllerian mixed tumor, with chondroblasts. H & E

The *müllerian adenosarcoma* (Figs. 215, 216) usually arises from the endometrium, but occasionally from the endocervix. It consists of sarcomatous endocervical stromal cells and fibroblasts focally intermingled with rhabdomyoblasts. The mitotic activity is moderate (Clement and Scully 1974; Zaloudek and Norris 1981). Round concentric hypercellular foci form perivascular nodules and periglandular cuffs. (Fig. 215). A few slitlike remnants of benign endocervical glands may be found surrounded by compact sarcoma cells. Long invaginations of the endocervical surface epithelium may produce fingerlike protrusions at the tumor periphery. Adult women with adenosarcoma have a more favorable prognosis than those with other types of sarcoma.

Differential Diagnosis. Distinguishing carcinosarcoma from malignant müllerian mixed tumor is possible by carefully evaluating the epithelial components. In the müllerian adenosarcoma, there are no carcinomatous cells; only benign glandular structures may be seen.

The *embryonal rhabdomyosarcoma* (*Sarcoma botryoides;* Figs. 217-220) has its peak incidence in young girls and adolescents (Brand et al. 1987). On gross examination, its grape-like protrusions may grow beyond the external cervical os and protrude into the vagina. Microscopically, it consists of immature rhabdomyoblasts of the embryonal type, which occasionally may be mature enough to form cross striations (Fig. 220). Cords of glandlike structures of carcinomatous cells may be found among the sarcomatous elements; mitoses are frequent. Prognosis is much less favorable than it is for adult women with adenosarcoma.

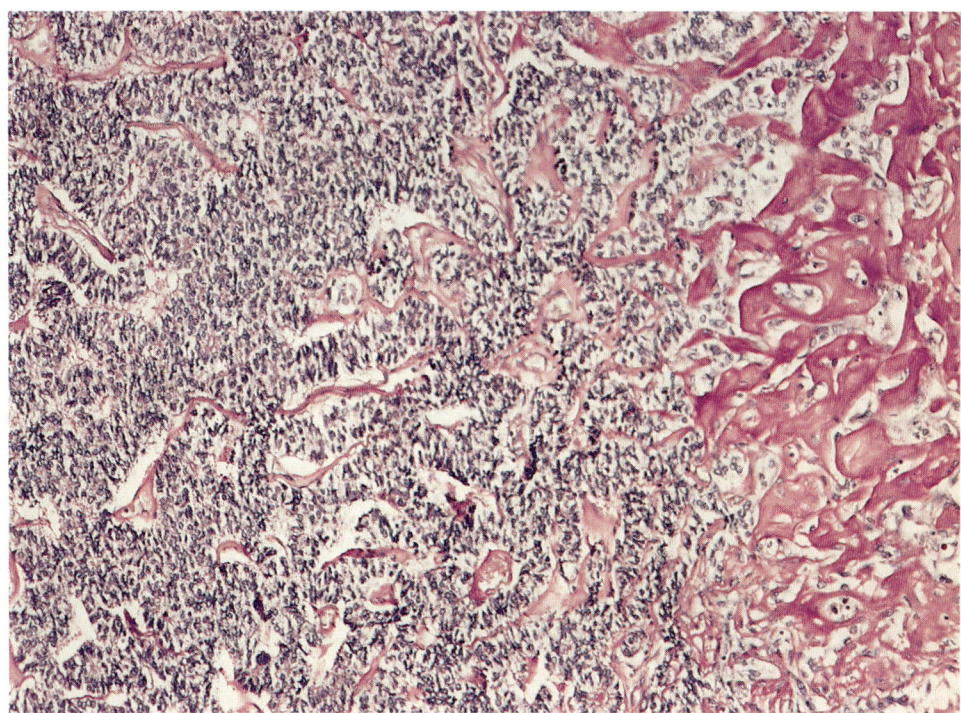

Fig. 214. Malignant müllerian mixed tumor, with osteoblasts. H & E

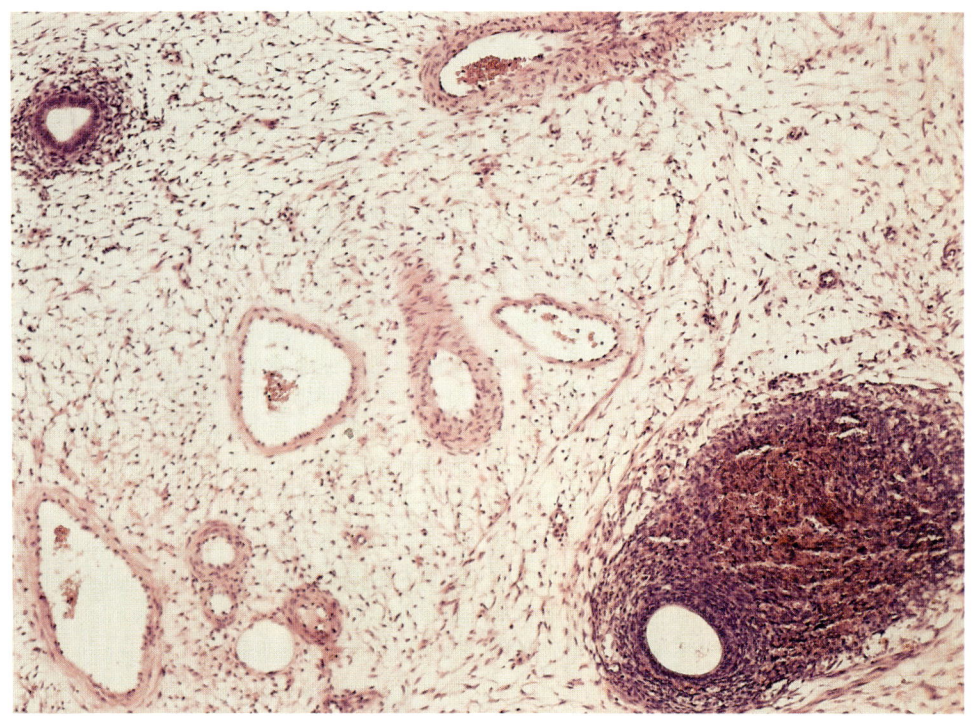

Fig. 215. Müllerian adenosarcoma. H & E

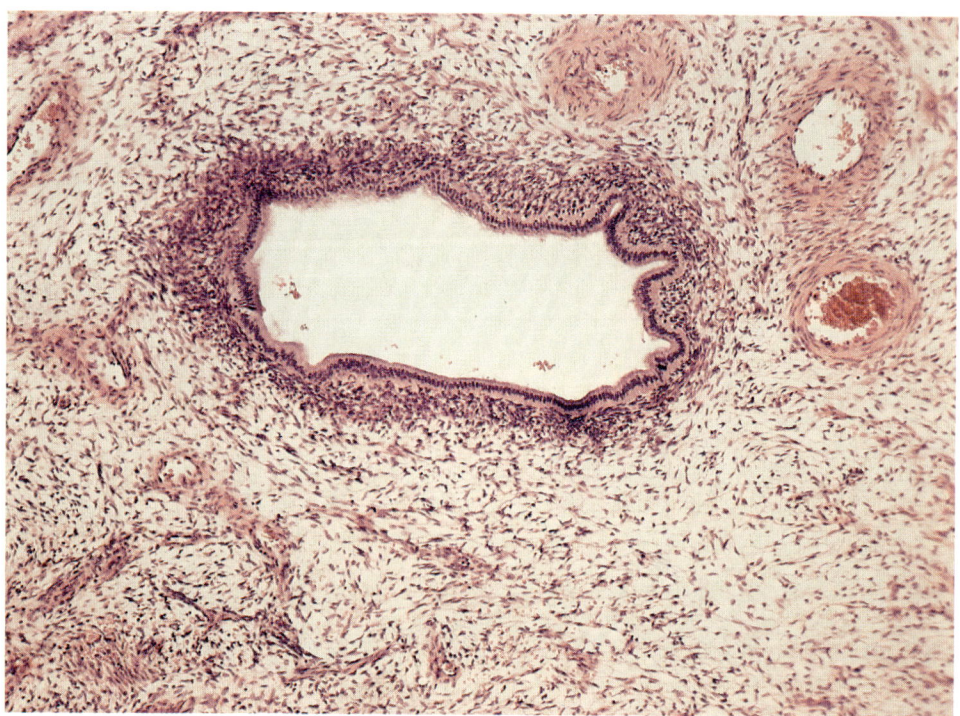

Fig. 216. Müllerian adenosarcoma. H & E

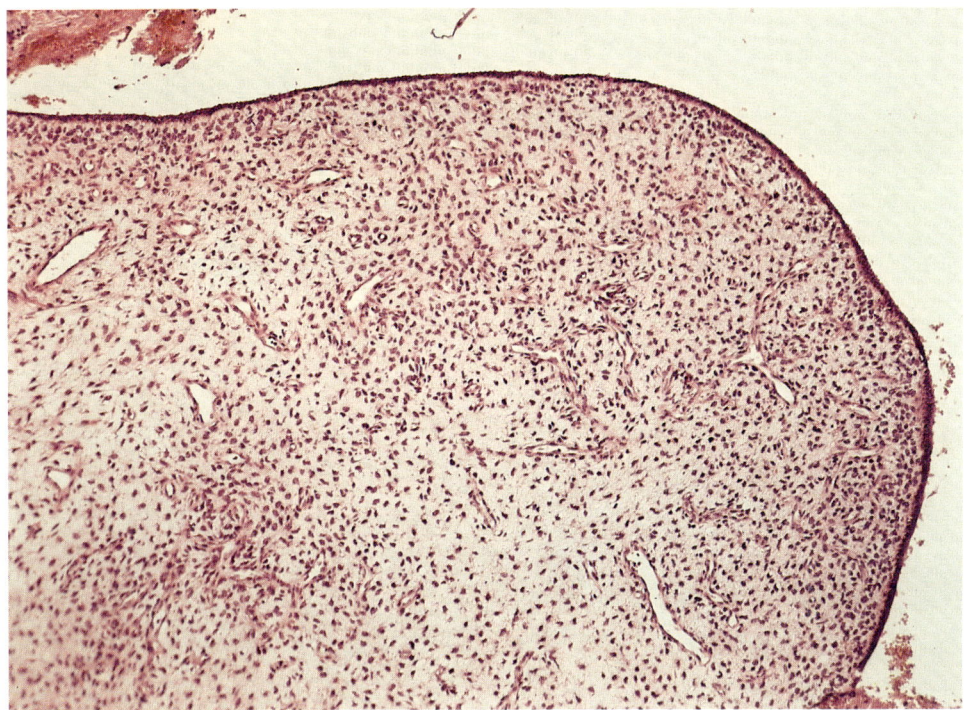

Fig. 217. Embryonal rhabdomyosarcoma. H & E

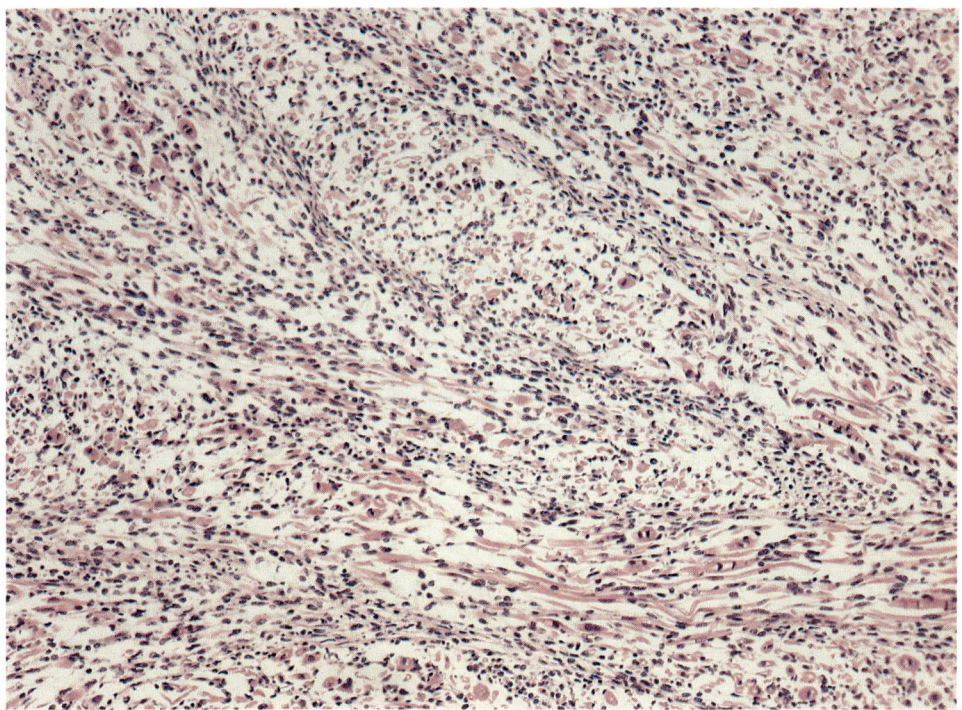

Fig. 218. Embryonal rhabdomyosarcoma. H & E

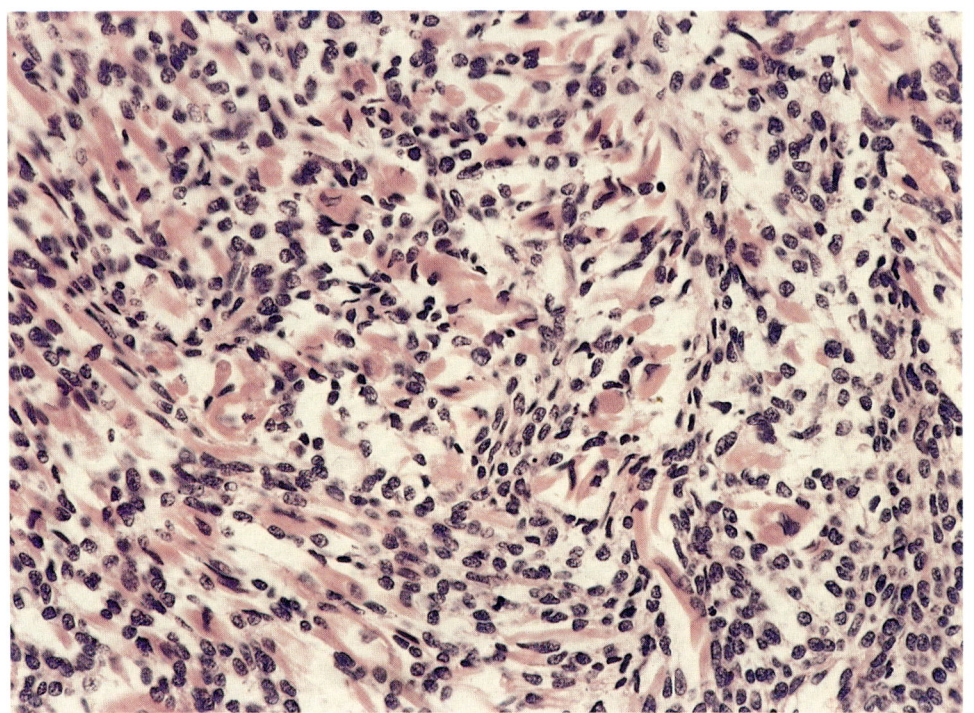

Fig. 219. Embryonal rhabdomyosarcoma. H & E, higher magnification

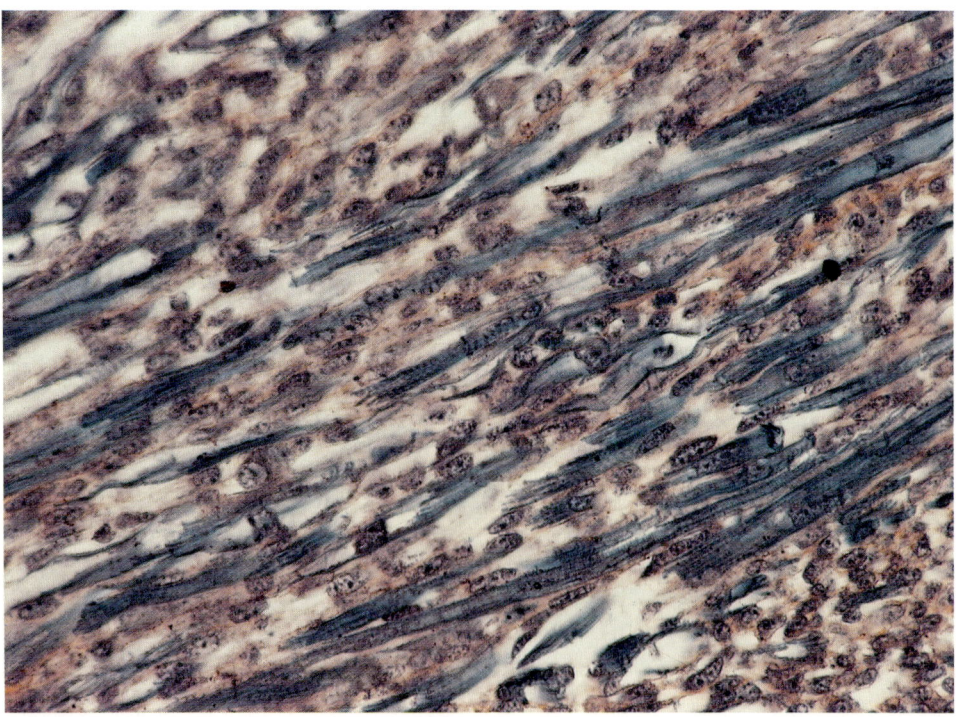

Fig. 220. Embryonal rhabdomyosarcoma. PTAH stain

Metastatic Tumors (Fig. 221)

Pelvic carcinomas, mainly those arising in the endometrium, ovary, rectum, and bladder, may extend into the cervix (Lemoine and Hall 1986). Distinguishing metastatic tumors from primary endocervical adenocarcinoma is often possible immunohistochemically (see p. 139). Metastases from distant primary tumors are rare. If they occur, the primary site most likely will be the breast (Fig. 221) or the gastrointestinal tract (Zhang et al. 1983).

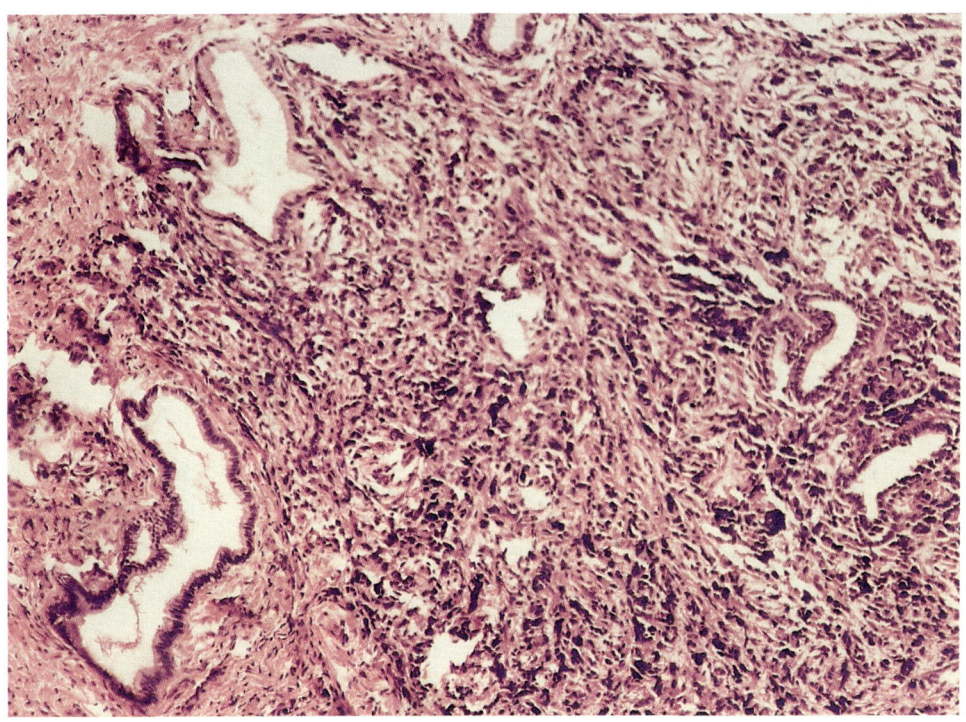

Fig. 221. Metastatic carcinoma from primary breast carcinoma. H & E

References

Abeler V, Kjørstad KE, Langholm R, Marton PF (1983) Granulocytic sarcoma (Chloroma) of the uterine cervix: report of two cases. Int J Gynecol Pathol 2: 88–92

Abell, MR (1971) Papillary adenofibroma of the uterine cervix. Am J Obstet Gynecol 110: 990–993

Abell MR, Gosling JRG (1962) Gland cell carcinoma (adenocarcinoma) of the uterine cervix. Am J Obstet Gynecol 83: 729–755

Adcock LL, Julian TM, Okagaki T, Jones TK, Prem KA, Twiggs LB, Potish RA, Phillips GL (1982) Carcinoma of the uterine cervix FIGO stage I-B. Gynecol Oncol 14: 199–208

Alva J, Lauchlan SC (1975) The histogenesis of mixed cervical carcinoma: the concept of endocervical columnar-cell dysplasia. Am J Clin Pathol 64: 20–25

Anderson SG, Linton EB (1967) The diagnostic accuracy of cervical biopsy and cervical conization. Am J Obstet Gynecol 99: 113–116

Aoyama C, Qualman SJ, Regan M, Shimada H (1990) Histopathologic Features of Composite Ganglioneuroblastoma: Immunohistochemical Distinction of the Stromal Component is Related to Prognosis. Cancer 65: 255–264

Ayroud Y, Gelfand MM, Ferenczy A (1985) Florid mesonephric hyperplasia of the cervix: a report of a case with review of the literature. Int J Gynecol Pathol 4: 245–254

Banik S, Grech A, Eyden B (1989) Granulocytic sarcoma of the cervix: an immunohistochemical, histochemical and ultrastructural study. J Clin Pathol 42: 483–488

Barter RA, Waters ED (1970) Cyto- and histomorphology of cervical adenocarcinoma in situ. Pathology 2: 33–40

Beecham JB, Halvorsen T, Kolbenstvedt A (1978) Histologic Classification, lymph node metastases and patient survival in stage 1 B cervical carcinoma: an analysis of 245 uniformly treated cases. Gynecol Oncol 6: 95–105

Benda JA, Platz CE, Buchsbaum H, Lifshitz S (1985) Mucin production in defining mixed carcinoma of the uterine cervix: a clinicopathologic study. Int J Gynecol Pathol 4: 314–327

Bistoletti P, Zellbi A, Moreno-Lopez J, Hjerpe A (1988) Genital Papillomavirus infection after treatment for cervical intraepithelial neoplasia (CIN) III. Cancer 62: 2056–2059

Bloch T, Roth LM, Stehman FB, Hull MT, Schwenk GR Jr (1988) Osteosarcoma of the uterine cervix associated with hyperplastic and atypical mesonephric rests. Cancer 62: 1594–1600

Boon ME, Baak JPA, Kurver PJH, Overdiep SH, Verdonk GW (1981a) Adenocarcinoma in situ of the cervix: an underdiagnosed lesion. Cancer 48: 768–773

Boon ME, Kirk RS, Rietveld-Scheffers PE (1981b) The morphogenesis of adenocarcinoma of the cervix - a complex pathological entity. Histopathology 5: 565–577

Boyes DA, Worth AH, Fidler HK (1970) The results of treatment of 4389 cases of preclinical cervical squamous carcinoma. J Obstet Gynaecol Br Commonw 77: 769–780

Brand E, Berek JS, Nieberg RK, Hacker NF (1987) Rhabdomyosarcoma of the uterine cervix: sarcoma botryoides. Cancer 60: 1552–1560

Brinton LA, Huggins GR, Lehman HF, Mallin K, Savitz DA, Trapido E, Rosenthal J, Hoover R (1986) Long-term use of oral contraceptives and risk of invasive cervical cancer. Int J Cancer 38: 339–344

Buntine DW (1979) Adenocarcinoma of the uterine cervix of probable wolffian origin. Pathology 11: 713–718

Burkman RT, Damewood MT (1985) Actinomyces and the intrauterine contraceptive device. In: Zatuchni GI, Goldsmith A, Sciarra J (eds) Intrauterine contraception. Advances and future prospects. Harper and Row, New York, pp 427–437

Campion MJ, Cuzich J, McCance DJ, Singer A (1986) Progressive potential of mild cervical atypia: prospective cytological, colposcopical and virological study. Lancet II: 237–240

Candy J, Abell MR (1968) Progesteron-induced adenomatous hyperplasia of the uterine cervix. J Am Med Assoc 203: 323–326

Chan JKC, Tsui WMS, Tung SY, Ching RCT (1989) Endocrine cell hyperplasia of the uterine cervix. Am J Clin Pathol 92: 825–830

Christopherson WM, Nealon N, Gray LA (1979) Noninvasive precursor lesions of adenocarcinoma and mixed adenosquamous carcinoma of the cervix uteri. Cancer 44: 975–983

Clement PB, Scully RE (1974) Müllerian adenosarcoma of the uterus. Cancer 34: 1138–1149

Clement PB, Scully RE (1982) Carcinoma of the cervix: histologic types. Sem Oncol 9: 251–264

Cohen C, Shulman G, Budgeon LR (1982) Endocervical and endometrial adenocarcinoma: an immunoperoxidase and histochemical study. Am J Surg Pathol 6: 151–157

Colgan TJ, Percy ME, Suri M, Shier RM, Andrews DF, Lickrish GM (1989) Human papilloma virus infection of morphologically normal cervical epithelium adjacent to squamous dysplasia and invasive carcinoma. Human Pathol 20: 316–319

Corey L (1984) Genital herpes. In: Holmes KK, Mardh PA, Sparling PF, Wiesner PJ (eds) Sexually transmitted diseases. McGraw-Hill, New York, pp 449–474

Crissman JD, Budhraja M, Aron BS, Cummings G (1987) Histopathologic prognostic factors in stage II and III squamous cell carcinoma of the uterine cervix: an evaluation of 91 patients treated primarily with radiation therapy. Int J Gynecol Pathol 6: 97–103

Crum CP, Mitao M, Winkler B, Reumann W, Boon ME, Richart RM (1984) Localizing chlamydial infection in cervical biopsies with the immunoperoxidase technique. Int J Gynecol Pathol 3: 191–197

Crum CP, Nagai N, Mitao M, Levine RU, Silverstein S (1985) Histological and molecular analysis of early cervical neoplasia. J Cell Biochem 9, Suppl: 70

Czernobilsky B, Moll R, Franke WW, Dallenbach-Hellweg G, Hohlweg-Majert P (1984) Intermediate filaments of normal and neoplastic tissues of the female genital tract with emphasis on problems of differential tumor diagnosis. Pathol Res Pract 179: 31–37

Dabbs DJ, Geisinger KR, Norris HT (1986) Intermediate filaments in endocervical carcinomas: the diagnostic utility of vimentin patterns. Am J Surg Pathol 10: 568–576

Dallenbach-Hellweg G (1981) Structural variations of cervical cancer and its precursors under the influence of exogenous hormones. In: Dallenbach-Hellweg G (ed) Cervical cancer. Springer, Berlin Heidelberg New York, pp 143–170

Dallenbach-Hellweg G (1984) On the origin and histological structure of adenocarcinoma of the endocervix in women under 50 years of age. Pathol Res Pract 179: 38–50

Dallenbach-Hellweg G (1985) Probleme der histopathologischen Untersuchung weiblicher Genitaltumoren. In: Wulf KH, Schmidt-Matthiesen H (eds) Klinik der Frauenheilkunde und Geburtshilfe, vol 10. Urban und Schwarzenberg, München, pp 87–98

Dallenbach-Hellweg G, Lang G (1990) Immunohistochemical studies on uterine tumors. I. Invasive squamous cell carcinomas of the cervix and their precursors. Pathol Res Pract (in press)

Dallenbach-Hellweg G, Poulsen H (1985) Atlas of endometrial histopathology. Munksgaard, Copenhagen

Dougherty CM, Moore WR, Cotten N (1962) Histologic diagnosis and clinical significance of benign lesions of the nonpregnant cervix. Ann NY Acad Sci 97: 683

Eide TJ (1987) Cancer of the uterine cervix in Norway by histology type, 1970–84. JNCI 79: 199–205

Elliott PM, Tattersal MHN, Coppleson M, Russell P, Wong F, Coates AS, Solomon HJ, Bannatyne PM, Atkinson KH, Murray JC (1989) Changing character of cervical cancer in young women. Br Med J 298: 288–290

Farnsworth A, Laverty C, Stoler MH (1989) Human papillomavirus messenger RNA expression in adenocarcinoma in situ of the uterine cervix. Int J Gynecol Pathol 8: 321–330

Fenoglio CM, Ferenczy A (1982) Etiologic factors in cervical neoplasia. Semin Oncol 9: 349–372

Fenoglio CM, Galloway DA, Crum CP, Levine RU, Richart RM, McDougall JK (1981) Herpes simplex virus and cervical neoplasia. In: Fenoglio CM, Wolff M (eds) Progress in surgical pathology. Masson, New York, pp 45–82

Ferenczy A (1987) Anatomy and Histology of the Cervix. In: Kurman RJ (ed) Blaustein's pathology of the female genital tract. Springer, Berlin Heidelberg New York

Ferenczy A, Winkler B (1987) Carcinoma and Metastatic Tumors of the Cervix. In: Kurman RJ (ed) Blaustein's Pathology of the female genital tract. Springer, Berlin Heidelberg New York, pp 218–256

Ferry JA, Scully RE (1988) "Adenoid Cystic" carcinoma and adenonid basal carcinoma of the uterine cervix: a study of 28 cases. Am J Surg Pathol 12: 134–144

Fetissof F, Berger G, Dubois MP, Arbeille-Brassart B, Lansac J, Sam-Gio M, Jobard P (1985) Endocrine cells in the female genital tract. Histopathology 9: 133–145

Fletcher S (1983) Histopathology of papilloma virus infection of the cervix uteri: the history, taxonomy, nomenclature and reporting of koilocytic dysplasias. J Clin Pathol 36: 616–624

Flint A, Gikas PW, Roberts JA (1985) Alveolar soft part sarcoma of the uterine cervix. Gynecol Oncol 22: 263–267

Franke WW, Moll R, Achtstaetter T, Kuhn C (1986) Cell typing of epithelial and carcinomas of the female genital tract using cytoskeletal proteins as markers. In: Peto R, zur Hausen H (eds) Viral etiology of cervical cancer. Cold Spring Harbor Labor, Cold Spring Harbor (Banbury Report No. 21) pp 121–148

Franquemont DW, Ward BE, Andersen WA,

Crum CP (1989) Prediction of "High-Risk" Cervical Papillomavirus Infection by Biopsy Morphology. Am J Clin Pathol 92, 577-582

Friedell GH, McKay DG (1953) Adenocarcinoma in situ of the endocervix. Cancer 6: 887-897

Fu YS, Reagan JW, Fu AS, Janiga KE (1982a) Adenocarcinoma and mixed carcinoma of the uterine cervix. II. Prognostic value of nuclear DNA analysis. Cancer 49: 2571-2577

Fu YS, Reagan JW, Hsiu JG, Storaasli JP, Wentz WB (1982b) Adenocarcinoma and mixed carcinoma of the uterine cervix. I. A clinicopathologic study. Cancer 49: 2560-2570

Fuchs PG, Girardi F, Pfister H (1988) Human papilloma virus DNA in normal, metaplastic, preneoplastic and neoplastic epithelia of the cervix uteri. Int J Cancer 41: 41-45

Fujii S, Konishi I, Ferenczy A, Imai K, Okamura H, Mori T (1986) Small cell undifferentiated carcinoma of the uterine cervix. Ultrastruct Pathol 10: 337-346

Gall SA, Bourgeois CH, Maguire R (1969) The morphologic effects of oral contraceptive agents on the cervix. J Am Med Assoc 207: 2243-2247

Gallup DG, Abell MR (1977) Invasive adenocarcinoma of the uterine cervix. Obstet Gynecol 49: 596-603

Gaton E, Zejdel L, Bernstein D, Glezerman M, Czernobilsky B, Insler V (1982) The effect of estrogen and gestagen on the mucus production of human endocervical cells. A histochemical study. Fertil Steril 38: 580-585

Gersell DJ, Mazoujian G, Mutch DG, Rudloff MA (1988) Small-cell undifferentiated carcinoma of the cervix: a clinicopathologic, ultrastructural and immunocytochemical study of 15 cases. Am J Surg Pathol 12: 684-698

Gilks CB, Young RH, Aguirre P, Delellis RA, Scully RE (1989) Adenoma malignum (minimal deviation adenocarcinoma) of the uterine cervix: a clinicopathological and immunohistochemical analysis of 26 cases. Am J Surg Pathol 9: 717-729

Gissmann L (1984) Papillomaviruses and their association with cancer in animals and in man. Cancer Surv 3: 162-181

Gloor E, Hurliman J (1986) Cervical intraepithelial glandular neoplasia (adenocarcinoma in situ and glandular dysplasia): a correlative study of 23 cases with histologic grading, histochemical analysis of mucins, and immunohistochemical determination of the affinity for four lectins. Cancer 58: 1272-1280

Gloor E, Ruzicka J (1982) Morphology of adenocarcinoma in situ of the uterine cervix: a study of 14 cases. Cancer 49: 294-302

Glücksmann A (1957) Relationships between hormonal changes in pregnancy and the development of "mixed carcinoma" of the uterine cervix. Cancer 10: 831-837

Groben P, Reddick R, Askin F (1985) The pathologic spectrum of small cell carcinoma of the cervix. Int J Gynecol Pathol 4: 42-57

Gusdon JT (1965) Hemangioma of the cervix. Am J Obstet Gynecol 91: 204-209

Hachitanda Y, Masazumi T, Enjoji M (1989) Expression of pan-Neuroendocrine protein in 53 neuroblastic tumors. An immunohistochemical study with neuron-specific enolase, chromogranin, and synaptophysin. Arch Pathol Lab Med 113: 381-384

Hall DJ, Schneider V, Goplerud DR (1980) Primary malignant melanoma of the uterine cervix. Obstet Gynecol 56: 525-529

Hamperl H, Kaufmann C (1959) The cervix uteri at different ages. Obstet Gynecol 14: 621-631

Harris NL, Scully RE (1984) Malignant lymphoma and granulocytic sarcoma of the uterus and vagina. Cancer 53: 2530-2545

Hart WR, McUsar M, Norris HJ (1972) Mesonephric adenocarcinomas of the cervix. Cancer 29: 106-113

Hellweg G (1957) Über Schleimbildung in Plattenepithelcarcinomen insbesondere an der Portio uteri (Mucoepidermoidcarcinome). Z Krebsforsch 61: 688-715

Helmerhorst TJM, Dijkhuizen GH, Veldhuizen RW, Stolk JG (1984) Microglandular hyperplasia - a complicating factor in the diagnosis of cervical intraepithelial neoplasia. Eur J Obstet Gynecol Reprod Biol 17: 53-59

Hiersche HD, Nagl W (1980) Regeneration of secretory epithelium in the human endocervix. Arch Gynecol 229: 83-90

Holmquist ND, Torres JT (1988) Malignant melanoma of the cervix. Acta Cytol 32: 252-256

Holzner JH (1981) Histologic verification of cervical cancer. In: Dallenbach-Hellweg G (ed) Cervical cancer. Springer, Berlin Heidelberg New York, p 67-78

Hopkins MP, Schmidt RW, Roberts JA, Morley GW (1988) Gland cell carcinoma (Adenocarcinoma) of the Cervix. Obstet Gynecol 72: 789-795

Hoskins WJ, Averette HE, Ng ABP, Yon SL (1979) Adenoid cystic carcinoma of the cervix uteri: report of six cases and review of the literature. Gynecol Oncol 7: 371-384

Hulka BS (1970) Punch biopsy and conization as diagnostic procedures after abnormal cervical smears. Obstet Gynecol 36: 54-61

Hurlimann J, Gloor E (1984) Adenocarcinoma in situ and invasive adenocarcinoma of the uterine cervix: an immunhistologic study with antibodies specific for several epithelial markers. Cancer 54: 103-109

Jaworski RC, Pacey NF, Greenberg L, Osborn RA (1988) The histologic diagnosis of adenocarcinoma in situ and related lesions of the cervix uteri: adenocarcinoma in situ. Cancer 61: 1171-1181

Kaku T, Enjoji M (1983) Extremely well-differentiated adenocarcinoma ("Adenoma malignum") of the Cervix. Int J Gynecol Pathol 2: 13-27

Kaminski PF, Norris HJ (1983) Minimal deviation carcinoma (adenoma malignum) of the cervix. Int J Gynecol Pathol 2: 141-152

Komaki R, Cox JD, Hansen RM, Gunn WG, Greenberg M (1984) Malignant lymphoma of the uterine cervix. Cancer 54: 1699-1704

Koss LG (1987) Carcinogenesis in the uterine cervix and human papilloma virus infection. In: Syrjünen K, Gissmann L, Koss LG (eds) Papilloma viruses and Human disease. Springer, Berlin Heidelberg New York, pp 235-267

Krimmenau R (1966) Adenocarcinoma in situ, beginnende adenocarcinomatöse Invasion und Microcarcinoma adenomatosum. Geburtshilfe Frauenheilkd 26: 1279-1305

Kurman RJ, Schiffman MH, Lancaster WD, Reid R, Jenson AB, Temple GF, Lorincz AT (1988) Analysis of individual human papillomavirus types in cervical neoplasia: A possible role for type 18 in rapid progression. Am J Obstet Gynecol 159: 293-296

Kyriakos M, Kempson RL, Knokov NF (1968) A clinical and pathological study of endocervical lesions associated with oral contraceptives. Cancer 22: 99-110

Lang G, Dallenbach-Hellweg G (1990) The Histogenetic origin of cervical mesonephric hyperplasia and mesonephric adenocarcinoma of the uterine cervix. Studied with immunohistochemical methods. Int J Gynecol Pathol 9: 145-157

Lauchlan SC (1984) Metaplasias and neoplasias of Müllerian epithelium. Histopathology 8: 543-557

Lemonine NR, Hall PA (1986) Epithelial tumors metastatic to the uterine cervix: a study of 33 cases and review of the literature. Cancer 57: 2002-2005

Levy R, Czernobilsky B, Geiger B (1988) Subtyping of epithelial cells of normal and metaplastic human uterine cervix, using polypeptide - specific cytokeratin antibodies. Differentiation 39: 185-196

Löning T, Kühler C, Caselitz J, Stegner HE (1983) Keratin and tissue polypeptide antigen profiles of the cervical mucosa. Int J Gynecol Pathol 2: 105-112

Lorincz AT, Temple GF, Kurman RJ, Jenson AB, Lancaster WD (1987) Oncogenic association of specific human papillomavirus types with cervical neoplasia. JNCI 79: 671-677

Makin CA, Bobrow LG, Bodmer WF (1984) Monoclonal antibodies to cytokeratin for use in routine histopathology. J Clin Pathol 37: 975-983

McGee CT, Cromer DW, Greene RR (1962) Mesonephric carcinoma of the cervix-differentiation from endocervical adenocarcinoma. Am J Obstet Gynecol 84: 358-366

McIndoe WA, McLean MR, Jones RW, Mullims PR (1984) The invasive potential of carcinoma in situ of the cervix. Obstet Gynecol 64: 451-458

Mestwerdt G (1947) Probeexzision und Kolposkopie in der Frühdiagnose des Portiokarcinoms. Zentralbl Gynäkol 69: 326-332

Michael H, Grawe L, Kraus FT (1984) Minimal deviation endocervical adenocarcinoma: clinical and histologic features, immunhistochemical staining for carcinoembryonic antigen, and differentiation from confusing benign lesions. Int J Gynecol Pathol 3: 261-276

Michael H, Sutton G, Hull MT, Roth LM (1986) Villous adenoma of the uterine cervix associated with invasive adenocarcinoma: a histologic, ultrastructural and immunohistochemical study. Int J Gynecol Pathol 5: 163-169

Moll RR, Levy R, Czernobilsky B, Hohlweg-Majert P, Dallenbach-Hellweg G, Franke WW (1983) Cytokeratins of normal epithelia and some neoplasms of the female genital tract. Lab Invest 49: 599-610

Moltz L, Becker K (1977) Cribriform polypoid adenomatous (atypical) hyperplasia of the endocervical glands of the uterus under hormonal contraception. Eur J Obstet Gynecol Reprod Biol 7/5: 331-336

Nagai N, Nuovo G, Friedman D, Crum CP (1987) Detection of papillomavirus nucleic acids in genital precancers with the in situ hybridization technique. Int J Gynecol Pathol 6: 366-379

Nanbu Y, Fujii S, Konishi I, Nonogaki H, Mori T (1988) Immunohistochemical localization of CA 125, carcinoembryonic antigen and CA 19-9 in normal and neoplastic glandular cells of the uterine cervix. Cancer 62: 2580-2588

Nasiell K, Nasiell M, Vaclavincova V (1983) Behaviour of moderate cervical dysplasia during long-term follow-up. Obstet Gynecol 61: 609-614

Noda K, Kimura K, Ikeda M, Teshima K (1983) Studies on the Histogenesis of cervical adenocarcinoma. Int J Gynecol Pathol 1: 336-346

Nuovo GJ, Nuovo MA, Cottral S, Gordon S, Silverstein SJ, Crum CP (1988) Histological correlates of clinically occult human papillomavirus infection of the uterine cervix. Am J Surg Pathol 12: 198-204

Okagaki T, Clark BA, Zachow KR (1984) Presence of human papillomavirus in verrucous carcinoma (Ackerman) of the vagina. Arch Pathol Lab Med 108: 567-570

Östör AG, Pagano R, Davoren RAM, Fortune DW, Chanen W, Rome R (1984) Adenocarcinoma in situ of the cervix. Int J Gynecol Pathol 3: 179-190

Paavonen J, Vesterinen E, Meyer B, Saksela E (1982) Colposcopic and histological findings in cervical chlamydial infection. Obstet Gynecol 59: 712-714

Patel DS, Bhagavan BS (1985) Blue nevus of the uterine cervix. Hum Pathol 16: 79–86

Pater MM, Hughes GA, Hyslop DE et al. (1988) Glucocorticoid-dependent carcinogenic transformation by type 16 but not type 11 papillomavirus DNA. Nature 335: 832–835

Peters RK, Chao A, Mack TM, Thomas D, Bernstein L, Henderson BE (1986) Increased frequency of adenocarcinoma of the uterine cervix in young women in Los Angeles County. JNCI 76: 423–428

Petersen O (1955) Precancerous changes of the cervical epithelium. Danish Science Press Ltd, Copenhagen

Pine L, Curtis EM, Brown JM (1985) Actinomyces and the intrauterine contraceptive device: aspects of the fluorescent antibody stain. Am J Obstet Gynecol 152: 287–290

Randall ME, Andersen WA, Mills SE, Kim JC (1986) Papillary squamous cell carcinoma of the uterine cervix: a clinicopathologic study of nine cases. Int J Gynecol Pathol 5: 1–10

Richard L, Guralnick M, Ferenczy A (1981) Ultrastructure of glassy cell carcinoma of cervix. Diagn Gynecol Obstet 3: 31–38

Richart RM (1987) Causes and management of cervical intraepithelial neoplasia. Cancer 60: 1951–1959

Rorat E, Benjamin P, Richart RM (1978) Verrucous carcinoma of the cervix: a problem in diagnosis and management. Am J Obstet Gynecol 130: 851–853

Sachs H, Ikeda J, Brachetti AKJ (1975) Mikroinvasives Adenokarzinom und Adenocarcinoma in situ der Cervix uteri. Med Welt 26: 1181–1183

Schneider V, Kay S, Lee HM (1983) Immunosuppression: high risk factor for the development of condyloma acuminata and squamous neoplasia of the cervix. Acta Cytol (Baltimore) 27: 220–224

Schwartz SM, Weiss NS (1986) Increased incidence of adenocarcinoma of the cervix in young women in the United States. Am J Epidemiol 124: 1045–1047

Scully RE, Aguirre P, DeLellis RA (1984) Argyrophilia, serotonin and peptide hormones in the female genital tract and its tumors. Int J Gynecol Pathol 3: 51–70

Seifert G, Löning T, Hoepfner I (1984) Morphologische Diagnostik bei Virusinfektionen, Pathohistologie, Immunhistologie, Hybridisierungstechnik, Elektronenmikroskopie. Pathologe 5: 326–342

Selim MA, So-Bosita JJ, Blair OM, Little BA (1973) Cervical biopsy versus conization. Obstet Gynecol 41: 177–182

Shah KH, Kurman RJ, Scully RE, Norris HS (1980) Atypical hyperplasia of mesonephric remnants in the cervix. Lab Invest 42: 149

Silverberg SG, Hurt WG (1975) Minimal deviation adenocarcinoma ("adenoma malignum") of the cervix: a reappraisal. Am J Obstet Gynecol 121: 971–975

Smotkin D, Berek JS, Fu YS, Hacker NF, Major FJ, Wettstein FO (1986) Human papillomavirus deoxyribonucleic acid in adenocarcinoma and adenosquamous carcinoma of the uterine cervix. Obstet Gynecol 68: 241–244

Southern EM (1975) Detection of specific sequences among DNA fragments separated by gel electrophoresis. J Mol Biol 98: 503–527

Speers WC, Picaso LG, Silverberg SG (1983) Immunohistochemical localisation of carcinoembryonic antigen in microglandular hyperplasia and adenocarcinoma of the endocervix. Am J Clin Pathol 79: 105–107

Stamm WE, Holmes KK (1984) Chlamydia trachomatis infections of the adult. In: Holmes KK, Mandh PA, Sparling PF, Weisher PS (eds) Sexually transmitted diseases. McGraw Hill Book Co, New York, pp 258–269

Steeper TA, Wick MR (1986) Minimal deviation adenocarcinoma of the uterine cervix ("Adenoma malignum"): an immunohistochemical comparison with microglandular endocervical hyperplasia and concentionalendocervical adenocarcinoma. Cancer 58: 1131–1138

Stegner HE (1959) Über melaninbildende Pigmentzellen und Pigmenttumoren der Portio vaginalis uteri. Zentralbl Gynäkol 81: 1686–1692

Stoll P (1969) Gynecologial vital cytology. Springer, Berlin Heidelberg New York

Syrjänen KJ (1979) Morphologic survey of the condylomatous lesions in dysplastic and neoplastic epithelium of the uterine cervix. Arch Gynecol 227: 153–161

Syrjänen K, Varynen M, Saarikoski S et al. (1985) Natural history of cervical human papillomavirus infection (HPV) based on prospective follow-up. Br J Obstet Gynaecol 92: 1086–1092

Talbert JR, Sherry JB (1969) Adenocarcinoma-like lesion of cervix: a pill-induced problem? Am J Obstet Gynecol 105: 117–120

Tam MR, Stamm WE, Handsfield HH, Stephens R, Kuo CC, Holmes KK, Ditzenberger K, Krieger M, Nowinski RC (1984) Culture-independent diagnosis of chlamydia trachomatis using monoclonal antibodies. N Engl J Med 310: 1146–1149

Tanaka T, Ohbayashi F, Shima H, Shimonaka G, Takahashi M (1984) Glassy cell carcinoma of the uterine cervix. Pathol Research Practice 178: 389–394

Tase T, Okagaki T, Clark BA, Manias DA, Ostrow RS, Twiggs LB, Faras AJ (1988) Human papillomavirus types and localization in adenocarcinoma and adenosquamous carcinoma of the uterine cervix: a study by in situ DNA hybridization. Cancer Res 48: 993–998

Tase T, Okagaki T, Clark BA, Twiggs LB, Ostrow RS, Faras AJ (1989) Human papillomavirus

DNA in adenocarcinoma in situ, microinvasive adenocarcinoma of the uterine cervix, and coexisting cervical squamous intraepithelial neoplasia. Int J Gynecol Pathol 8: 8-17

Taylor HB, Irey NS, Norris HJ (1967) Atypical endocervical hyperplasia in women taking oral contraceptives. J Am Med Ass 202: 637-639

Teshima S, Shimosato Y, Kishi K, Kasamatsu T, Ohmi K, Uei Y (1985) Early stage adenocarcinoma of the uterine cervix: histopathologic analysis with consideration of histogenesis. Cancer 56: 167-172

Tsukamoto N, Kaku T, Matsukuma K, Matsuyama T, Kamura T, Saito T, Suenaga T (1989) The problem of stage I a (FIGO, 1985) carcinoma of the uterine cervix. Gynecol Oncol 34, 1-6

Tsutsumi Y, Nagura H, Watanabe K (1984) Immunohistochemical observations of carcinoembryonic antigen (CEA) and CEA-related substances in normal and neoplastic pancreas. Am J Clin Pathol 82: 535-542

Ueda G, Shimizu C, Shimizu H, Saito J, Tanaka Y, Inoue M, Tanizawa O (1989) An Immunohistochemical study of small-cell and poorly differentiated carcinomas of the cervix using neuroendocrine markers. Gynecol Oncol 34: 164-169

Ulbright TM, Gersell DJ (1983) Glassy cell carcinoma of the uterine cervix: a light and electron microscopic study of five cases. Cancer 51: 2255-2263

Ulich TR, Liao SY, Layfield L, Romansky R, Cheng L, Lewin KJ (1986) Endocrine and tumor differentiation markers in poorly differentiated small-cell carcinoids of the cervix and vagina: Arch Pathol Lab Med 110: 1054-1057

van Dinh T, Woodruff JD (1985) Adenoid cystic and adenoid basal carcinomas of the cervix. Obstet Gynecol 65: 705-709

Villiers de EM, Schneider A, Miklaw H, Papendick U, Wagner D, Wesch H, Wahrendorf J, Zurhausen H (1987) Human papillomavirus infections in women with and without abnormal cervical cytology. Lancet II: 703-706

Wagner EK (1974) The replication of herpesvirus. Am Sci 62: 584

Walker AN, Mills SE, Tylor P (1988) Cervical neuroendocrine carcinoma: a clinical and light microscopic study of 14 cases. Int J Gynecol Pathol 7: 64-74

Walker J, Bloss JD, Liao SY, Berman M, Bergen S, Wilczynski SP (1989) Human papillomavirus genotype as a prognostic indicator in carcinoma of the uterine cervix. Obstet Gynecol 74: 781-785

Wells M, Brown LJR (1986) Glandular lesions of the uterine cervix: the present state of our knowledge. Histopathology 10: 777-792

Werner R, Waidecker F (1975) Adenocarcinoma in situ und mikroinvasives Adenokarzinom der Cervix uteri. Öesterr Z Onkol 2: 154-157

Wilczynski SP, Walker J, Liao SY, Bergen S, Berman M (1988) Adenocarcinoma of the cervix associated with human papillomavirus. Cancer 62: 1331-1336

Willett GD, Kurman RJ, Reid R, Greenberg M, Jenson AB, Lorincz AT (1989) Correlation of the histologic appearance of intraepithelial neoplasia of the cervix with human papillomavirus types: emphasis on low grade lesions including so-called flat condyloma. Int J Gynecol Pathol 8: 18-25

Winkler B, Crum CP (1986) Chlamydia trachomatis infection of the female genital tract: pathogenetic and clinicopathologic considerations. In: Sommers SC, Fechner RE, Rosen PP (eds) Pathology annual. Appleton-Century-Crofts, Norwalk, CT

Winkler B, Crum PC, Fujii T, Ferenczy A, Boon M, Braun L, Lancaster WD, Richart RM (1984) Koilocytotic lesions of the cervix: the relationship of mitotic abnormalities to the presence of papillomavirus antigens and nuclear DNA content. Cancer 53: 1081-1087

Yamasaki M, Tateishi R, Hongo J, Ozaki Y, Inoue M, Ueda G (1984) Argyrophil small cell carcinoma of the uterine cervix. Int J Gynecol Pathol 3: 146 152

Young RH, Scully RE (1988) Mucinous Ovarian tumors associated with mucinous adenocarcinomas of the cervix. Int J Gynecol Pathol 7: 99-111

Young RH, Scully RE (1989) Atypical forms of microglandular hyperplasia of the cervix simulating carcinoma: a report of five cases and review of the literature. Am J Surg Pathol 13: 50-56

Young RH, Scully RE (1989) Villoglandular papillary adenocarcinoma of the uterine cervix. A clinicopathologic analysis of 13 cases. Cancer 63: 1773-1779

Young RH, Kleinman GM, Scully RE (1981) Glioma of the uterus. Am J Surg Pathol 5: 695-699

Young RH, Harris NL, Scully RE (1985) Lymphoma-like lesions of the lower female genital tract: a report of 16 cases. Int J Gynecol Pathol 4: 289-299

Zaloudek CJ, Norris HJ (1981) Adenofibroma and adenosarcoma of the uterus: a clinicopathologic study of 35 cases. Cancer 48: 354-366

Zhang YC, Zhang PF, Wei YH (1983) Metastatic carcinoma of the cervix uteri from the gastrointestinal tract. Gynecol Oncol 15: 287-290

Subject Index

actinomycosis 64, 65
adenocarcinoma 44, 47, 77, 78, 128ff.
-, clear cell 140, 141, 144
-, endometrioid type 138f.
-, intestinal type 137
-, mesonephric 26, 144ff.
-, minimal deviation type 129, 133
-, mucinous 130ff.
- in situ 44, 76ff., 101ff.
- -, anti-CEA 107
- -, differential diagnosis 106
adenofibroma, papillary 74, 75
adenoid basal carcinoma 154
- cystic carcinoma 152, 153
adenoma 69
-, benign 69
- malignum: see adenocarcinoma, minimal deviation type
-, villous 69
adenomatous hyperplasia 42ff., 106
adenomyoma 74
adenosarcoma 74, 165, 166
- Müllerian 165, 166
adenosquamous carcinoma 77, 137, 148, 149
alveolar soft part sarcoma 158
angiomatous polyps 50
angiosarcoma 158
anti-CEA: see CEA
anticytokeratin: see cytokeratin
argyrophile cells 155
Arias-Stella reaction 40, 142
ascending repair 10ff., 35

B-cell non-Hodgkin lymphoma 161
bacterial infections 61ff.
basal layer 9, 17
- -, gland formation 9
- -, protrusions 9
- membrane 7
benign tumors 69ff.
biopsy, methods of 1
blot hybridization, southern 78, 82
blue nevus 72, 73

candida albicans 64
carcinogenic progression 108
carcinoid 125, 155, 157
carcinoma, adenoid 152ff.
-, - basal 154

-, - cystic 152, 153
-, adenosquamous 77, 137, 148, 149
-, clear cell 47, 77, 140, 141, 144
-, gestational changes 148
-, heterotopic type 155ff.
-, invasive 77, 114, 116ff., 121
-, large cell 116, 119ff.
-, - - keratinizing 122ff.
-, - - -, reserve cell type 124
-, - - nonkeratinizing 116, 119, 121
-, - - pleomorphic 127
-, microinvasive: see microinvasive carcinoma (MIC)
-, mixed type 148ff.
-, mucoepidermoid 148ff.
-, neuroendocrine 125, 155, 157
-, papillary squamous cell 128
-, reserve cell type 114, 121, 124, 125
-, serous papillary 142f.
- in situ 76ff., 95ff., 101, 108
- -, biological behavior 108
- -, differential diagnosis 100
- -, etiology and pathogenesis 76ff.
- -, histopathology 78ff.
- -, immunohistochemistry 78ff.
- -, reserve cell type 78, 95ff., 101
- -, squamous cell type 86, 87
-, small cell 116ff., 157
-, - -, of neuroendocrine origin 155, 157
-, squamous cell type 121, 125
-, verrucous 128
carcinosarcoma 162, 163
CEA, positive reaction for 26, 44, 82, 100, 101, 106, 107, 114, 120ff., 131, 135, 136, 139, 142, 148
cells, hobnail 26, 47, 141
-, signet-ring 47
cervical cone, precise orientation 3
- conization 2
- curettage 2
cervicitis: see also ecto- and endocervicitis
-, chlamydial 61ff.
- emphysematosa 66, 67
-, trichomonas 64
-, tuberculous 61
chlamydia trachomatis 58, 62, 63
- cervicitis 61ff.
chondrosarcoma 158, 159
clear cell adenocarcinoma 47, 77, 140, 141, 144
- - change 88, 91

177

condylomatous papilloma 71
conization, cervical 2
–, methods of 2
conus, orientation 3
–, sectioning, techniques of 3
curettage, cervical 2
cyst(s), dermoid 33
–, epidermoid 32, 33
–, nabothian 24
–, retention 24
cystic hyperplasia 35, 38 ff.
– – during pregnancy 41
– polyps 49
cytokeratins 6 ff., 16, 17, 19, 20, 80, 82, 87, 100, 114, 120, 121, 126
cytomegaly virus 76
cytoplasmic inclusions 62

decidua, ectopic 40
dermoid cyst 33
descending repair 18 ff., 24, 48, 49
desmoplakin 6, 7
desmoplastic stromal reaction 26
duct, Gartner's 26
– hyperplasia, mesonephric 26, 27, 146
– remants, mesonephric 26, 27
– –, Müllerian 28, 29
dyskaryosis 56
dysplasia 76 ff., 81, 108
–, etiology 76
–, histopathology 78 ff.
–, immunohistochemistry 78 ff.
–, koilocytic 58, 77, 79, 81 ff., 88 ff., 92
–, mucoid 88, 91
–, non-koilocytic 81, 84
–, papillary type 88, 94
–, pathogenesis 76
–, postirradiation 66
–, reserve cell type 82, 88 ff., 95
–, squamous cell type 79 ff.

echinococcosis 64
ectocervical polyps 50
– squamous epithelium, regenerating 12 ff., 18, 35, 76
ectocervicitis 51 ff.
–, acute 52
–, emphysematosa 66, 67
–, erosive 51, 52
–, nonspecific 51 ff.
–, specific 56 ff.
–, ulcerative 51, 52, 60
ectocervix, hyperkeratosis 35, 37, 69
–, normal 4 ff.
–, parakeratosis 35 f., 56, 69, 85
ectopic decidua 40
ectropium: see eversion
embryonal neuroblastoma 156 f.
– rhabdomyosarcoma 165, 167, 168
endocervical eversion 11, 40, 48
– glands, koilocytes 89

– polyps 48 ff., 74
endocervicitis 51 ff.
–, follicular 54, 55
–, nonspecific 51 ff.
–, specific 56 ff.
–, subacute 53
–, ulcerative 55
endocervix, adenocarcinoma 128 ff.
–, eversion of 11, 40, 48
–, normal 14 ff.
–, –, during gestation 40, 41
endometriosis 28 ff.
– in the cervical wall 30
endosalpingeal metaplasia 28, 31
entamoeba histolytica 58, 64
epidermoid cyst 32, 33
epithelial tumors 69 ff.
epithelium, regenerative 12 ff., 18, 35, 76
erosive ectocervicitis 51, 52
estrogenic hormonal stimulation 18, 35 ff.
estrogens 18
eversion, endocervical 11, 40, 48
–, glandular papillary 48

fixation, techniques of 2
follicular endocervicitis 54, 55
foreign body granuloma 61
– – reaction 33
fungal infections 64

Gartner's duct: see mesonephric duct
gestagenic hormonal stimulation 18, 40 ff., 128
gestagens, synthetic 42 ff., 128
–, –, mucine formation under 42, 44, 45
gestation(al) changes 40, 41
– – in carcinomas 148
–, normal endocervix during 40, 41
gland formation in basal layer 9
– –, sebaceous 33, 34
glandular atypia 44
– differentiation, potential for 8, 9
– hyperplasia 40, 41
– – during pregnancy 40, 41
– papillary ectropium 11, 40, 48
gonorrhea 62
granulocytic sarcoma 160
granuloma inguinale 61, 64
–, foreign body 61
–, tuberculous 61

hemangioma 72, 73
herpes simplex virus 76
– –, infection 56, 58 ff., 76
– – –, intranuclear inclusions 59
heterotopic tissues 26 ff.
– type carcinoma 155 ff.
hobnail cells 26, 47, 141
hormonal stimulation 35 ff., 76, 77, 148
– –, estrogenic 18, 35 ff.
– –, gestagenic 18, 40 ff., 128

human papilloma virus (HPV), infection 56 ff., 69, 76 ff., 88 ff., 100, 125, 128, 148
- - -, progression rates 108
- - -, in situ hybridization 3, 78, 82, 83, 92, 100
- - -, types 77, 78, 108
hybridization, in situ 3, 78, 82, 83, 92, 100
-, southern blot 78, 82
hyperkeratosis 35, 37, 69
hyperplasia, adenomatous 42 ff., 106
-, cystic 35, 38 ff.
-, glandular 40, 41
-, mesonephric duct 26, 27, 146
-, microglandular 46, 47, 106
-, reserve cell 19, 20, 22, 35, 42, 46 ff., 50, 76

immunohistochemical methods 3
inclusions, intracytoplasmic 61 ff.
-, intranuclear 59
-, viral 58
infection(s), bacterial 61 ff.
-, fungal 64
-, herpes virus 56, 58 ff., 76
-, human papilloma virus (HPV) 56 ff., 69, 88 ff., 100, 125, 128, 148
-, parasitic 64
-, trichomonal 62
-, viral 56 ff.
inflammatory lesions 51 ff.
- -, non-specific 51 ff.
- -, specific 56 ff.
in situ hybridization 3, 78, 82, 83, 92, 100
intestinal metaplasia 28, 137
intracytoplasmic inclusions 61 ff.
intraepithelial vesicles 58
intranuclear inclusions 59
- - of herpes virus 59
invasive carcinoma: see carcinoma
irradiation changes 66, 67
isthmic mucosa 14, 15

junction, squamocolumnar 1, 17, 22 ff., 80, 87

keratinization 35, 88, 121, 125, 148
-, monocellular 56, 121, 148, 151
koilocyte(s) 56 ff., 69, 77 ff., 81 ff., 85, 88 ff., 92
-, in endocervical glands 89
koilocytic dysplasia 58, 77, 79, 81 ff., 88 ff., 92

large cell carcinoma 116, 119 ff.
- - keratinizing carcinoma 122 ff.
- - nonkeratinizing carcinoma 116, 119, 121
- - pleomorphic carcinoma 127
layer, basal 9, 17
leiomyoma 72
leiomyosarcoma 158, 159
lipoma 72
lues 61
lymphatic invasion 112, 116, 118, 153
lymphogranuloma venereum 61, 64
lymphoma 54, 160, 161

malignant lymphoma 54, 160, 161
- melanoma 158
- Müllerian mixed tumors 162 ff.
- tumors 109 ff.
mesenchymal tumors 72, 73, 158 ff.
mesodermal mixed tumors 162 ff.
mesonephric adenocarcinoma 26, 144 ff.
- duct hyperplasia 26, 27, 146
- - remnants 26, 27
metaplasia, endosalpingeal 28, 31
-, intestinal 28, 137
-, Müllerian 28, 29, 137
-, neuroendocrine 155
-, sebaceous 33, 34
-, squamous 18, 20, 21, 23 ff., 35, 48, 139
metastatic tumors 169
microglandular hyperplasia 46, 47, 106
microinvasive carcinoma (MIC) 109 ff.
- -, definition 109
- -, netlike infiltration 110, 111
- -, plump infiltration 112 ff.
- -, stromal invasion 111
mixed tumors 74, 75, 162 ff.
- -, benign 74, 75
- -, malignant 162 ff.
monocellular keratinization 56, 121, 148, 151
mucin formation, monocellular 18, 21, 88, 91, 131, 148, 151
- - under synthetic gestagens 42, 44, 45
mucinous adenocarcinoma 130 ff.
mucoepidermoid carcinoma 148 ff.
mucoid dysplasia 88, 91
mucosa, isthmic 14, 15
-, third 24
Müllerian adenosarcoma 165, 166
- duct remants 28, 29
- metaplasia 28, 29, 137
- mixed tumors 162 ff.

nabothian cyst 24
neometaplasia 33
neurinoma 72
neuroblastoma 156, 157
neuroectodermal tumor 156, 157
neuroendocrine carcinoma 125, 155, 157
- metaplasia 155
neurofibroma 72
nevus, blue 72, 73
non-koilocytic dysplasia 81, 84

osteosarcoma 158
ovula Nabothi 24

papillary adenofibroma 74, 75
- polyps 49
- squamous cell carcinoma 128
- type dysplasia 88, 94
papilloma 69 ff., 77, 88, 128
- condylomatous 71
- virus: see human papilloma virus
parakeratosis 35, 36, 56, 69, 85

parasitic infections 64
polyarteriitis nodosa 66, 67
polyp(s) 48 ff.
-, angiomatous 50
-, cystic 49
-, ectocervical 50
-, endocervical 48 ff., 74
-, papillary 49
postirradiation dysplasia 66
pregnancy changes: see gestational changes
pregnant women, invasive cervical carcinoma 148
premalignant lesions 76 ff.
- -, biological behavior 108
- -, etiology 76 ff.
- -, histopathology 78 ff.
- -, immunohistochemistry 78 ff.
- -, pathogenesis 76 ff.
- -, risk factors 77
psammoma bodies 142
punch biopsy 1

radiation changes 66, 67
regeneration 4 ff.
regenerative epithelium 12 ff., 18, 35, 76, 78
repair 4 ff.
-, ascending 10 ff., 35
-, descending 18 ff., 24, 48, 49
reserve cell(s) 16 ff., 19, 22, 41, 42
- - carcinoma 114, 121, 124, 125
- - dysplasia 82, 88 ff., 95
- - hyperplasia 19, 20, 22, 35, 42, 46 ff., 50, 76
retention cysts 24
rhabdomyosarcoma 158
-, embryonal 165, 167, 168

sarcoidosis 61
sarcoma(s) 158 ff.
-, alveolar soft part 158
- botryoides 165, 167, 168
-, granulocytic 160
schistosomiasis 61, 64
sebaceous glands, formation 33, 34
sectioning conus, techniques of 3
serous papillary carcinoma 142 f.

signet-ring cells 47
small cell carcinoma 116 ff., 157
- - -, lymphatic invasion 118
- - - of neuroendocrine origin 155, 157
southern blot hybridization 78, 82
squamocolumnar junction 1, 17, 22 ff., 80, 87
- -, location 1
squamous cell carcinoma 121, 125
- - dysplasia 79 ff.
- metaplasia 18, 20, 21, 23 ff., 35, 48, 139
staining, methods 3
steroid hormones: see hormonal stimulation
stromal invasion 26, 111 ff.
- reaction, desmoplastic 26

third mucosa 24
transformation zone 24 ff.
trichomonal infection 62
- cervicitis 64
trichomonas vaginalis 58, 62, 64, 65
tuberculous cervicitis 61
- granulomas 61
tumors, benign 69 ff.
-, epithelial 69 ff.
-, malignant 109 ff.
-, mesenchymal 72, 73, 158 ff.
-, metastatic 169
-, mixed 74, 75, 162 ff.
-, - mesodermal 162 ff.
-, - Müllerian 162 ff.
-, neuroectodermal 156, 157

ulcerative ectocervicitis 51, 52, 60
- endocervicitis 55

verrucous carcinoma 128
vesicles, intraepithelial 58
vestigial and heterotopic tissues 26 ff.
villous adenoma 69
viral inclusions 58
- infections 56 ff.
- -, herpes 56, 58 ff., 76
virus, cytomegaly 76
-, HPV 56 ff.

149.00
52295-b